Micromanipulation of Human Gametes and Embryos

Micromanipulation of Human Gametes and Embryos

Jacques Cohen, Ph.D.

*Associate Professor of Embryology
in Gynecology and Obstetrics
Scientific Director of Assisted Reproduction
Gamete and Embryo Research Laboratory
The Center for Reproductive Medicine
and Infertility
The New York Hospital—
Cornell University Medical College
New York, New York*

Henry E. Malter, B.S.

*Doctoral Program
Division of Medical Genetics
Eggleston Hospital
Emory University
Atlanta, Georgia*

Beth E. Talansky, Ph.D.

*Assistant Professor of Gynecology
and Obstetrics
Gamete and Embryo Research
Laboratory
The Center for Reproductive Medicine
and Infertility
The New York Hospital—
Cornell University Medical College
New York, New York*

Jamie Grifo, M.D., Ph.D.

*Assistant Professor of Gynecology
and Obstetrics
Gamete and Embryo Research
Laboratory
The Center for Reproductive Medicine
and Infertility
The New York Hospital—
Cornell University Medical College
New York, New York*

Raven Press ☙ New York

Raven Press Ltd., 1185 Avenue of the Americas, New York, New York 10036

Made in the United States of America

Library of Congress Cataloging-in-Publication Data

Micromanipulation of human gametes and embryos / Jacques Cohen . . . [et al.]
    p. cm.
    Includes bibliographical references and index.
    ISBN 0-88167-835-X
    1. Fertilization in vitro, Human. 2. Micrurgy. 3. Microsurgery.
I. Cohen, Jacques.
    [DNLM: 1. Fertilization in Vitro–methods. 2. Genetic Techniques.
3. Mammals–embryology. 4. Microinjection. 5. Micromanipulation—
methods. 6. Microsurgery—methods.   WQ 205 M626]
RG135.M53 1992
618.1'78059—dc20
DNLM/DLC
for Library of Congress   91—32567
                                                                       CIP

9 8 7 6 5 4 3 2 1

Contents

Preface

Micromanipulation of preimplantation embryos, although only recently applied to assisted human reproduction, has been practiced for decades by developmental biologists and animal scientists. Introduction of this well-established technological field to the human in vitro fertilization laboratory has met with resistance because of the limited clinical benefit of most experimental micromanipulation approaches. Although fascinating, techniques such as the reconstruction of zygotes and blastocysts, embryo splitting, and cloning may appear superfluous to those involved in treatment of infertile couples using assisted reproductive technology. Moreover, such invasive research into early human developmental phases may face ethical and political constraints.

Two main reasons exist for the recent changes regarding the application of micromanipulation techniques to human in vitro fertilization. First, an overwhelming need for more precise control of the fertilization process has developed: in some cases, infertile men with few functional spermatozoa have previously been deemed hopeless for therapeutic fertilization; in other cases, spermatozoa are present in sufficient numbers but are unable to penetrate oocytes. Second, the advent of safe and reliable preconception and preimplantation genetic diagnostic methods that pose no risk to embryonic viability may now allow for replacement of genetically fit embryos in couples at risk for genetic disease.

We are witnessing a coordination of molecular biology and clinical fertilization technology, which in the near future may mark a turning point in our ability to control reproductive mechanisms. The ever increasing sensitivity of biochemical assays, especially those involving genes and gene products, may enable us to perform preimplantation diagnosis at the single-cell level. These techniques may initiate new prospects for molecular gene therapy, with gamete and embryonic genomes as potential targets. Surprisingly, such scientific progress has not been entirely accompanied by corresponding changes in the human embryo laboratory. Rather than evaluating the fertilization process by interpreting interactions between thousands of sperm cells and oocytes, we can now observe individual gametes through the use of micromanipulation. The ability to perform a biopsy on an embryo not only allows us to undertake clinical evaluation but also provides a vehicle by which to study cell differentiation and totipotency.

The impetus for this book arose from the need to update exciting recent developments in reproductive micromanipulation technology as well as from the desire to provide a comprehensive textbook for colleagues considering incorporation of micromanipulation in the in vitro fertilization laboratory. Consequently, this book is directed foremost to the clinical embryologist as well as students of several disciplines, including molecular genetics, developmental physiology, and animal science, and those interested in the application of novel preconception and preimplantation technology.

Micromanipulation does not constitute an independent discipline. Rather, it should be considered as a sophisticated tool for manipulating cells and cell components. Nevertheless, its introduction into the field of human fertilization and preimplantation development is important, both from a clinical and a scientific point of view, and it warrants in-depth documentation. This book is one of the first attempts to describe both the background and the current practice of those fields involving micromanipulation of human gametes and embryos. The first chapter discusses the historical evolution of micromanipulation technology. This is followed in Chapters 2 and 3 by a description of those two fields in reproductive science to which micromanipulation technology has been widely applied: developmental reproduction and animal husbandry. Chapters 4 through 7 are dedicated to the development and application of assisted fertilization. Correction of aberrant fertilization necessitates an understanding of the processes involved in normal fertilization and early embryonic development (Chapter 4). These subjects are then discussed independently from an overview of the development of microsurgical fertilization in animal models (Chapter 5). Clinical results and implications of microfertilization methodology are subsequently outlined in Chapters 6 and 7. The effect of micromanipulation techniques on gamete and embryo viability is treated in Chapter 8. Preimplantation genetic diagnosis and techniques such as polar body, blastomere, and trophoblast biopsy methods are discussed separately (Chapter 9). Chapter 10 is a technical guide to microsurgical instruments and toolmaking. Finally, a short glimpse into the immediate future is provided in Chapter 11, with emphasis on the application of clinical micromanipulation.

Jacques Cohen
Henry E. Malter
Beth E. Talansky
Jamie Grifo

Acknowledgments

This handbook was written during the first quarter of 1991 at The Center for Reproductive Medicine and Infertility, Department of Gynecology and Obstetrics, The New York Hospital—Cornell Medical Center. We are grateful to Drs. Zev Rosenwaks and William Ledger for giving us the opportunity to pursue this effort. Our special thanks for providing the information contained in Chapters 7 and 8 go to embryologists Mina Alikani, Alexis Adler, and Adrienne Reing at The Center for Reproductive Medicine and Infertility in New York and Michael Tucker, Graham Wright, and Sharon Wiker at Reproductive Biology Associates in Atlanta. We are also indebted to our many colleagues listed in Table 7.1 from other in vitro fertilization programs who provided us with current data on the progress of clinical microsurgical fertilization efforts in their institutes.

We are grateful to Janet Trowbridge for literature searches, editing, and general organization during the preparation of this book. Dr. Michael Bedford is acknowledged for his advice on several scientific aspects. The Cornell University Medical Archives and Adele Lerner are thanked for the opportunity to study and photograph Dr. Chambers' historical micromanipulation apparatus. Drs. Ralph Brinster, Steen Willadsen, Ben Brackett, and Robert Godke are thanked for providing additional information. Henry Malter was given partial support by the Redel Foundation.

1

Early Development of Micromanipulation

Henry E. Malter

Since the development of the first microscopes in the 17th century, biologists looking into a new world of tissues and cells probably desired the ability to physically manipulate the tiny specimens they observed. As the field of cell biology expanded and matured, scientists perceived conundrums that could be solved only by gaining access to individual cells and probing them for their secrets. What were the true physical characteristics of the living protoplasm and the nucleus? What were the cellular pH and chemical makeup? Gametes and embryos were perhaps the most tantalizing subjects for observation. How did the sperm and egg interact during fertilization? What was the meaning of the various nuclear changes during the inception of embryonic development and, moreover, how could development proceed from single cell to starfish or human? We are still in the process of answering these and other questions.

Since the early years of this century, cell biologists have been developing methods that allow microscopic living cells to be directly manipulated. For perhaps hundreds of years, organisms and tissues were routinely studied by dissection, biopsy, and invasive measurements and injections. With the birth of micromanipulation, these techniques were modified and reduced to the microscopic scale to allow a similar analysis of individual cells.

THE FIRST EXPERIMENTS

Tracing the history of this field in their seminal book on cell biology technique, Chambers and Chambers (1) allude to the work of Dujardin (2). In 1835, he published a monograph in which perhaps the first cellular microdissection was described. Dujardin used a cotton fiber, which was present under the coverglass of a slide he was studying, as a tool for microsurgery. When a protozoan moved into position under the fiber; the coverglass was depressed against the slide causing the fiber to pinch off a portion of cytoplasm! No doubt, other early cell biologists performed similar spontaneous experiments.

In 1859, H. D. Schmidt (3) published the first description of a device and a method for the microdissection of tissue. Schmidt was a Philadelphia physician interested in mammalian anatomy. In studying the fine structure of the liver, he was frustrated by the limits of simple dissection in revealing the pathways of the smallest vessels and ducts. His paper, published in the *American Journal of Medical Sciences,* was entitled: *On the minute structure of the hepatic lobules, particularly with reference to the relationship between the capillary blood vessels, the hepatic cells, and the canals which carry off the secretion of the latter.* Shown in Fig. 1.1, Schmidt's apparatus, which he termed the "microscopic dissector," consisted of a special microscope stage that held a specimen of tissue and provided three screw-controlled positioners for operating a variety of microscopic dissection instruments. Tiny metal needles, scissors, and scalpels could be fitted into these holders (see Figs. 1.1–1.3). By turning the screws, a corresponding fine motion of the instrument was obtained.

L. Chabry (4) performed perhaps the first true embryological micromanipulation in 1887. These experiments were similar to the work of Roux (5), who studied embryonic development by destroying individual blastomeres of cleaving frog embryos. Chabry developed an ingenious methodology, based on capillary tubing, to perform this type of experiment with the much smaller embryos of ascidians and other marine animals. Basically, the embryo was stabilized by placing it within the lumen of a section of glass capillary tubing of the appropriate inner diameter. This tubing was placed into a holder on the microscope stage fitted with a lever mechanism that controlled the insertion of a very fine glass needle (Fig. 1.2). The needle was introduced into the end of the capillary tubing and used to precisely pierce selected blastomeres. Chabry commented on the elasticity of the embryonic membranes that made needle penetration difficult. He devised a simple spring apparatus to provide the quick movement necessary for successful penetration. As we will see, Chabry was the first of many scientists who had to solve the problem of needle insertion into resilient membranes. Chabry also developed a technique for the fabrication of the ultrafine glass needles needed for this procedure, which will be discussed in a later section on the development of microtools. Chabry made prolific use of his apparatus in obtaining a large body of developmental observations. He attempted to relate the abnormal cleavage patterns obtained following experimental manipulation to previously identified embryonic "monsters."

The credit for the first practical cellular micromanipulation experiments should go to M. A. Barber. Barber was an early bacteriologist working at the

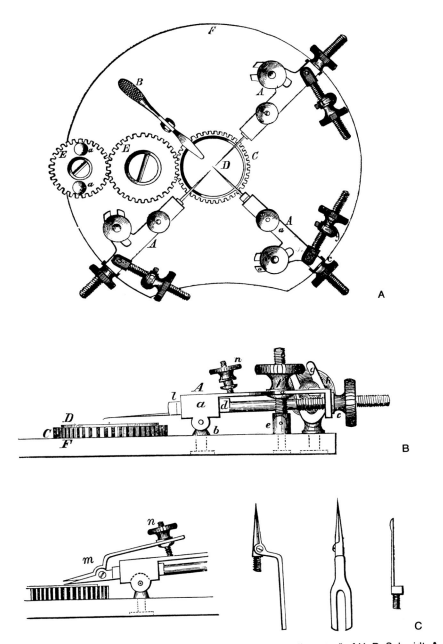

FIG. 1.1. The first microsurgical apparatus: the "microscopic-dissector" of H. D. Schmidt. **A:** Top view showing three manipulators *(A)* positioned around the specimen holder *(D)*, which could be turned by the gear mechanism *(E)*. **B:** A side view of the mechanism. **C:** Various microdissection instruments could be fitted into the manipulators including tiny scissors *(m)* and scalpel blades. (From Schmid HD. On the minute structure of the hepatic lobules, particularly with reference to the relationship between the capillary blood vessels, the hepatic cells and the canals which carry off the secretions of the latter. *Am J Med Sci* 1859;37:13–40, with permission.)

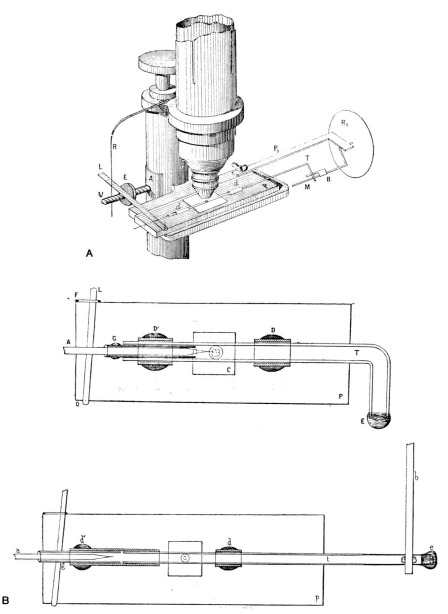

FIG. 1.2. The micromanipulation apparatus of L. Chabry. **A:** The basic setup. A capillary tube *(T)*, containing the embryo, is placed in a holder on the microscope stage. The tube can be adjusted and rotated by using the mechanism at the *right* (P_0, R_0, B, M). On the *left* is a lever that controls the insertion of a fine needle into the capillary tube. A spring *(R)* provides force for rapid needle movement, as restricted by the adjustable wheel *(E)*. **B:** A closeup of the capillary tube chambers. The *upper* chamber *(T)* is used for larger ascidian embryos. The needle *(A)* is shown with the point inserted into a blastomere of the embryo. The *lower* chamber *(t)* was used for species with smaller embryos.

University of Kansas at about the turn of the century. In 1904, Barber (6) described preliminary experiments with a screw-driven "pipette holder," which he used to handle individual bacteria under high-power magnification. Four years later, Barber published a major paper (7) describing his techniques by which individual bacteria could be isolated. Barber wanted to study the reproductive rate of bacteria under different temperature regimens. Rather than rely on the classic methods of dilution to obtain a base concentration of cells, he wanted to achieve a new level of accuracy by starting his culture with a single bacterium. To separate a single cell, he devised the first practical micromanipulation apparatus. A glass pipette was pulled in a flame to reduce its diameter to the appropriate size for picking up the bacteria. He attached his pulled glass pipette to a simple mechanism consisting of screw-driven metal bars. As a screw was turned, the bar would move proportionally. He devised a special microscope stage from which a coverslip was suspended. Drops hanging from the coverslip could be accessed from below by the micropipette. A mouthpiece was connected to

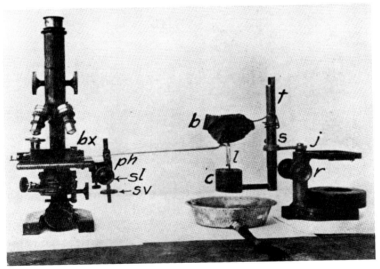

FIG. 1.3. The micromanipulation–microinjection setup of M. A. Barber. On the *left* is the microscope, with a hanging-drop chamber *(bx)* and stage-mounted micropipette holder *(ph)* with vertical and lateral screw controls *(vs,vl)*. The micropipette extends from the pipette holder and terminates with a 90°+ bend, forming a mercury-containing loop *(l)* on the *right*. An old microscope rack-and-pinion drive *(r)* is arranged so that it can position a bag *(b)* or cup *(c)* containing warm and cold water, respectively. By adjusting the position of the bag and cup the temperature of the mercury column was altered to control pressure in the micropipette. (Reprinted with permission from Barber MA. A technic for the inoculation of bacteria and other substances into living cells. *J Infect Dis* 1911;8:348–360. Courtesy of the University of Chicago Press.)

the pipette and, by looking through the microscope, Barber could position his pipette and easily aspirate a single bacterium, which was transferred to another adjacent drop and from there on to an appropriate culture vessel. Three years later (8), Barber discussed the first microinjection of living plant cells and single-cell organisms, using his apparatus and a microneedle made from glass capillary tubing. The microneedle was fabricated with a loop that contained mercury. Pressure within this pipette was adjusted by altering the temperature of the loop section. Vessels containing hot and cold water were attached to an old microscope mechanism, such that as the focus control was raised or lowered, the loop of the pipette was exposed to hot or cold temperature. With this apparatus, injection and aspiration of cellular contents was possible with some precision. Barber's cell injection setup is illustrated in Fig. 1.3. In Barber's ground-breaking experiments, the basics of micromanipulator and microtool construction, as well as the basic techniques of cell injection and the hanging-drop technique, were established. Barber would be at home in any modern micromanipulation laboratory. In fact, many workers still use a simple mouthpiece for controlling aspiration and injection in their only slightly more sophisticated microtools!

IMPROVEMENTS AND ADVANCEMENTS

Apparatus for Micromanipulation

Barber's work in the area of bacteriology excited great interest in several of his contemporaries. George Lester Kite took the methods of Barber and applied them to some basic cell biology experiments. In a 1911 lecture at the Woods Hole institute, Kite discussed a nuclear dissection experiment in which he attempted to use a microneedle to separate the pronuclei in a newly fertilized zygote (9). In the years that followed, many workers began the pursuit of improved mechanisms, microtools, and methods. This section will concern advances in the development of apparatus and methods. Robert Chambers, working first with Kite and then independently, produced the first modern high-precision micromanipulator (10). The Chambers' manipulator became the standard instrument used by a multitude of researchers for 20 years or more. Barber's micromanipulator was a simple screw-driven positioner, which was subject to the fluctuation and vibration of the threaded mechanism. Chambers expanded on the ideas of Barber to forge a practical and productive scientific methodology. The Chambers' micromanipulator was based on the principle of levers. Basically, three metal bars, connected by spring hinges, were placed under the control of very finely machined micrometer screws. By rotating the screws, the bars were alternatively forced apart or drawn back together, imparting a proportional motion to an apically positioned microtool holder. A commercial version of the Chambers' manipulator, manufactured by the Leitz corporation, is illustrated in Fig. 1.4. This mechanism provided very fine control and could be used at high magnification to provide stable, precise, and repeatable placement of the microtools. Later models incorporated a form of remote control, in that knobs were connected to the actual micrometer drives by flexible shafts. This provided a more convenient control setup and isolated the actual micromanipulator mechanism, to some extent, from the vibrations of the operator's hands.

The Chambers' micromanipulator was still based on a three-axis, screw-driven system. The motion of the microtool was derived from the separate adjustment of three individual controls. In 1928, Emmerson described the first micromanipulator to use the joystick design (11). This innovation provided a much more natural technique. Rather than having to mentally translate the desired motion into the adjustment of a rotary control, the operator of a joystick instrument could perform the movement directly. The Emmerson system was purely mechanical and was based on a sliding stage-type mechanism. In 1934, de Fonbrune (12), working at the Pasteur Institute in Paris, developed an ingenious joystick manipulator that used the

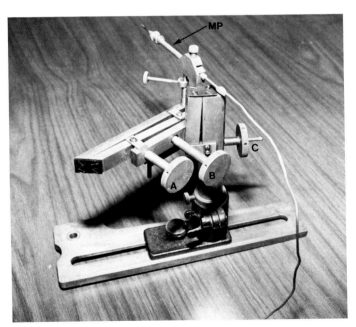

FIG. 1.4. The Chambers' micromanipulator. This is a commercial model manufactured by the Leitz company. The three screws (*A, B,* and *C*) control the expansion of three hinged bars to which the micropipette holder *(MP)* is connected. (Courtesy of the Cornell University Medical College Archive.)

principles of hydraulics. Dunn (13) had reported on hydraulic micromanipulators as early as 1927, but these required the adjustment of separate hydraulic cylinders to position the microtool. By connecting two pneumatic cylinders together with a joystick linkage to derive the X-Y motion and incorporating a screw-driven vertical drive on the joystick itself, the de Fonbrune manipulator provided true simultaneous three-dimensional control. The joystick mechanism was connected by pneumatic tubing to a remote receiver unit, which was placed adjacent to the microscope. Motion of the joystick cylinders resulted in a reduced proportional motion by the corresponding diaphragms of the receiver unit, which were connected by a linkage with the microtool holder. An added advantage of this scheme was that any vibration of the operator's hands was completely isolated from the microtool. A modern version of the de Fonbrune unit is illustrated in Fig. 1.5. This unit provided the microsurgeon with the precise and intuitive control necessary for the most critical procedures. With use of this new mechanism, the first nuclear transfer (in *Amoeba*) was accomplished (14). de Fonbrune made another great contribution in describing the first microforge and a body of microtool-making techniques that are still in use today. These are discussed in a later section.

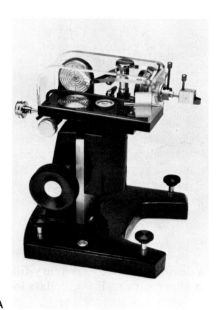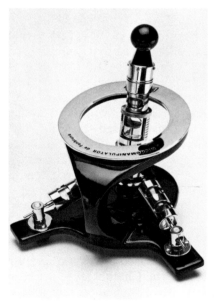

A   B

FIG. 1.5. The de Fonbrune micromanipulator. The joystick control unit **(B)** with three pneumatic cylinders is connected by rubber tubing to the receiver unit **(A)** that drives the microtool. (Courtesy of Technical Products International, St.Louis, Missouri.)

In the 1950s, the Leitz company introduced their famous mechanical micromanipulator, and in 1983, Nikon-Narishige of Japan released their excellent hydraulic model. Because these are currently the most popular units for embryological work, they are discussed in Chapter 10 in the section on current equipment. There were a multitude of other early micromanipulator designs. For a complete review of the early technical development of micromanipulators, the interested reader is directed to El Badry's excellent book (11).

One problem with micromanipulators was that as the extent of microtool motion was reduced by the mechanism, so was the velocity. This reduced velocity was not a great drawback until workers desired the ability to pierce cell membranes with microelectrodes for electrophysiological experiments. Membranes would often simply deform around the "slow-moving" needle. Chabry dealt with this problem in the development of his apparatus in 1887. To provide rapid controlled motion to microtools, piezoelectric devices were introduced. These devices are based on the property of certain crystals to deform in response to an electric stimulus. The reverse phenomenon (physical deformation of the crystal resulting in an electrical signal) has been used for many years in the operation of phonograph cartridges. Pascoe (15) reported the first use of a piezoelectric crystal in microelectrode placement in 1955. The microelectrode was fitted in a holder that incorporated a piezoelectric transducer. When an electric signal was sent through the transducer, a rapid deformation occurred that drove the needle into the cell membrane. In 1962, Ellis (16) reported on the construction of a three-dimensional micromanipulator based on piezoelectric transducers (actually taken from phonograph and record-cutting units). This joystick-controlled system not only provided smooth, stable control of the microtool, but also allowed the high-velocity movement necessary to perform microelectrode placement. This complicated and cumbersome unit was popular for a brief period and was used for highly critical procedures, such as the microdissection of chromosomes. Piezoelectric devices are still used in modern electrophysiological experiments, usually as an accessory unit connected to a conventional micromanipulator; not unlike the original design of Pascoe. These will be briefly discussed in Chapter 10.

Apparatus for Microinjection

Barber devised the first microinjection device based on a mercury-filled glass pipette. Chambers (17) suggested an alternative to Barbers glass loop pipette by using a screw-driven clamp to apply and release pressure to a metal vessel containing mercury. This vessel was connected with the micropipette through flexible metal tubing. Later, Chambers (18) developed the concept of the microsyringe injector which remains the method of choice for microinjection to this day. A simple 2-mL glass syringe was connected pneumatically with the micropipette holder through a section of flexible metal tubing. The syringe and tubing were carefully filled with water, ensuring that no trapped air remained. For noncritical procedures, the plunger could be operated by hand. Chambers, borrowing an idea from Barber's more primitive unit, used an old microscope drive to obtain precise control over the syringe plunger. The base of the microscope tube was placed over the plunger, such that when the focus control was turned, the plunger was depressed. In this way, both coarse and fine control of injection pressure were obtained. Chambers found that for most procedures the pressure within the system was enough that when the focus drive was retracted, the plunger slid back as well. Later modifications included a spring to provide reverse tension on the plunger. One of these units is illustrated in Fig. 1.6. In modern units, the syringe plunger is usually physically connected with the micrometer drive, such that precise bidirectional movement is possible. Chambers (19) also described a holder for glass capillary pipettes with a "chuck" consisting of a resilient rubber washer that was

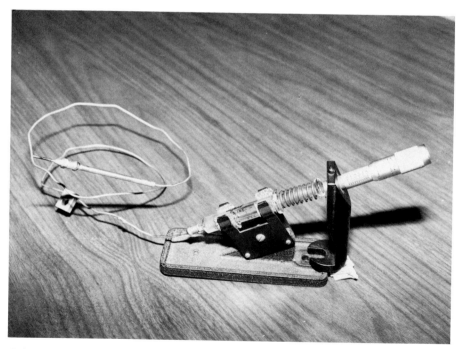

FIG. 1.6. The Chambers' microsyringe, which uses a micrometer drive and spring tension with the attached metal tubing and micropipette holder. (Courtesy of the Cornell University Medical College Archive.)

tightened around the capillary to provide a pneumatic seal. This design is incorporated into most modern micropipette holders.

Microtool Fabrication

Barber's micropipettes for the transfer of bacteria and the injection of cells were formed by hand over the small flame of a microburner (8). This burner was made from a piece of constricted glass tubing. Barber described the conditions with which the finest needle points were derived. The capillary was heated in the small flame and, when the glass became soft, it was raised out of the flame while being pulled apart. Barber pointed out the difficulty in describing the "feeling" of proper pulling. When there was a slight feeling of tension in the glass before the two sections of tubing separated, this resulted in the formation of the best needle points. This apparently indicated the proper degree of cooling, without which long "wispy" tips were produced. Present day researchers can well appreciate Barber's discussion. The production of hand-pulled microtools is a skill that requires much practice.

Chambers refined this hand-pulling technique and suggested the use of a microburner fabricated from a hypodermic needle (19). In 1932, du Bois (20) published a description of the first apparatus for pulling micropipettes. As illustrated in Fig. 1.7, this unit consisted of two spring-driven arms that provided the pulling force and an electric filament that provided the heat to partially melt the glass. For pulling, a capillary was held under the tension of the springs while electric current was applied to the filament, heating the

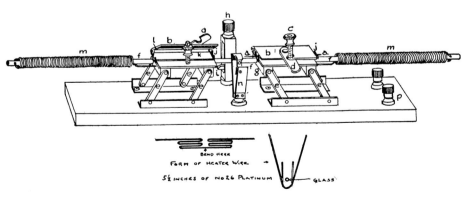

FIG. 1.7. The micropipette puller of Delafield du Bois. The glass capillary is held by two clamps *(b)*, lined with leather and rubber pads *(k,l)*, by a locking nut *(c)*. Two springs *(m)* provide tension for pulling with a platinum electric filament *(n)* for heat. (Reprinted with permission from du Bois D. A machine for pulling glass micropipettes and needles. *Science* 1931;73:344–345. Copyright 1931 by the AAAS.)

glass until it became soft. When the glass was sufficiently heated, the spring tension pulled apart the two arms, drawing the glass out into two sharp tips. This design was apparently derived from observing the technique of a master hand-puller at work. As the arms pulled apart, the glass was drawn up and away from the hot filament by the hinged pantograph mechanism of the puller. This action cooled the glass and allowed the creation of fine needle tips with relatively short pulled sections. This basic design of an electric filament for heating the glass, coupled with a source of force for pulling, has been used with a variety of modifications over the years in the development of modern pipette pullers. Twenty years later, Alexander and Nastuck (21) produced the first pipette puller in which the pulling force was derived and adjusted electrically through a solenoid. In this way, the amount of force could be precisely controlled by selecting the current applied to the solenoid. This puller also permitted a change in the degree of force during a pulling cycle. By beginning the cycle with a weaker pull and then increasing the pull strength, fine-tipped pipettes with relatively short shank sections could be created. In this unit, the pulling force came only from one side. Thus, one pipette was drawn out and away from the hot filament, while the other pipette remained in place. This design has been used in most modern pullers. Numerous improvements have been incorporated into the design of micropipette pullers, including air jets to precisely cool the glass during pulling, sensors for measuring the glass temperature, high-velocity pull mechanisms with rapid acceleration, improved filament designs, and microprocessor control of the pulling process. Many advances in pipette puller design have been in response to the need for extremely fine-tipped pipettes for electrophysiological purposes. These will be discussed in Chapter 10. The evolution of micropipette puller design is discussed thoroughly by Brown and Flaming (22), who were instrumental in the development of this field (22).

As stated before, one of de Fonbrune's greatest contributions to this field was the description of the first practical microforge (12). Before this development, workers could make some modifications to their pulled needles, using the flame of the microburner. For instance, bends were placed near the tip of microtools to permit proper placement in the hanging-drop chamber. In 1887, Chabry (4) described a technique that, in anticipation of microforge techniques, used a hot platinum wire to pull minute, sharp points from the tip of glass microneedles. The tool, stabilized by a grooved holder, was slowly brought into contact with the heated wire and then quickly withdrawn. The tip of the tool adhered to the hot wire and was pulled out into a sharp point. With the microforge, the apical section of the microneedle could be modified by using the precise heat of an electric filament to produce a variety of new tools. The de Fonbrune-type microforge, which is basically unchanged today, consisted of a simple micromanipulator that controls the position of a microtool during the forging procedures. The electric filament was provided as a source of heat, under the control of an adjustable rheostat. Procedures were observed at high magnification with a microscope that was fitted to the forge and focused on the filament and microtool. To more precisely control the temperature of the glass during forging, air jets were provided for cooling the filament area. This ensured that hot air current emanating from the filament did not affect the glass temperature during critical forging procedures. With this apparatus, de Fonbrune developed a spectrum of techniques for modifying micropipettes, some of which are illustrated in Fig. 1.8. When warmed, the glass of the microtool could adhere to the filament or to a ball of glass placed on the filament. Ultrafine needle points could be pulled from the tip of pipettes, as in the Chabry method. The extreme apical section of microneedles could be broken off or bent back into a variety of hooks and loops. Secondary needle tips could be pulled from the end of a pipette by depending small weights from a temporary apical hook and applying heat with the filament. Techniques for microglassblowing were even explored to produce tiny cup-type vessels on the tip of micropipettes. Many of these techniques are still in use for modern micropipette construction. Later advances in microtool fabrication involved such techniques as beveling and chemical treatment. These will be discussed fully in Chapter 10.

Electrophysiology

In the 1940s, interest in the ionic character of cell physiology resulted in the development of micromanipulation for electrophysiological analysis. Hodgkin and Huxley (23) had reported on macroscopic electrophysiology of the "giant" neurons in the squid in 1939. Later, Graham and Gerard (24) were the first to describe the use of a micromanipulator to position a glass microelectrode into an individual sarcomere of frog muscle. Preliminary experiments toward determining the resting and action potential were

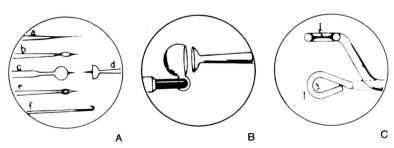

FIG. 1.8. Various microtools and fabricating techniques developed by de Fonbrune, including different types of micropipettes **(A)**, a microcup **(B)**, and a microspatula **(C)**. (Courtesy of Technical Products International, St. Louis, Missouri.)

undertaken. Later work by Nastuk and Hodgkin (25) defined these potentials in this tissue and showed that an increase in membrane sodium permeability was involved. This work has developed into an entirely new field of cell biology, which cannot be covered within the limited scope of this book. Some early electrophysiological experiments involving gametes and embryonic development will be discussed in a later section.

Laser Micromanipulation

Shortly after the invention of the laser, experiments in the early 1960s showed that laser-generated radiation could be used in a variety of cellular microsurgical techniques (26,27). The laser beam, when focused though the optics of a high-power microscope, proved to be a precise "scalpel" for the microdissection of cellular organelles, such as mitochondria and the cytoskeleton. Early work relied on the use of photosensitizing agents (vital stains such as Janus green or acridine orange) to permit the absorption of laser energy and the formation of lesions (28,29). Later work showed that laser energy could have the desired effect without prestaining (30). Much of the research toward the development of laser micromanipulation was conducted by M. W. Berns, who continues this work at the Beckman Laser Institute (of which he was the cofounder) at the University of California, Irvine. Laser techniques will be discussed in later sections and in Chapter 11.

EARLY SCIENTIFIC INVESTIGATION USING MICROMANIPULATION

Chambers and others performed a variety of experiments involving simple cellular dissection. Sharp needle probes were used to pierce the cell and tease away portions of cytoplasm (31,32). A variety of salt solutions were injected into the protoplasm (33). In 1920, Taylor (34) studied ciliate motion in *Euplotes* by using a microneedle to cut through different sections of the cell. In 1925, Needham and Needham (35) used a modification of Chambers' system to study intracellular pH and redox potential in *Amoeba proteus.* Their method involved the cytoplasmic injection of a variety of indicator dyes. In later experiments, more precise dyes were used to determine the pH of the nucleus, protoplasm, and vacuoles (36).

A popular technique was the use of oil drops in examining the nature of the cell's membrane and extraneous coats (1). A drop of oil was expelled from the tip of a micropipette adjacent to the cell under observation. The oil drop would, under certain conditions, coalesce with the cell. By evaluating the interaction between the cell and the oil drop through such characteristics as drop size and timing of coalescence, various treatments and cell types (such as unfertilized and fertilized eggs) could be compared. For instance, fertilized *Arbacia* eggs (devoid of their fertilization membranes) were found to have a "determinant of coalescency" ten times higher than unfertilized eggs (37). After fertilization, the value dropped to zero as a new exterior layer was formed. Another technique involved the injection of oil drops into the cytoplasm to study and quantify cellular protein (9,38). Protein molecules would apparently be adsorbed on the surface of these oil drops. If a drop was allowed to equilibrate within the cell and then was partially aspirated (to reduce its size and surface area) the degree of protein adsorption could be determined by the size at which a distortion of the drop surface was observed owing to the Devaux (crinkling) effect, as illustrated in Fig. 1.9 (39). Also, the crinkling effect was observed when oil drops were introduced immediately around the time of cytolysis, indicating a potential difference between proteins in the living or disrupted cytoplasm.

M. J. Kopac was an outstanding cell biologist who worked with Chambers on the development of the oil drop technique and other studies. He went on to perform a variety of ambitious experiments, using specialized high-precision equipment developed in his laboratory, which extended the limits of micromanipulative techniques. In 1953 (40), he reported on a technique for performing microenzymatic analysis on minute volumes of cytoplasm. With use of a complex micromanipulation and microsyringe system, aliquots of cytoplasm were removed with a microneedle. Volumes as small

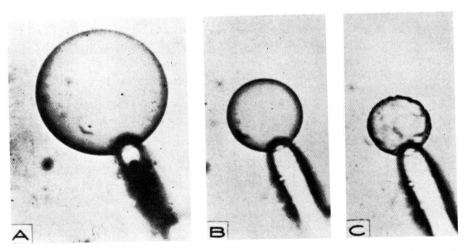

FIG. 1.9. The oil-drop retraction method. An oil drop is introduced into the cytoplasm and allowed to equilibrate **(A)**. As the drop is retracted **(B)**, at some point the diameter/surface area is reduced to the point that the Devaux effect (crinkling) occurs **(C)**. The diameter of the drop at this point can be related to cytoplasmic protein characteristics. (From Kopac MJ. The surface chemical properties of cytoplasmic proteins. *Ann NY Acad Sci* 1950;50:870–909, with permission.)

as 0.3 pL could be obtained. By using centrifugation, cellular contents could be stratified, thereby allowing sampling of specific components of the cytoplasm. The cytoplasmic aliquots were placed on a special coverglass, and the micromanipulator was then used to add a similar microvolume of "substrate" solution. The complete reaction slide was then immersed in a microvolumetric column (dilatometer) so that the enzymatic reaction could proceed. The progress of the reaction was quantified by a volumetric change in the reaction column.

Berns and coworkers (30) used laser microbeams to study contractility in cardiac cells. The laser was used to selectively damage individual mitochondria producing an abnormal contractile response. It was postulated that a release of calcium from the damaged mitochondria caused the contractile response. Later work showed that a similar response was obtained after laser irradiation of myofibrils and the cell membrane and that this response was, indeed, dependent on extracellular calcium (41). Interestingly, this effect was not observed when skeletal muscle cells were used.

Micromanipulation of the Cell Nucleus

From the earliest cell biology experiments with microsurgery, the nucleus was an attractive target for analysis. In one of the first cell biology experiments following Barber's work, Kite and Chambers, in 1912 (42), dissected the nuclei of insect testicular cells and pulled out individual chromosomes. They commented on the glutinous and adherent nature of nuclear material—a fact well appreciated by gene injectors today! Taylor and Farber (43) reported on the effect of removing the "micronucleus" in *Euplotes* by aspiration with a micropipette. Organisms in which this structure was removed survived only a few days and did not exhibit proper cell division. When the micronucleus was removed and then immediately replaced, survival and proliferation were normal. This work, done in 1924, was perhaps the first report of the successful removal and replacement of a cellular organelle. Comandon and de Fonbrune (14) reported on the first nuclear transfer in the ameba in 1939. With use of the new joystick manipulator, nuclei were simply "pushed," using a blunt probe, from one organism to another. In the 1950s, Kopac (44) reported on dramatic work involving the controlled dissection of nuclear structures. Using microsurgical techniques of amazing precision, the transfer of individual nucleoli with attached chromosomes from the nucleus of one cell to the anaphase spindle of another cell (in adenocarcinoma cells of the frog) was accomplished, as illustrated in Fig. 1.10. Following transfer, the nucleoli were shown, upon completion of mitosis, to be incorporated into the new nucleus of the recipient cell. In a review of his work on the eve of his retirement as president of the New York Academy of Sciences in 1960, Kopac (45) even alluded to

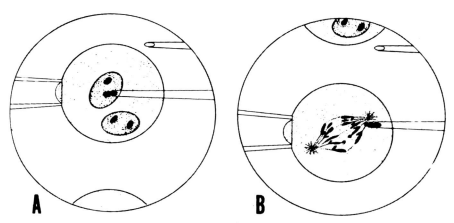

FIG. 1.10. Nucleolar transplantation. **(A)**: A binucleate donor cell is held with a holding pipette while a micropipette is introduced into the nucleus and one of the nucleoli is aspirated. **B:** This micropipette is then introduced into another anaphase-stage cell behind one of the sets of chromosomes. (From Kopac MJ. Exploring living cells by microsurgery. *Trans NY Acad Sci* 1960;23:200–214, with permission.)

preliminary experiments on the microsurgical alteration of individual chromosomes. This work was undertaken to produce a chromosome having two nucleolar-organizing regions. With ultrafine microneedles, leptotene chromosomes of the cells of certain plant species were cut, producing the desired fragment containing a nucleolar-organizing region. This fragment was then moved into proximity with an adjacent chromosome and positioned next to the telomere. The promotion of fusion between the fragment and the telomere was attempted by the general application of ribonuclease and ATP or the microneedle directed application of an alkylating agent to the telomeric region. This heroic work was apparently never taken further, but it is a tribute to the skill and ingenuity of the scientists involved and to the vast potential of micromanipulative technique.

Berns and coworkers (27) used laser irradiation to damage chromosomal segments associated with nucleolar organization. This resulted in cells that lacked one or more of the normal complement of nucleoli. In an extension of this research, the laser was used to destroy selected nucleoli. Cells in which nucleoli had been destroyed exhibited a diminished rate of uridine incorporation, providing evidence for the role of nucleoli in RNA synthesis.

Micromanipulation has been used since the early 1950s in elucidating the nature of chromosomal movement during mitosis. In earlier experiments, Chambers (46) reported that chromosomes could be "easily" removed from the mitotic apparatus. This cast doubt on the definite attachment of chromosomes to the spindle fibers. In 1952, Carlson (47) carefully examined chromosomal attachment, using a microneedle probe on living insect spermatocyte cells and found evidence of a firm connection. This work was continued and expanded by Niklas and coworkers (48,49) starting in the mid-1960s. By probing with a fine microneedle connected to the new Ellis piezoelectric micromanipulator, definite chromosome–spindle attachment was established. In a series of experiments, chromosomal movement was examined. Single chromosomes were "held back" from the normal mitotic movement, without any effect on spindle attachment or the motion of the other chromosomes. When the chromosome was released, it continued its spindle-mediated movement. Later micromanipulation experiments, including the use of laser microsurgery, have made great progress in elucidating the physiology and physics of mitotic movement (50,51).

In the 1960s, Lowenstein and others (52) performed electrophysiological measurements on the nucleus in amphibian eggs. In these experiments, the nucleus was shown to have an ionic resting potential. This was an unexpected finding, since the nuclear membrane was known to be traversed by large pores that would seem to permit a free flow of ionic constituents. In a modern extension of this work, the patch-clamping technique was used on isolated murine pronuclei to demonstrate the presence of ion channels in the nuclear membrane (53).

Early Work with Gametes and Embryos

Gametes had always been prime subjects for microscopic study. In a story attributed to one of van Leeuwenhook's students, human spermatozoa were observed and, with the preformatist bias of the day, he claimed to have seen a homunculus inside each sperm cell (54).

With the onset of micromanipulation, a variety of experiments were undertaken. First oocytes were subjected to the basic microdissection procedures and injection studies outlined earlier. Eventually, experiments were conducted to elucidate two basic areas of interest: the nature of gamete interaction at fertilization, and the nature of early embryonic development. The bulk of this work will be discussed in greater detail in later sections of this book. At this time, a few early experiments will be discussed.

As early as 1923, Chambers (55) studied the mechanism of fertilization in the starfish. He found that the sperm could form a strong association with the oocyte membrane. Casual contact could be broken by the action of a microneedle. However, if tight binding took place, the sperm could not be teased away. Ten years later, he reported on a more extensive study (56). Similar microdissection experiments were performed in the sea urchin, various annelids, and other marine organisms. Chambers demonstrated the rigid nature of the fertilization membrane and the extraprotoplasmic nature of the jelly coats.

Hiramoto (57) showed that when the aster was removed from fertilized sea urchin eggs, cleavage could still occur. The new electrophysiological techniques were applied to fertilization in the mid-1950s in the continuing study of echinoderm fertilization. Tyler and coworkers (58) wanted to measure the electrical potential of eggs of the starfish, *Asterias forbesii.* Previous experiments had failed to demonstrate a potential in marine eggs (59,60), despite evidence of a large potassium concentration difference in relation to sea water (61). However, previous microinjection experiments by Tyler and Monroy (62) demonstrated the great difficulty with which the egg membrane was penetrated by micropipettes. It was found that a sudden vibration, such as provided by a tap to the microscope table, could assist in penetration. This technique can be seen as a primitive precursor of the piezoelectric microdrive. With the experience and techniques developed in their microinjection experiments, Tyler and coworkers successfully inserted microelectrodes into *Asterias* eggs and found an electrical potential that varied between −10 and −50 millivolt (mv) in different eggs. They also did further experiments to measure the potential of eggs during fertilization. Eggs were impaled on the electrode and a steady-state reading was obtained. Sperm were then added to the medium surrounding the egg. When a sperm cell made contact with the egg membrane, the potential suddenly increased by 5 to 10 mv. The potential then slowly increased, reaching a maximum (5 to 20 mv higher than in the unfertilized egg) with the completion of the fertilization membrane. They discussed the membrane potential changes in relation to visual and physiologic changes such as the propagation of a color change across the oocyte, the block to polyspermy, and ion concentrations in unfertilized and fertilized eggs. These outstanding preliminary experiments established the basis for the continuing biophysical study of the events of fertilization.

In 1954, Duryee (63) published a report on preliminary microdissection studies with human eggs. Ovarian tissue was obtained through routine surgical procedures and dissected to obtain the cumulus masses and eggs. The eggs were placed in a hanging-drop chamber and dissected with microneedles. Duryee described the connections between the corona cells (numbered at 3,000 to 4,000 per egg) and the vitellus, and he commented on the jellylike consistency of the zona pellucida. He dissected out a few germinal vesicles and described their physical structure and volume. In examining some of the more mature eggs, he thought he perceived a displacement of the nucleus, perhaps indicating the beginning of an "animal–vegetal" axis of polarity. He properly questioned this assumption, however, because of the lack of a corresponding cytoplasmic gradient.

Hiramoto (64,65), working at the famous Stazione Zoologica in Naples, performed several micromanipulation experiments on fertilization in the sea urchin. With a micropipette, he removed the sperm immediately after contact with the egg. The events associated with activation were observed to

occur despite the absence of the sperm, thereby demonstrating that preliminary contact by the gametes was enough to trigger these events (64). In a
related experiment, Hiramoto (65) injected spermatozoa directly into the
starfish egg, bypassing any surface interaction between the gametes. There
was no evidence of activation following injection. In fact, sperm-injected
eggs could later be fertilized. These experiments established the need for
gamete contact to initiate activation during the fertilization process. This

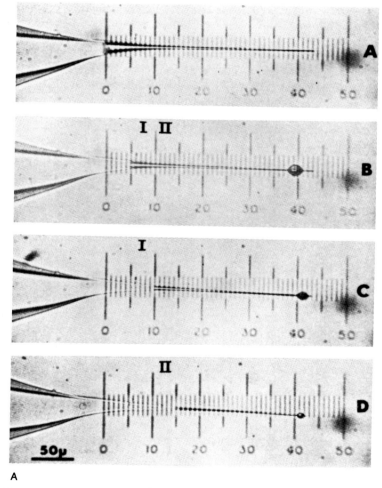

A

FIG. 1.11. Microinjection of murine eggs. **A:** The micropipette is calibrated using an ocular
micrometer. Drop size is related to the volume of various segments of the pipette tip as deline-
ated with the micrometer (I, II).

was also the first reported instance of successful sperm injection, although Kite had apparently attempted the identical experiment 50 years earlier (66). The basic system described by Hiramoto became the standard for later sperm injection work. He used a bolus of mercury loaded into the apical section of his microneedle to provide more precise control over the aspiration and injection pressure. He also described the technique of applying brief suction to the needle during insertion to help break through the vitelline membrane.

In 1966, Lin (67) reported on the first successful microinjection in mouse zygotes. Zygotes were injected with up to 3 μL of a solution of bovine gamma globulin. Injection volume was determined through calibration of the terminal portion of the microneedle by the measurement of drop size with an ocular micrometer, as illustrated in Fig. 1.11. After the transfer of injected embryos to pseudopregnant recipients, normal, living fetuses were obtained and evaluated on day 17. In this work, the basics of critical mammalian cell injection were determined, paving the way for the later development of pronuclear injection for gene transfer.

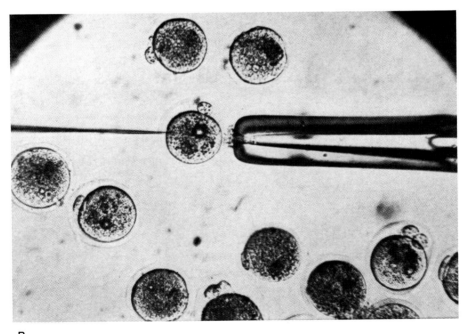

B

FIG. 1.11 *(Continued).* **B:** A mouse egg is being injected with an oil droplet. The holding pipette is on the *right* with the injection needle on the *left.* Several previously injected eggs are seen *below.* (Reprinted with permission from Lin TP. Microinjection of mouse eggs. *Science* 1966;151:333–337. Copyright 1966 by the AAAS.)

Ito and Hori (68) used electrophysiological methods to analyze cleavage in early newt embryos. In this work, membrane coupling between cleaving blastomeres was demonstrated. In later experiments (69), a stimulation microelectrode was inserted into a single cell within a newt morula while two other electrodes measured the voltage within the stimulated cell and in adjacent cells. With this technique, clear evidence of electrical coupling between blastomeres was provided. Blastomeres were separated and then allowed to readhere. Upon separation, coupling was terminated, but it was quickly reestablished when cells came into contact again. More recent experiments in this area will be discussed in the next chapter.

Micromanipulation has come a long way from the microdissection of Schmidt, to the cellular micromanipulation of Barber, Chambers, and their followers, to the complex electrophysiological analysis and laser microsurgery of today. Since the time of Chabry, micromanipulation has proved to be of great value in the field of developmental biology. These experiments will be discussed in detail in the next chapter.

REFERENCES

1. Chambers R, Chambers EL. *Investigations into the nature of the living cell.* Cambridge, Mass.: Harvard University Press; 1961.
2. Dujardin F. Recherches sur les organismes infe'rieurs. *Ann Sci Nat Zool* 1835;4:343–377.
3. Schmidt HD. On the minute structure of the hepatic lobules, particularly with reference to the relationship between the capillary blood vessels, the hepatic cells and the canals which carry of the secretion of the latter. *Am J Med Sci* 1859;37:13–40.
4. Chabry L. Contribution a l'embryologie normal et teratologique des ascidies simples. *J Anat Physiol* 1887;23:167.
5. Roux W. Contributions to the development mechanics of the embryo (origionally published, 1888). In: Willier BH, Oppenheimer JM, eds. *Foundations of experimental embryology.* New York: Hafner Press; 1964:3–37.
6. Barber MA. A new method of isolating micro-organisms. *J Kan Med Soc* 1904;4:487.
7. Barber MA. The rate of multiplication of *Bacillus coli* at different temperatures. *J Infect Dis* 1908;5:379–400.
8. Barber MA. A technic for the inoculation of bacteria and other substances into living cells. *J Infect Dis* 1911;8:348–360.
9. Chambers R. The micromanipulation of living cells. In: *The cell and protoplasm.* American Association for the Advancement of Science publication no. 14; 1940:20–30.
10. Chambers R. A simple apparatus for micromanipulation under the highest magnifications of the microscope. *Science* 1921;54:411–413.
11. El Badry HM. *Micromanipulators and micromanipulation.* New York: Academic Press; 1963.
12. de Fonbrune P. Demonstration d'un micromanipulateur pneumatique et d'un appareil pour la fabrication des microinstruments. *Ann Physiol Physiochem* 1934;10:4.
13. Dunn FL. The use of hydraulic devices for obtaining micromanipulation. *J Infect Dis* 1928;40:383–398.
14. Comandon J, de Fonbrune P. Greffe nucleaire totale, simple ou multiple, chez une amibe. *C R Soc Biol* 1939;130:183–197.
15. Pascoe JE. A technique for the introduction of intracellular electrodes. *J Physiol* 1955;128:26–27.
16. Ellis GW. Piezoelectric micromanipulators. *Science* 1962;138:84–91.
17. Chambers R. A simple micro-injection apparatus made of steel. *Science* 1921;54:522.

18. Chambers R. New apparatus and methods for the dissection and injection of living cells. *Anat Rec* 1922;24:1–19.
19. Chambers R. Methods for the study of fresh material. Physical agents: microdissection, micro-injection. In: *Handbook of microscopical technique*. New York: Hoeber; 1929:39–73.
20. Du Bois D. A machine for pulling glass micropipettes and needles. *Science* 1931;73: 344–345.
21. Alexander JT, Nastuck WL. An instrument for the production of microelectrodes used in electrophysiological studies. *Rev Sci Inst* 1953;24:528–531.
22. Brown, KT, Flaming DG. *Advanced micropipette techniques for cell physiology*. New York: J Wiley and Sons; 1986.
23. Hodgkin AL, Huxley AF. Action potential recorded from inside a single nerve fiber. *Nature* 1939;144:710–711.
24. Graham J, Gerard RW. Membrane potentials and excitation of impaled single muscle fibers. *J Cell Comp Physiol* 1946;28:99–117.
25. Nastuk WL, Hodgkin AL. The electrical activity of single muscle fibers. *J Cell Comp Physiol* 1950;35:39–73.
26. Bessis M, Gires F, Mayer G, Nomarski G. Irradiation des organites cellularies l'aide d'un laser a Rubis. *C R Acad Sci* 1962;255:1010–1012.
27. Berns MW, Rounds DE. Cell surgery by laser. *Sci Am* 1970;222(2):98–110.
28. Amy RL, Storb R, Fauconnier B, Wertz RK. Ruby laser micro-irradiation of single tissue culture cells vitally stained with Janus green B. *Exp Cell Res* 1967;45:361.
29. Berns MW, Olson RS, Rounds DE. Argon laser micro-irradiation of nucleoli. *J Cell Biol* 1969;43:621–626.
30. Berns MW, Gamaleja N, Olson R, Duffy C, Rounds DE. Argon laser micro-irradiation of mitochondria in rat myocardial cells in tissue culture. *J Cell Physiol* 1970;76:207–214.
31. Chambers R. Microdissection studies on the germ cell. *Science* 1915;41:290–293.
32. Chambers R. Microdissection studies; I. The visible structure of protoplasm and death changes. *Am J Physiol* 1917;43:1–12.
33. Chambers R, Reznikoff P. Micrurgical studies in cell physiology; I. The action of the chlo- rides of Na, K, Ca, and Mg on the protoplasm of *Amoeba proteus. J Gen Physiol* 1926;8:369–401.
34. Taylor CV. Demonstration of neuromotor apparatus in *Euplotes* by the method of micro- dissection. *Univ Calif Publ Zool* 1920;19:403–470.
35. Needham J, Needham DM. The hydrogen-ion concentration and the oxidation–reduction potential of the cell-interior: a micro-injection study. *Proc R Soc Lond* 1925;98:259–286.
36. Chambers R. Intracellular hydrion concentration studies; I. The relation of the environ- ment to the pH of protoplasm and its inclusion bodies. *Biol Bull* 1928;55:369–376.
37. Chambers R, Kopac MJ. The coalescence of living cells with oil drops; I. *Arbacia* eggs immersed in sea water. *J Cell Comp Physiol* 1937;9:331–343.
38. Kopac MJ. The Devaux effect at oil–protoplasm interfaces. *Biol Bull* 1938;75:351.
39. Kopac MJ. The surface chemical properties of cytoplasmic proteins. *Ann NY Acad Sci* 1950;50:870–909.
40. Kopac MJ. Submicro methods in enzymatic cytochemistry. *Trans NY Acad Sci* 1953; 16:290–297.
41. Strahs KR, Burt JM, Berns MW. Contractility changes in cultured cardiac cells following laser microirradiation of myofibrils and the cell surface. *Exp Cell Res* 1978;113:75–83
42. Kite GL, Chambers R. Vital staining of chromosomes and the function and structure of the nucleus. *Science* 1912;35:639–641.
43. Taylor CV, Farber WP. Fatal effects of the removal of the micronucleus in *Euplotes. Univ Calif Publ Zool* 1924;26:131–144.
44. Kopac MJ. Transplantation of subcellular particles by micrurgy. *Ann NY Acad Sci* 1957;68:380–393.
45. Kopac MJ. Exploring living cells by microsurgery. *Trans NY Acad Sci* 1960;23:200–214.
46. Chambers R. Some physical properties of the cell nucleus. *Science* 1914;40:824–827.
47. Carlson JG. Microdissection studies of the dividing neuroblast of the grasshopper, *Chorto- phaga vieridifasciata. Chromosoma* 1952;5:199–220.
48. Niklas RB, Staehly CA. Chromosome micromanipulation I. The mechanics of chromo- some attachment to the spindle. *Chromosoma* 1967;21:1–16.

49. Niklas RB. Chromosome micromanipulation. II. Induced reorientation and the experimental control of segregation at meiosis. *Chromosoma* 1967;21:17–50.
50. Aist JR, Berns MW. Mechanics of chromosome separation during mitosis in *Fusarium* (Fungi imperfecti): new evidence from ultrastructural and laser microbeam experiments. *J Cell Biol* 1981;91:446–458.
51. Hiramoto Y, Nakano Y. Micromanipulation studies of the mitotic apparatus in sand dollar eggs. *Cell Motil Cytoskel* 1988;10:172–184.
52. Kanno Y, Lowenstein WR. A study of the nucleus and cell membranes of oocytes with an intra-cellular electrode. *Exp Cell Res* 1963;31:149–166.
53. Mazzanti M, DeFelice LJ, Cohen J, Malter H. Ion channels in the nuclear envelope. *Nature* 1990;343:764–767.
54. Hartsoeker N. *Essai de dioptrique.* Paris; 1694.
55. Chambers R. The mechanism of the entrance of sperm into the starfish egg. *J Gen Physiol* 1923;5:821–829.
56. Chambers R. The manner of sperm entry in various marine ova. *J Exp Biol* 1933; 10:130–141.
57. Hiramoto Y. Cell division without the mitotic apparatus in sea urchin eggs. *Exp Cell Res* 1956;11:630–636.
58. Tyler A, Monroy A, Kao CY, Grundfest H. Membrane potential and resistance of the starfish egg before and after fertilization. *Biol Bull* 1956;111:153–177.
59. Rothschild Lord. The biophysics of the egg surface of *Echinus esculentus* during fertilization and cytolysis. *J Exp Biol* 1938;15:209–216.
60. Scheer BT, Monroy A, Santangelo M, Riccobono G. Action potentials in sea urchin eggs at fertilization. *Exp Cell Res* 1954;7:284–287.
61. Rothschild Lord, Barnes H. The inorganic constituents of the sea-urchin egg. *J Exp Biol* 1953;30:534–544.
62. Tyler A, Monroy A. Apparent and real micro-injection of echinoderm eggs. *Biol Bull* 1955;109:370.
63. Duryree WR. Microdissection studies on human ovarian eggs. *Trans NY Acad Sci* 1954;17:103–108.
64. Hiramoto Y. An analysis of the mechanism of fertilization by means of enuclation of sea urchin eggs. *Exp Cell Res* 1962;28:323–324.
65. Hiramoto Y. Microinjection of the live spermatozoa into sea urchin eggs. *Exp Cell Res* 1962;27:416–426.
66. Lillie FR. Studies of fertilization. VI. The mechanism of fertilization in *Arbacia. J Exp Zool* 1914;16:523–590.
67. Lin TP. Microinjection of mouse eggs. *Science* 1966;151:333–337.
68. Ito S, Hori N. Electrical characteristics of *Triturus* egg cells during cleavage. *J Gen Physiol* 1966;49:1019–1027.
69. Ito S, Lowenstein WR. Ionic communication between early embryonic cells. *Devel Biol* 1969;19:228–243.

2

Micromanipulation: A Tool for Studying Preimplantation Development

Jacques Cohen and Beth E. Talansky

For nearly a century, micromanipulation of embryos has been used in invertebrates and lower vertebrates to elucidate patterns of early development. It is largely through such investigations that cellular interactions, the role of individual blastomeres, and the organization of the preimplantation embryo, in general, have been established. Studies involving early mammalian embryos, aimed at monitoring processes that control embryonic organization and early differentiation, have only recently begun. Developmental embryology studies frequently involve the use of micromanipulation (possibly with the exception of studies evaluating growth and metabolism). A review of all such studies and micromanipulation techniques used by developmental embryologists is not necessarily appropriate, especially considering the scope of this book. However, some of the techniques, such as blastocyst reconstitution, may be implemented clinically in the near future (see Chap. 11). The present chapter is limited to subjects that are of immediate interests to those practicing assisted reproductive technology. Some of the subjects are obviously interrelated, such as totipotency and cell-to-cell communication (the onset of communicational links usually determines differentiation, limiting the totipotency of individual cells). Other processes, such as chimera production and genomic imprinting, are of individual import.

TOTIPOTENCY

Among the earliest experiments involving micromanipulation of mammalian embryos were those of Nicholas, in 1932 (1), who transplanted isolated blastomeres from two-cell rat embryos to the kidney capsule and observed various degrees of development. A few years later, Pincus (2) transplanted single blastomeres from two-cell rabbit embryos to the oviducts of pseudopregnant does and obtained normally differentiating, but small-sized blastocysts. In a similar experiment, Nicholas and Hall (3) showed that rat blastomeres, isolated at the two-cell stage, were capable of forming complete embryos. These results were confirmed and extended when Seidel (4) and Tarkowski (5) obtained viable offspring in the rabbit and in the mouse, respectively, from two-cell embryos in which one of the blastomeres had been destroyed by microneedle puncture. This technique of selective destruction did not necessarily justify the true developmental capability of individual blastomeres, since the degenerate cell may have affected the developing embryo. However, it did demonstrate that early mammalian embryos produce an excess of cells.

The options, later described by Willadsen (6), were more elegant, involving all the original cells of the embryo, separated from each other and housed temporarily in donor zonae. Investigations aimed at studying the developmental potential of each blastomere necessitated the removal of the zona pellucida. This also applied to investigations involving the aggregation of blastomeres from different embryos. Such experiments depended mainly on effective culture of embryos in vitro, since early cleavage stages in mammals are generally unable to survive in the female genital tract if the zona has been removed or extensively damaged (see Chap. 8)

In cleaving mouse embryos, all blastomeres belonging to the same cell generation are not only morphologically similar, but they also possess essentially the same developmental potential. The contribution made by the progeny of individual cells in younger embryos to the inner cell mass and trophectoderm is influenced by the presence of fellow blastomeres and governed by positional relationships within the late morula. Those cells that are completely surrounded by others at the time of blastulation give rise to the inner cell mass, while the rest form trophectoderm (7). This is generally described as the "inside–outside" model. A slight asynchrony in cell cycle between early blastomeres appears to be perpetuated in their daughter cells. This results in a disproportionately high representation in the inner cell mass of cells deriving from one of the first two blastomeres to enter mitosis (8).

If mouse blastomeres are separated early, each of them will continue to develop, eventually giving rise to a diminutive blastocyst or a trophectodermal vesicle (7). The latter form, which contains no inner cell mass and is not viable, is the result of an embryo consisting of so few cells at cavitation that none is completely enveloped by fellow blastomeres. In the mouse, single blastomeres from two-cell embryos and pairs of blastomeres from four-cell embryos are capable of developing into normal concepti, whereas single blastomeres from four-cell embryos lack such ability (9). The normal developmental potential of individual precompacted embryonic cells is dependent on the total number of cell cycles needed to achieve polarity and differentiation. In the rabbit, for instance, individual blastomeres of four- and eight-cell embryos may occasionally form viable offspring (10). There is no experimental evidence to prove that these basic principles and patterns of early embryonic development in most eutherian mammals differ from those observed in rodents.

The time of cavitation is correlated with the cell generation, rather than with cell number (11). In the mouse, blastulation usually occurs after five cell cycles, when the embryo consists of approximately 32 cells, whereas, in the rabbit, blastulation normally takes place after about seven cell cycles. Accordingly, a single mouse blastomere from a four-cell embryo will cavitate at the eight-cell stage, consequently, producing an embryo with hardly any inside cells. By contrast, following the same principles, a quarter embryo from the rabbit will consist of 32 cells, certainly sufficient for incorporation of several cells surrounded by fellow cells. Chimeric blastocysts, produced by fusing two intact embryos, will produce blastocysts with twice the number of inner mass cells. The highest number of genotypes recorded in chimeric mice is three, which suggests that the actual fetus is produced from only three inner cells, irrespective of the bulk of inner cell mass (12).

Totipotency was relatively impossible to study in embryos of larger domestic species until Willadsen (6) introduced several improvements. The problems previously encountered not only involved the culture of precompacted embryos, but progress was also hampered by the virtual impossibility of maintaining transferred micromanipulated embryos in the reproductive tract. Such studies were feasible only after Willadsen devised a method of culturing micromanipulated split embryos in the ligated oviduct of temporary recipients, by surrounding them with a protective agar coating. The method of agar embedding is described in Chapter 3.

Willadsen's approach of embryo splitting has, as yet, not been implemented in human embryology, although, as will be discussed later, it may be applicable in specific patients. Selective destruction of individual blastomeres, as proposed by Seidel and Tarkowski (4,5), has also not been applied to the human embryo. Hence, totipotency has not been actively investigated in the human. However, selective blastomere destruction may be the inadvertent result of embryo cryopreservation. Half and three-quarter intact four-cell embryos with two or three blastomeres, respectively, frequently implant and develop into normal fetuses. Survival and transfer of a single quarter four-cell embryo is relatively rare, but live births have anecdotally been reported. In one instance, one-quarter four-cell and one-half four-cell, resulted in viable dizygotic twins (Fehilly CB, personal communication). Further evidence suggesting relatively late formation of inside cells (after five cell cycles) in the human embryo, is based on the formation of gap junctions (13). It appears, in the human, that these intercellular bridges arise at later stages than those developing in mouse embryos. Thus, it is likely that individual blastomeres of human embryos are still totipotential after two or maybe three cleavage divisions.

INDUCTION OF CHIMERIC DEVELOPMENT

Biology as well as mythology provide examples of composite associations between different species. Such chimeras occur naturally in a variety of species of mammals, including humans. *Chimera* is a term used to describe any composite animal or plant in which the different cell populations are derived from more than one egg or from the union of more than two gametes (14). In *primary chimerism,* the genetically different cell populations coexist from a very early stage of embryogenesis. In *secondary chimerism,* tissues from different fetuses or adults are combined after organogenesis. Examples of the latter include individuals undergoing blood transfusion or organ transplants. A known example of a gestational secondary chimera is a bovine twin sharing a common placental circulation. When the twins are of opposite sexes, the female nearly always develops as a sterile freemartin, and the male cotwin is also affected, leading both to the mixing of blood cells and to female germ cells in the testes of the male fetus. Chimeras are extremely useful in investigations of embryogenesis. Before the experimental induction of chimerism in preimplantation embryology, limited chimerism was achieved by injecting tissue into mouse fetuses shortly before term. Obviously, many experimental situations have been developed whereby adult animals or humans can undergo tissue transplants. A related phenomenon, *mosaicism,* is the result of a composite individual from a single unfertilized egg, in which, for instance, an X chromosome in an early two-cell blastomere would be lost, giving rise to a genetically different cell line.

Embryonic chimerism has been achieved by aggregating zona-free embryos of two or three different mouse strains, using fusogenic materials or by aggregating the embryos in reduced culture volumes (15,16). Adult chimeric mice were first described by Mintz (17). An alternative method giving rise to so-called injection chimeras, was devised by Gardner (18), using micromanipulation techniques. Foreign blastocyst cells were injected into the blastocoelic cavity of mouse blastocysts, and chimerism was verified by genetic markers. The experiments involved disaggregation of blastocyst donor cells (with a color marker and a T6 translocation) in calcium- and magnesium-free medium and inserting them into albino recipient blastocysts. Injection chimeras have also been produced in sheep and rabbits (19,20).

An injection chimera is produced by holding the recipient blastocyst with a suction pipette, which is then penetrated through the trophoblastic region with two very fine glass needles (Fig. 2.1) (21). A slit is formed in the trophoblast wall by separating the needles with the scissor action on the double

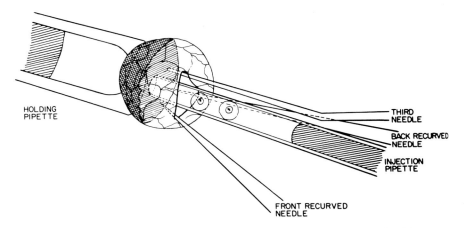

FIG. 2.1. Diagrammatic representation of cell injection into the blastocyst as it might appear when viewed obliquely from the above right to show the deployment of the five micro-instrument tips. (From Gardner RL. Production of chimeras by injecting cells or tissues into the blastocyst. In: Daniel JC, ed. *Methods in mammalian reproduction.* New York: Academic Press;1978:137–163, with permission.)

instrument head of a Leitz micromanipulator. A fourth micromanipulator is used to introduce a pipette filled with the donor cells. The rate of chimeric efficiency has been shown to be 14%. Difficulties encountered with this procedure were related to the relatively large size of the donor cells, the escape of injected cells through the artificial opening, and the resistance to disaggregation. A major technical problem inherent in this type of micro-manipulation technique is a contraction response, leading to collapse of the blastocoelic cavity. Patience may be required, since the blastocyst will usually re-expand after a few hours.

Although aggregation and injection chimeras have been made between rodent embryos of different species, live birth of such interspecific chimeras has not been reported (22,23). Viable interspecific chimerism between two related mouse species (*Mus musculus* and *M. caroli*) has been reported, but these species can also be hybridized (24). Hybridization between sheep and goat does not spontaneously occur, but interspecific chimerism has been successfully accomplished (25). Sheep and goat blastomeres were combined to form interspecific blastocysts, some of which were viable and produced sheep–goat chimeras (Fig. 2.2). The experiments also showed that a goat fetus can develop to term in a sheep and, similarly, that a sheep fetus can develop to term in a goat. However, the abortion rate was considerable, indicating incompatibility between recipient ewes and the goat component of the embryos. The incompatibility between chimeric conceptus and recipient may be neutralized by constructing the chimeric embryos in such a way

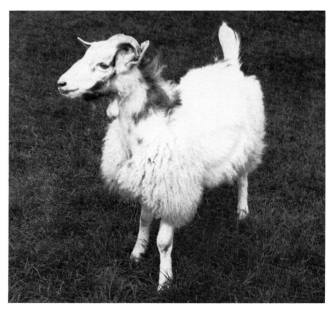

FIG. 2.2. A sheep–goat chimera produced by combining one eight-cell sheep embryo with three eight-cell goat embryos. It exhibits various characteristics confirming its chimeric nature—a mixture of hairy and woolly areas in its coat, goatlike horns, twisted like sheep horns, and blood containing sheep and goat red blood cells (25). (Courtesy of Dr. Steen Willadsen and Dr. Carole Fehilly. Reprinted by permission from NATURE vol. 307, cover photograph. Copyright © 1985 Macmillan Magazines Ltd.)

that the trophectoderm and, hence, the chorionic epithelium consist entirely of tissue belonging to the same species as the recipient. This can be accomplished by injecting a goat inner cell mass into the blastocoelic cavity of a sheep. The two inner cell masses may aggregate to form an interspecific embryo, which when transferred to a recipient ewe, may implant with high efficiency owing to the unique presence of sheep trophectoderm.

STEM CELLS

During the past two decades, several methods have been developed to alter the genetic constitution of embryos. Integration of simian virus 40 (SV40) into blastocysts was performed by Jaenisch and Mintz (26). Subsequently, Jaenisch and coworkers (27) described successful germline integration of Moloney murine leukemia virus. Micromanipulation methodology involving the direct microinjection of cloned DNA into the pronucleus of mouse zygotes, leading to the formation of *transgenic* offspring, provided an alternative method to achieve genomic alteration (28).

Embryonic stem cells represent yet another important vector by which to introduce foreign genetic material into the germline. Stem cells are *pluripotential;* that is, they are cells that possess the ability to differentiate into a variety of cell types as a result of changes in their environmental conditions. Totipotential embryonal stem cell lines may originate either from teratocarcinomas or early embryos. Both cell types are derived from early embryonic cells that are removed either spontaneously or artificially from the constraints of normal embryonic development. The first method of stem cell isolation results in the formation of embryonal carcinoma cells. These cell lines originate from naturally occurring tumors or malignant tumors induced by methods involving grafting of early embryos onto nonuterine sites (29,30). The tumor-derived genotype of the embryonal carcinoma cells and the extended periods of in vitro culture frequently render the cells karyotypically abnormal. A method of producing pluripotential stem cells from normal embryonic material was described by several investigators (31,32). These EK or ES stem cells were generated using one of two methodologies, involving either isolation of undifferentiated "teratocarcinoma-type" stem cells from blastocysts in which normal implantation was interrupted (33) or by the rescue of embryonic stem cells from the inner cell masses of late blastocysts, followed by culture in medium conditioned by teratocarcinoma cell lines. Since these embryonic stem cell lines are derived from "normal" embryonic material, they are typically euploid and have inherent genetic advantage over the embryonal carcinoma lines in terms of their usefulness for genetic manipulation and long-term study. Undifferentiated stem cell lines may be maintained for long periods in culture and have the ability to resume a defined developmental program either after modification of their in vitro conditions, or more importantly, after reintroduction into a host embryo.

The generation of undifferentiated stem cell lines has particular applicability for production of chimeras. The initial methods for production of chimeric animals (15,16) involved aggregation of zona-denuded embryos, followed by replacement into pseudopregnant foster females. These early methodologies were followed by modifications involving the use of micromanipulation. As described earlier, Gardner (21) created chimeric individuals by microinjecting cells or pieces of tissues into the blastocoelic cavity of mouse embryos. Since it involved direct placement of cells into the blastocoelic cavity, micromanipulation alleviated the need for removal of the zona pellucida, as is required in embryo aggregation (Fig. 2.3). The limitations of this particular technique were mentioned earlier in this chapter. It was of interest to utilize the easily manipulated pluripotential stem cells as vehicles for introducing new genetic material into blastocysts. Embryonal carcinoma stem cells have limited use for chimera formation owing to their unstable characteristics after culture and their relatively rare incorporation into the germline of the resulting offspring. On the other hand, the advan-

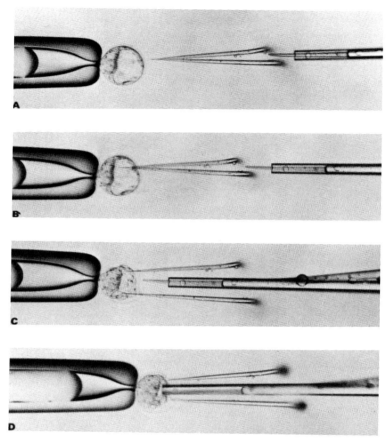

FIG. 2.3. Stages in the cell injection operation. **A:** The inner cell mass is at the 9 o'clock position and the instruments are aligned. **B:** The apposed tips of the recurved needles are pushed well into the blastocoele toward 12 o'clock. **C:** A fairly wide slit is made in the zona and trophectoderm into which the third needle is pushed. **D:** The injection pipette is then moved into the blastocoele relative to the third needle, and the cell injected. (From Gardner RL. Production of chimeras by injecting cells or tissues into the blastocyst. In: Daniel JC, ed. *Methods in mammalian reproduction*. New York: Academic Press;1978:137–163, with permission.)

tages conferred by microinjection of embryonic-derived cell lines have been demonstrated by Evans et al. (33), who created chimeric mice with the introduction of EK cells into blastocysts. These investigators obtained chimeric offspring with high efficiency. In addition, this study involved the use of host blastocysts carrying alleles that rendered them subfertile. This resulted in a significantly elevated percentage of chimeric offspring with an EK-derived germline.

Thus, the ability to produce the genetic chimera, a very powerful tool for the study of mammalian development, has been greatly enhanced with the use of micromanipulation technology in conjunction with undifferentiated embryonic stem cell lines. Increasingly sophisticated gene expression studies may be performed as it becomes possible to introduce a variety of genes into embryonic stem cell lines by techniques such as electroporation (34), retroviral transfer (35), and calcium phosphate precipitation (36). Additionally, genetic chimeras, produced by micromanipulated ES cells, afford the opportunity to study mammalian development by analysis of insertional mutations (37).

THE INNER CELL MASS, TROPHECTODERM, AND BLASTOCYST RECONSTITUTION

Gardner (38) separated the blastocyst into its two constituent tissues and compared their properties both in culture and after uterine transfer. Interestingly, manipulations were carried out at room temperature, to diminish the increased adherence of cells and debris to the instruments at 37°C. Gardner used the so-called hanging-drop micromanipulation method, which is described in Chapter 10. Although this method is rather cumbersome for direct clinical application, it is efficient for maintaining stable metabolic conditions.

Blastocysts were placed in a drop of medium hanging from the coverslip of a chamber filled with heavy liquid paraffin. Trophoblast tissue was freed from the inner cell mass by holding the blastocyst against the underside of the hanging drop. A piece of the cutting edge of a razor blade attached to a mounted needle with Araldite (CIBA) was arranged vertically on one micromanipulator unit such that its cutting surface was parallel with the coverslip of the chamber. By raising the blade slowly, the blastocyst can be divided parallel to the surface of the inner cell mass, either equatorially (to yield small trophoblastic fragments) or close to the embryonic pole (to yield maximal trophoblastic vesicles) (Fig. 2.4). Equatorial division is relatively easy, but polar sectioning could cause the embryo to rotate on the holding device. A third needle instrument was then used to immobilize the embryo. Inner cell masses were isolated by penetrating expanded blastocysts from opposite sides with fine needles, tearing the trophoblast open and pinning it out against the coverslip. The inner cell mass was scraped from the trophoblast. Solter and Knobil (39) developed an alternative method, using immunosurgery for efficient removal of the inner cell mass.

The results of Gardner's investigations revealed that trophoblastic fragments did not aggregate like morulae, probably owing to the junctional bridges between cells. Inner cell masses resembled cleaving embryos, since they were able to fuse with each other. Trophoblastic vesicles caused decidual reactions and continued to have an active blastocoelic pump. These were the three major biological differences between the two types of tissues. Implanted trophoblastic vesicles did not develop an embryo,

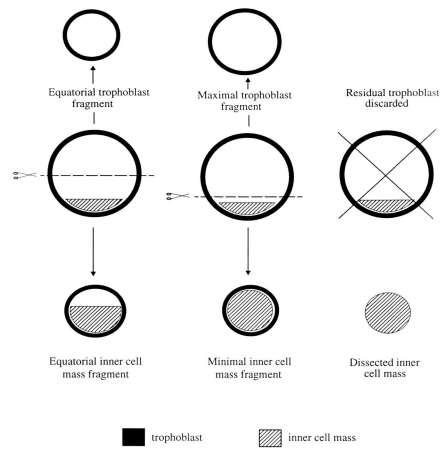

FIG. 2.4. Scheme of manipulations carried out on the mouse blastocyst to obtain trophoblast and inner cell mass tissue. (Adapted from Gardner RL. An investigation of inner cell mass and trophoblast tissues following their isolation from the mouse blastocyst. *J Embryol Exp Morphol* 1972;28:279–312, with permission.)

amnion, allantois, yolk sac, or Reichert's membrane, indicating that these structures were dependent on the presence of inner cell mass precursor cells. The differentiation of morula cells into trophectoderm and inner cell mass coincides with major changes in cell polarity and communication.

CELL-TO-CELL COMMUNICATION

Developmental information in the early embryo may be transferred via direct cell-to-cell pathways, such as gap junctions and cytoplasmic bridges, or through ligand–receptor mechanisms at the cell surface (40). Gap junctions are present in both vertebrate and invertebrate embryos; however, their distribution and permeability properties vary according to developmental stage and species (41). In many embryos, cells of specific developmental fate often form communication compartments, thereby limiting information flow to other cell groups (42,43), whereas, in others, such as the squid, gap junctions are uniformly distributed over the cells (44). Gap junctions play an important role in embryogenesis. Microinjection of antibody or antisense RNA to a 27-kd gap junction protein into amphibian or mammalian embryos reduced dye and electrical coupling between blastomeres and caused developmental defects (45).

Ionic coupling is based on the principle that, after the perforation of two contacting cells with microelectrodes, the injection of current into one cell can be detected as a voltage deflection in the second cell. It was also observed that cells in culture were able to transfer low–molecular-weight metabolites (metabolic cooperation). These processes are correlated morphologically with the presence of a specialized intercellular contact, the gap junction. Almost all cells can communicate, as indicated by ionic coupling, metabolic coupling, or dye transfer, or as inferred from the morphological presence of gap junctional structures. Ducibella and coworkers (46) found that during compaction, junctional processes are formed between the cells, like tight and gap junctions. This is also the approximate time during which the first differentiation event occurs in the mouse embryo (47).

Gap junctions in the mouse embryo occur at the onset of compaction at the eight-cell stage (48). Early mouse blastomeres are also linked in a syncytial network (49) and, slightly later, tight junction and desmosome formation begins (50).

Lo and Gilula (48) studied the extent to communication between cells in mouse embryos between the two-cell and blastocyst stage. Three assays were performed to investigate the nature of communication between blastomeres. The presence of ionic coupling, the transfer of injected fluorescein (molecular weight 330), and the transfer of injected horseradish peroxidase (HRP) (molecular weight 40,000). In the two-cell, four-cell, and precompacted eight-cell embryos, cytoplasmic bridges between sister blastomeres were responsible for ionic coupling and the transfer of injected fluorescein as well as the transfer of injected horseradish peroxidase. In contrast, no communication was observed between blastomeres from different sister pairs. Junction-mediated intercellular communication was unequivocally detected at the early compaction stage (late eight-cell embryo) (Fig. 2.5). At that stage, ionic coupling was present, and fluorescein injected into one cell spread to all other cells of the embryo. Injected horseradish peroxidase was passed to only one other cell, however, again indicating the presence of cytoplasmic bridges between blastomeres. Junctional communication for both ionic coupling and dye transfer was retained between all the cells throughout

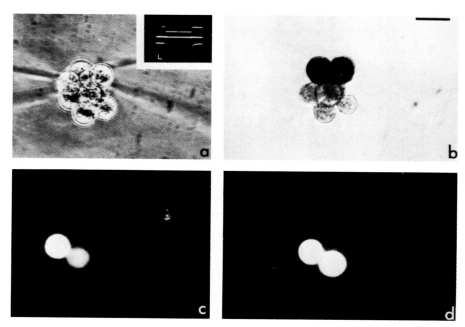

FIG. 2.5. Intercellular communication in the precompacted eight-cell embryo by cytoplasmic bridges. **A:** Two blastomeres of an early eight-cell embryo impaled with microelectrodes. **Inset:** As a current pulse *(top trace)* was injected into the impaled cell on the *right,* a voltage deflection was detected in that blastomere *(bottom trace),* but none was detected in the impaled blastomere on the *left (middle trace).* **B:** (HRP) Horseradish peroxidase was injected into the impaled blastomere on the right. The two dark HRP-reacted cells represent the injected cell and an adjacent cell. **C, D:** Fluorescein injected into right blastomere and images recorded after 4 minutes **(C)** and 25 minutes **(D).** (Reprinted with permission from Lo CW, Gilula NB. Gap junctional communication in the preimplantation mouse embryo. *Cell* 1979;18:399–409. © Cell Press.)

compaction. Ionic coupling with microelectrodes was performed on zona-free embryos adhered to the petri dish after a short culture period (holding pipette replacement).

Recently, Dale et al. (13) studied intercellular communication in early human embryos, using dye-coupling techniques and electron microscopy (Fig. 2.6). Lucifer yellow was injected through a micropipette of 1 to 2 μm diameter and approximately 10 Mohm resistance. Following contact with the cell surface a Gohm (giga=10^9) seal was obtained, and the pipette potential was lowered to break the seal. The holding potential was then altered to give zero current and the lucifer yellow solution was allowed to diffuse into the blastomere. Blastomeres were injected between the four-cell and blastocyst stage. Dye spread, indicating the status of gap junction formation, was observed only when blastocysts were formed. Electron microscopic studies revealed that blastomeres were loosely associated until the

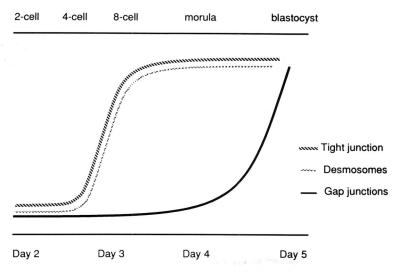

2-cell   4-cell   8-cell   morula   blastocyst

Day 2   Day 3   Day 4   Day 5

〜〜〜 Tight junction

〜〜〜 Desmosomes

—— Gap junctions

FIG. 2.6. Formation of intracellular mechanisms in human preimplantation embryos. (Based on Dale et al., 1991 (ref. 13).)

four-cell stage, and only microvilli extended into the intercellular space. The diameter of these spaces reduced by a factor of five to ten from the six-cell stage onward. Desmosome-like structures were found in deeply located planes, but rarely peripherally. Focal points of apparent membrane fusion, resembling tight junctions, were often seen in six- to ten-cell stages, associated with desmosome-like structures. These communicational structures can be observed mechanically during biopsy procedures in the precompacted human embryo. Blastomeres from four-cell embryos are more easily loosened from their sibling blastomeres than blastomeres from eight-cell embryos. The safe removal of blastomeres of eight-cell embryos requires preincubation in a Ca^{2+}/Mg^{2+}-free medium to eliminate junctional structures.

Intercellular devices appear to develop later in the human than in other mammalian embryos. The formation of tight junctions coincides with embryonic gene expression in the human embryo (51). Whether these two processes are related is not yet known.

CELL FUSION

Fusion studies between complete cells or anucleate fragments can reveal processes involved in the organization of oogenesis and embryogenesis. An example of this type of study is provided by the work of Czolowska et al. (52). Interphase blastomeres from two- to eight-cell mouse embryos were fused in a volume ratio of 1:1 with karyoplasts or cytoplasts from metaphase

II oocytes. The ability of the introduced material to induce premature chromosomal condensation in the fusion product was evaluated. Surgical procedures were either carried out by hand or micromanipulation. Bisection of oocytes was carried out according to the method of Tarkowski (53) on an agar-coated petri dish, using a glass needle. Microsurgery was performed following cytochalasin B exposure, using an inverted scope with a Zeiss micromanipulator (54). The karyoplasts were obtained by aspiration into a sharply pointed pipette (20 μm in diameter) the region in which the metaphase II spindle was previously localized with the smallest possible amount of the cytoplasm. Karyoplasts thus obtained were about one-eighth the oocyte volume. Cytoplasts were produced as a by-product of enucleation, or small cytoplasts were obtained by a similar technique. After preincubation in phytohemagglutinin, fusion was either induced with polyethylene glycol or with the use of electrofusion (55), with modifications made for use with mouse blastomeres (56). The investigators assessed the presence and frequency of premature chromosomal condensation after fusion between interphase blastomeres and karyoplasts (hybrids). Also, they evaluated the ability of anucleate fragments or cytoplasts to induce chromosomal condensation following fusion with interphase blastomeres (cybrids).

In most hybrids, the nucleus in the fusion product had undergone premature chromosomal condensation. The phenomenon occurred, regardless of the karyoplast size used for fusion, the postovulatory age of the contributing oocyte, or the cleavage stage of the embryo from which the blastomere was obtained. In contrast, extensive premature chromosomal condensation in cybrid fusion products was observed only when cytoplasts were derived from recently ovulated oocytes (14.5 to 15 hours post-HCG). This value was significantly decreased as the interval after ovulation was increased. Interestingly, the effect of aging could be counteracted if the size of the cytoplasts was increased to as much as seven-eighths that of the original contributing oocyte. From these experiments, it was postulated that nuclear condensation activity is predominantly bound to the nuclear apparatus (most probably to the chromosomes) and that, in the cytoplasm of metaphase II mouse oocytes, the activity decreases with postovulatory age.

Recently, another method of micromanipulation was used to elucidate the effect of cytoplasmic factors on nuclear activities, such as oocyte maturation and fertilizing ability. Flood et al. (57) based their investigation on the fact that immature, germinal vesicle-stage oocytes could be matured in vitro, but even if they are fertilized, this rarely leads to pregnancy. This notion can be especially problematic in the context of clinical in vitro fertilization (IVF), since immature oocytes are frequently retrieved after routine methods of follicular stimulation. The investigators postulated that factors from mature oocytes, if introduced into the cytoplasm of germinal vesicle eggs, would induce normal oocyte maturation that more closely resembled the in vivo process. Unlike the previous study described in this section, cytoplasm was not introduced by fusion techniques, but instead, was directly microinjected into the cytoplasm of the recipient oocyte. The basic procedure involved aspiration of small volumes of cytoplasm from metaphase II oocytes and microinjection of this ooplasm into prophase I monkey oocytes. Micromanipulation was followed by in vitro incubation of the oocytes and, finally, transfer into the fallopian tubes of mated recipients. Of 24 oocytes that were replaced, four pregnancies resulted, and three live births were reported. Forty-three oocytes that did not receive metaphase II ooplasm were transferred, and no pregnancies resulted. These results suggested that a factor transferred from the mature oocyte was effective in stimulating maturational events in the germinal vesicle oocytes necessary for fertilization and implantation. Additionally, the fact that pregnancies did not result when the transferred cytoplasm was subjected to heat and RNase indicates that mRNA might be involved (57). The use of micromanipulation technology will, no doubt, allow further characterization of important cytoplasmic factors that are significant in early mammalian development.

EMBRYO RECONSTRUCTION AND CHROMOSOMAL IMPRINTING

Certain alleles can function differently, depending on whether they are located on paternal or maternal chromosomes. Functional differences between homologous alleles are called *genomic imprinting,* an epigenetic programming process that occurs in the germline and that has important consequences for embryonic development (58,59). The presence of two maternal or two paternal copies of particular chromosomes can cause abnormal development in mice (60). A link between imprinting and malignant disease has been suggested in humans, following the finding that maternal chromosomes are lost in some embryonal tumors (61). Such observations may provide information on the import of differences of imprinted paternal and maternal alleles and the expression of recessive tumors. The processes responsible for germline modification of homologous chromosomes and the wide-ranging implications for mammalian development have yet to be fully defined.

The discovery, during the last decade, that the parental genomes are not functionally equivalent during embryogenesis has been made primarily by application of novel experimental techniques to mouse eggs and embryos. The most significant advances have been made by altering the genetic constitution of zygotes by pronuclear and nuclear transplantation, as well as by the introduction of specific cloned genes into eggs and embryos. In conjunction with other experimental reconstruction techniques, such as embryonic fusion and trophoblast transplantation, a number of important developmental aspects have been revealed. In the mouse, eggs can be artificially altered to contain either paternal or maternal genomes alone, and experiments have been designed—mainly by the team of Dr. Surani in Cambridge—for the reconstruction of embryos from tissues of different genotypes.

Neither activated uniparental mammalian eggs, such as parthenogenones, nor reconstituted biparental eggs, with either maternal or paternal nuclei, can develop to term. Although asexual reproduction is a relatively efficient mode for multiplication, sexual reproduction confers greater genetic flexibility, probably more beneficial for the species, and allows adjustment to changing environments. In mammals, remnants of parthenogenetic reproduction remain in the LT/Sv strain of mice, and activated eggs are common, although none of them implant (62). Artificial activation of the egg can be achieved in most species, including humans (63). It is also possible to produce zygotes from which the male pronucleus has been replaced with a second maternal pronucleus (64). These gynogenetic eggs are biparental and heterozygous.

Over a decade ago, researchers postulated that there were two explanations for the demise of parthenogenetic embryos in mammals. First, since parthenogenones are usually homozygous, it was suggested that recessive lethal genes were expressed frequently. Second, activated embryos lack "essential" extragenetic sperm factors. Surani and Barton (65) performed experiments to distinguish between these two possible theories. Triploid zygotes were obtained by suppressing second polar body formation with cytochalasin B. When one female pronucleus was removed, consequently restoring diploidy, normal development to term was possible. However, removal of the single male pronucleus, consequently rendering the diploidized embryo gynogenetic, was incompatible with normal development. Like parthenogenones, some of the gynogenetic embryos implanted, and a few even reached the 25-somite stage; however, none developed to term. This result eliminated the possibility that nonnuclear sperm components were important. This was also confirmed by others, who obtained live mice after transplantation of male and female pronuclei into enucleated parthenogenetic eggs (66).

The significance of homozygosity for failure of parthenogenetic eggs was ruled out by another interesting set of experiments (64). Diploidy in parthenogenetic eggs with a single haploid pronucleus was restored by transfer of the male or female pronucleus from normal donor zygotes. Whereas those with a male pronucleus (and the haploid parthenogenetic pronucleus) developed normally, those with a female pronucleus (heterozygous biparental gynogenesis) did not (Fig. 2.7) (67). Even when fertilized eggs were used for the two heterozygous female pronuclei, embryos failed to reach term (68). The most obvious characteristic of these gynogenetic, and also parthenogenetic, embryos was the chronic lack of placental tissue.

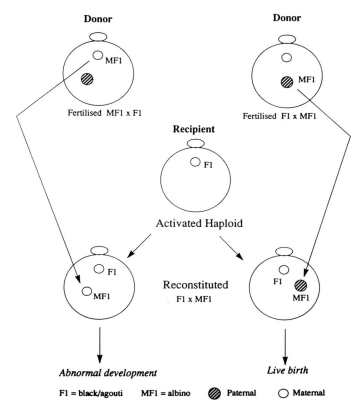

FIG. 2.7. Development of parthenogenetic haploid recipient eggs after introduction of male or female donor pronucleus. (Adapted from Surani MAH, et al. Experimental reconstruction of mouse eggs and embryos: an analysis of mammalian development. *Biol Reprod* 1987; 36:1–16.)

Several types of androgenetic embryos have been produced by micromanipulation (54,69). For instance, one can suppress the first cleavage division following the removal of the female pronucleus from normal zygotes to yield a uniparental homozygous variety. Alternatively, one can produce biparental heterozygous androgenones by introducing a second male pronucleus into a haploid androgenetic egg. A very small proportion of such varieties will implant, and development is always arrested at the early somite stage. However, in contrast with gynogenetic embryos, androgenetic fetuses have well-developed placental tissue. In the human, diploid androgenetic embryos can occur spontaneously by one spermatozoon that becomes diploid or by two different spermatozoa; in both cases the maternal genome is excluded (70). These so-called hydatidiform moles develop trophoblastic hyperplasia, similar to artificial mouse androgenones.

Trophoblast deficiency in parthenogenetic and gynogenetic embryos has been investigated with the use of reconstructed blastocysts (Fig. 2.8). Trophoblast failure persisted after transfer of normal inner cell masses to gynogenetic and parthenogenetic trophectodermal vesicles. However, trophectodermal vesicles from normal embryos were able to support inner cell masses from gynogenetic and parthenogenetic variants up to the 40-somite stage (day 12) of gestation.

The use of aggregation chimeras is especially beneficial for the study of

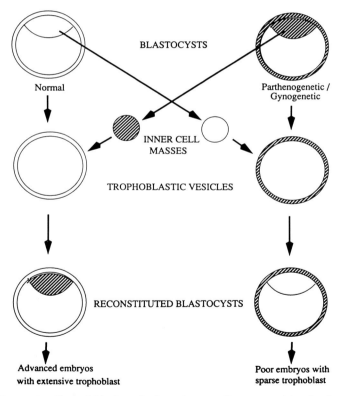

FIG. 2.8. Reconstruction of blastocysts from inner cell mass and trophectoderm tissue obtained from parthenogenetic/gynogenetic and fertilized embryos. (Adapted from Surani MAH, et al. Experimental reconstruction of mouse eggs and embryos: an analysis of mammalian development. *Biol Reprod* 1987;36:1–16.)

androgenetic and gynogenetic tissue. When parthenogenetic embryos were aggregated with normal embryos, adult animals with parthenogenetic cells could be obtained (71). By using similar techniques, androgenetic cells did not survive. Further experiments, using combinations of androgenetic and parthenogenetic embryos, indicated that, even when chromosomes from both parents are present, the resulting embryos fail to reach term unless both sets of chromosomes are present inside the same cells (58). Interestingly, parthenogenetic cells were confined to the fetus, whereas androgenetic cells were predominantly found in the trophoblast. This preferential localization could be attributed to specific information contained in parental chromosomes resulting from modifications of homologous alleles in the germline.

The ability to produce chimeric adults with cells from embryos that would otherwise not develop to term provided an opportunity to obtain unique gametes (72). Hence, it was found that maternal genetic information could be transferred to the next generation in the absence of a paternal contribution. However, androgenetic gametes could not be obtained in the absence of a maternal component.

Nuclear transplantation techniques (transfer of blastomere nuclei into enucleated zygotes) have also been applied to the study of egg reconstitution. For instance, haploid embryonic nuclei have been transplanted into partially enucleated fertilized eggs, from which either the male or female pronucleus was removed. Normal development was restored when haploid nuclei from two- to four-cell androgenetic embryos were transferred into fertilized eggs with a single female pronucleus (69). Transfer of these androgenetic nuclei into zygotes in which the female pronuclei were removed yielded the usual androgenetic pattern. Similar mechanisms were observed when gynogenetic haploid nuclei were transferred into partially enucleated zygotes.

The foregoing studies indicate that gender-specific programming of homologous chromosomes in the germline has profound consequences throughout development. This is confirmed by studies on uniparental disomy in certain abnormal mice. Evidence for heritable molecular differences between maternally and paternally derived alleles on mouse chromosomes was obtained by inserting random DNA into transgenic mice to probe the genome for modified regions (73). One of the autosomal loci showed a difference in DNA methylation, with the paternally derived copy being relatively undermethylated.

Considering these results, Surani et al. (58) have proposed a model of four different classes of genes for controlling gene expression in parental chromosomes. The first class consists of housekeeping genes, which are independent of their parental origin. The second class of regulatory *s* genes are activated only when they are maternally derived. These first two classes of genes—both active in parthenogenones—determine embryonal and fetal development, but do not regulate extraembryonic tissue. The next class of regulatory *w* genes are important for the development of the trophoblast and are modified in the paternal germline. The fourth group of *z* genes are probably only activated when chromosomes from both parents are present within the same cell. The existence of this last group of genes would explain the failure of androgenetic parthenogenetic biparental chimeras to develop normally.

REFERENCES

1. Nicholas JS. Development of transplanted rat eggs. *Proc Soc Exp Biol Med* 1932;30:1111.
2. Pincus, G. *The eggs of mammals*. New York: Macmillan; 1936.
3. Nicholas JS, Hall BV. Experiments on developing rats. II. The development of isolated blastomeres and fused eggs. *J Exp Zool* 1942;90:441–459.
4. Seidel F. Die Entwicklogspotenzen einen isolierton Blastomere des Zweizellenstadiums in Saugetierei. *Naturwissenschaften* 1952;39:355–356.
5. Tarkowsky AK. Experiments on the development of isolated blastomeres of mouse eggs. *Nature* 1959;184:1286–1287.
6. Willadsen SM. A method for culture of micromanipulated sheep embryos and its use to produce monozygotic twins. *Nature* 1979;277:298.
7. Tarkowski AK, Wroblewska J. Development of blastomeres of mouse eggs isolated at the 4- and 8-cell stage. *J Embryol Exp Morphol* 1967;18:155–180.
8. Graham CF, Lehtonen E. Formation and consequences of cell patterns in preimplantation mouse development. *J Embryol Exp Morphol* 1979;49:277.
9. Rossant J. Postimplantation development of blastomeres from 4- and 8-cell mouse eggs. *J Embryol Exp Morphol* 1976;36:283–290.
10. Moore NW, Adams CE, Rowson LEA. Developmental potential of single blastomeres of the rabbit egg. *J Reprod Fertil* 1969;17:527–531.
11. Tarkowski AK. Embryonic and postnatal development of mouse chimaeras. In: Wolstenholme GEW, O'Connor M, eds. *Preimplantation stages of pregnancy.* (A CIBA Symposium). London: Churchill; 1965:183–193.
12. Markert CL, Petters RM. Manufactured hexaparental mice show that adults are derived from three embryonic cells. *Science* 1978;202:56.
13. Dale B, Talevi R, Gualtiere R, et al. Intercellular communication in the early human embryo. *Mol Reprod Dev* 1991;29:22–28.
14. McLaren A. *Mammalian chimareas*. Cambridge: Cambridge University Press;1976.
15. Tarkowsky AK. Mouse chimaeras developed from fused eggs. *Nature* 1961;190:857–860.
16. Mintz B. Experimental study of the developing mammalian egg: removal of the zona pellucida. *Science* 1962;138:594–595.
17. Mintz B. Experimental genetic mosaicism in the mouse. In: Wolstenholme GEW, O'Connor M, eds. *Preimplantation stages of pregnancy.* (A CIBA Symposium). London: Churchill; 1965:194–207.
18. Gardner RL. Mouse chimaeras obtained by the injection of cells into the blastocyst. *Nature* 1968;220:596–597.
19. Tucker EM, Moor RM, Rowson LEA. Tetraparental sheep chimaeras induced by blastomere transplantation. Changes in blood type and age. *Immunology* 1974;26:613–621.
20. Gardner RL, Munroe AJ. Successful construction of chimaeric rabbit. *Nature* 1974; 250:146–147.
21. Gardner RL. Production of chimeras by injecting cells or tissue into the blastocyst. In: Daniel JC, ed. *Methods in mammalian reproduction*. New York: Academic Press; 1978:137–163.
22. Zeilmaker G. Fusion of rat and mouse morulae and formation of chimaeric blastocysts. *Nature* 1973;242:115–116.

23. Gardner RL, Johnson MH. Investigation of early mammalian development using inter-specific chimaeras between rat and mouse. *Nature* 1973;246:86–89.
24. Rossant J, Mauro VM, Croy BA. Importance of trophoblast genotype for survival of inter-specific murine chimaeras. *J Embryol Exp Morphol* 1982;69:141–149.
25. Fehilly CB, Willadsen SM, Tucker E. Interspecific chimaerism between sheep and goat. *Nature* 1984;307:634–636.
26. Jaenisch R, Mintz B. Simian virus 40 DNA sequences in DNA of healthy adult mice derived from preimplantation blastocysts injected with viral DNA. *Proc Natl Acad Sci USA* 1974;71:1250–1255.
27. Jaenisch R, Harbars K, Schnieke A, et al. Germ line integration of Moloney murine leukemia virus at the *Mov 13* locus leads to recessive mutation and early embryonic death. *Cell* 1983;32:209–216.
28. Gordon JW, Scangos GA, Plotkin DJ, Barbosa JA, Ruddle FH. Genetic transformation of mouse embryos by microinjection of purified DNA. *Proc Natl Acad Sci USA* 1980; 77:7380–7384.
29. Stevens LC Jr. The development of transplantable teratocarcinomas from intratesticular grafts of pre- and postimplantation mouse embryos. *Dev Biol* 1970;21:364.
30. Solter D, Damjanov I, Koprowski H. In: Ball M, Wild AE., eds. *The Early development of mammals.* Cambridge: Cambridge University Press;1975:243–264.
31. Evans MJ, Kaufman MH. Establishment in culture of pluripotantial cells from mouse embryos. *Nature* 1981;292:154–156.
32. Martin GR. Isolation of a pluripotential cell line from early mouse embryos cultured in medium conditioned with teratocarcinoma cells. *Proc Natl Acad Sci USA* 1981;78: 7634–7639.
33. Evans M, Bradley A, Robertson E. EK cell contribution to chimeric mice: from tissue culture to sperm. In: Constantini F, Jaenisch R, eds. *Genetic manipulation of the early mammalian embryo.* Banbury Rep 1985;20:93–102.
34. Thomas K, Capecchi MR. Site directed mutagenesis by gene targeting in mouse embryo-derived stem cells. *Cell* 1988;51:503–512.
35. Robertson EJ, Bradley A, Kuehn M, Evans M. Germ line transmission of gene sequences introduced into cultured pluripotential cells by a retroviral vector. *Nature* 1986; 323:445–448.
36. Scangos GA, Ruddle FA. Mechanism and application of DNA-mediated gene transfer in mammalian cells—a review. *Gene* 1981;14:1–10.
37. Robertson EJ. Using embryonic stem cells to introduce mutations into the mouse germ line. *Biol Reprod* 1991;44:238–245.
38. Gardner RL. An investigation of inner cell mass and trophoblast tissues following their isolation from the mouse blastocyst. *J Embryol Exp Morphol* 1972;28:279–312.
39. Solter D, Knowles BB. Immunosurgery of mouse blastocysts. *Proc Natl Acad Sci USA* 1975;72:5099–5102.
40. Slack J. *From egg to embryo.* Cambridge: Cambridge University Press;1983.
41. Warner A. The gap junctions. *J Cell Sci* 1988;89:1–7.
42. Warner A, Lawrence P. Permeability of gap junctions at the segmental border in insect epidermis. *Cell* 1982;28:243–252.
43. Serras F, van den Biggelaar J. Is a mosaic embryo also a mosaic of communication compartments? *Dev Biol* 1987;120:132–138.
44. Marthy H, Dale B. Dye-coupling in the early squid embryo. *Roux Arch Dev Biol* 1990;198:211–218.
45. Lee S, Gilula NB, Warner AE. Gap junctional communication and compaction during preimplantation stages of mouse development. *Cell* 1987;51:851–860.
46. Ducibella T, Albertini DF, Anderson E, Biggers JD. The preimplantation mammalian embryo: characterization of intercellular junctions and their appearance during develop-ment. *Dev Biol* 1975;45:231–250.
47. Gardner RL, Rossant J. Determination during embryogenesis. In: *Embryogenesis in mammals. Ciba Found Symp* 1976;40:5–25.
48. Lo CW, Gilula NB. Gap junctional communication in the preimplantation mouse embryo. *Cell* 1979;18:399–409.
49. Goodhall H, Johnson MH. The nature of intercellular coupling within the preimplantation mouse embryo. *J Embryol Exp Morphol* 1984;79:53–76.

50. Fleming TP, Johnson MH. From egg to epithelium. *Annu Rev Cell Biol* 1988;4:459–485.
51. Braude P, Bolton V, Moore S. Human gene expression first occurs between the four and eight cell stages of preimplantation development. *Nature* 1988;332:459–461.
52. Czolowska R, Waksmundzka M, Kubiak JZ, Tarkowski AK. Chromosome condensation activity in ovulated metaphase II mouse oocytes assayed by fusion with interphase blastomeres. *J Cell Sci* 1986;84:129–138.
53. Tarkowski AK. *In vitro* development of haploid mouse embryos produced by bisection of one-cell fertilized eggs. *J Embryol Exp Morphol* 1977;38:187–202.
54. McGrath J, Solter D. Nuclear transplantation in the mouse embryo by microsurgery and cell fusion. *Science* 1983;220:1300–1302.
55. Zimmermann U. Electric field-mediated fusion and related phenomena. *Biochim Biophys Acta* 1982;694:227–277.
56. Kubiak JZ, Tarkowsky AK. Electrofusion of mouse blastomeres. *Exp Cell Res* 1985; 157:561–566.
57. Flood JT, Chillik CF, van Uem JFHM, Iritani A, Hodgen GD. Ooplasmic transfusion: prophase germinal vesicle oocytes made developmentally competent by microinjection of metaphase II egg cytoplasm. *Fertil Steril* 1990;53:1049–1054.
58. Surani MAH, Barton SC, Norris ML. Influence of parental chromosomes on spatial specificity in androgenetic ⟷ parthenogentic chimeras in the mouse. *Nature* 1987;326: 395–397.
59. Reik W, Surani MAH. Genomic imprinting and embryonal tumours. *Nature* 1989; 338:112–113.
60. Cattanach BM, Krik M. Differential activity of maternally and paternally derived chromosome regions in mice. *Nature* 1985;315:496–498.
61. Toguchida J, Ishizaki K, Sasaki MS, et al. Preferential mutation of paternally derived *RB* gene as the initial event in sporadic osteosarcoma. *Nature* 1989;338:156–158.
62. Stevens LC. Teratocarcinogenesis and spontaneous parthenogenesis in mice. In: Markert CL, Papaconstantinou J, eds. *Developmental biology of reproduction.* New York: Academic Press;1975:13–106.
63. Malter HE, Cohen J. Partial zona dissection of the human oocyte: a nontraumatic method using micromanipulation to assist zona pellucida penetration. *Fertil Steril* 1989;51: 139–148.
64. Surani MAH, Barton SC, Norris ML. Development of reconstituted mouse eggs suggests imprinting of the genome during gametogenesis. *Nature* 1984;307:548–550.
65. Surani MAH, Barton SC. Development of gynogenetic eggs in the mouse: implications for parthenogenetic embryos. *Science* 1983;222:1034–1036.
66. Mann JR, Lovell-Badge RH. Inviability of parthenogenones is determined by pronuclei, not egg cytoplasm. *Nature* 1984;310:66–67.
67. Surani MAH, Barton SC, Norris ML. Experimental reconstruction of mouse eggs and embryos: an analysis of mammalian development. *Biol Reprod* 1987;36:1–16.
68. McGrath J, Solter D. Completion of mouse embryogenesis requires both maternal and paternal genomes. *Cell* 1984;37:179–183.
69. Barton SC, Surani MAH, Norris ML. Role of paternal and maternal genomes in mouse development. *Nature* 1984;311:374–376.
70. Jacobs PA, Wilson C, Sprenkle T. Mechanism of origin of complete hydatiform moles. *Nature* 1980;286:714–716.
71. Surani MAH, Barton SC, Kaufman MH. Development to term of chimaeras between diploid parthenogenetic and fertilized embryos. *Nature* 1977;270:601–602.
72. Stevens LC. Totipotent cells of parthenogenetic origin in a chimaeric mouse. *Nature* 1978;276:266–267.
73. Reik W, Collick A, Norris ML, Barton SC, Surani MAH. Genomic imprinting determines methylation of parental alleles in transgenic mice. *Nature* 1987;328:248–251.

3

Micromanipulation in Animal Husbandry: Gene Alteration and Cloning

Henry E. Malter

In the previous chapter, we examined how micromanipulation techniques have been used to elucidate many important aspects of developmental biology. Experiments on the totipotency of individual blastomeres, as well as those concerning nuclear transfer and reprogramming, demonstrated the plasticity of the early embryo. Animal scientists have taken advantage of this plasticity in developing a variety of techniques for improving animal husbandry. As knowledge about the embryonic genome was gained through a variety of viral and recombinant DNA experiments, the concept of using the new techniques of molecular biology to introduce genetic alterations at the embryonic stage was developed. Using several techniques, the transfer of genes has been successfully completed, creating animals with novel genetic complements. These techniques have not only had a tremendous effect on basic genetic research but also show great promise for use in the improvement of agricultural animals, in the production of vital proteins, and possibly in the treatment of genetic disease. This chapter deals with the application of embryological micromanipulation to genetic alteration, genome extension, and other practical aspects of animal husbandry.

GENETIC ENGINEERING OF ANIMALS: EARLY EXPERIMENTS

Over the past 15 years a variety of strategies have been suggested for the genetic transformation of gametes and early embryos. Theoretically, only by introducing a new gene at the embryonic stage, could it become incorporated into the genome of the developing organism and be appropriately expressed.

Brackett et al. (1) attempted to use sperm as a carrier for foreign DNA. Rabbit sperm was incubated with simian virus (SV) 40 in the presence of dimethyl sulfoxide (DMSO). The sperm was then used to fertilize rabbit eggs. When examined by autoradiography, the eggs were shown to contain the virus. There was, however, no evidence of integration into the embryonic genome. This seductive idea of using sperm as a vector for gene transfer is currently under reevaluation by several laboratories, as discussed later in this section.

In 1974, Jaenisch and Mintz (2,3) produced perhaps the first truly genetically transformed animals by using a micromanipulator to inject a solution of retrovirus into the blastocoele of mouse embryos. Mice that developed following this procedure exhibited viral DNA sequences apparently integrated into their genomes. This showed that stable integration of foreign DNA into a mammalian genome could occur at the embryonic stage. However, for true gene transfer to be accomplished, the DNA to be inserted would ideally be a specific gene, rather than viral DNA. Advances in molecular biology now permit the isolation and cloning of individual genes. Work with *Xenopus* oocytes showed that purified mRNA and DNA could be injected and subsequently transcribed (4,5). This experiment was successfully repeated in the mouse by Brinster et al. (6,7) using globin mRNA. Several laboratories were experimenting with the injection of a solution of cloned genes directly into the pronuclei of mouse zygotes. In 1980, Gordon and coworkers (8) reported the birth of the first animals with a new gene transferred to their genome by gene injection. Other laboratories soon followed with reports of not only successful gene integration, but positive gene expression as well (9–12). Brinster et al. (12) injected a fusion construct consisting of the promoter region of the mouse metallothionein gene combined with the thymidine kinase gene from herpes simplex virus (*HSV-tk*) into the pronuclei of mouse zygotes. Mice were born following the transfer of these injected embryos. The construct was shown to be incorporated into the genome of some of these mice, and several mice demonstrated expression of the transferred gene and thymidine kinase activity. In this experiment, integration efficiency was approximately 20%, with an expression efficiency of 10%.

Gordon and Ruddle (13) suggested the term *transgenic* for genetically engineered animals produced by gene injection. Over the past 10 years, great advancement has been made in the development and application of this technique. The method is now fairly standard, and transgenic rabbits, sheep, pigs, and cows have been produced, as well as perhaps thousands of transgenic mouse lines (14–16).

PRODUCTION OF TRANSGENIC ANIMALS

Gene Injection

During the gene injection procedure, several hundred to several thousand copies of a specific DNA fragment are introduced into the pronucleus of a zygote. A fine glass needle is loaded with an aqueous solution of the DNA to be injected. The zygote is stabilized with a holding pipette while the needle is inserted into the male pronucleus. The procedure is illustrated in Fig. 3.1. The male pronucleus is selected for its larger size. It has been suggested that owing to the DNA alterations that take place during sperm pronuclear formation and at *syngamy* (protamine–histone replacement and DNA repair), that integration may be enhanced by placement of the transgene into the sperm pronucleus (10,17). A volume of solution is expelled and the pronucleus is observed for expansion. Often an approximate doubling in size is used as a gauge for the maximum safe injection volume, which corresponds to approximately 2 pL. The needle is then quickly withdrawn. The procedure is straightforward and relatively nontraumatic. With practice, several hundred zygotes can be injected in a day's experiment, with approximately 70% to 90% survival. Zygotes are cultured until the desired stage for transfer to a pseudopregnant female.

In examining the efficiency of various gene injection protocols, Brinster et al. (18) determined that the optimum DNA concentration for maximum efficiency was approximately 1 ng/mL; higher concentrations were toxic. In the same study, the optimum DNA form was found to be linear molecules with standard ("sticky") ends. The highest integration efficiency obtained was 25% to 30%, for an overall efficiency of approximately 6%.

The timing of pronuclear injection can be important to success. Injections are best performed shortly after pronuclear formation. Mice are bred overnight and pronuclear zygotes can be collected and injected during the late morning or early afternoon. This timing was evaluated by Walton et al. (19) in discussing various aspects related to zygote viability during gene injection in the mouse and sheep. Zygote survival was particularly reduced when injections were done late in the day. At this time, when the pronuclear membranes become indistinct in advance of syngamy and cleavage, susceptibility to damage is apparently quite high. Ultrastructural analysis of damage to the oocyte membrane resulting from the insertion of the micropipette was also provided. They found that, as might be expected, survival of the procedure was related to the size of the micropipette used for injection. They used both "large" and "small" pipettes, both with 0.7 μm tips, but the small pipette had a more rapid taper. The smaller pipette, thus produced substantially smaller holes in the plasma membrane and resulted in increased zygote survival, especially in the sheep zygotes. Variations in

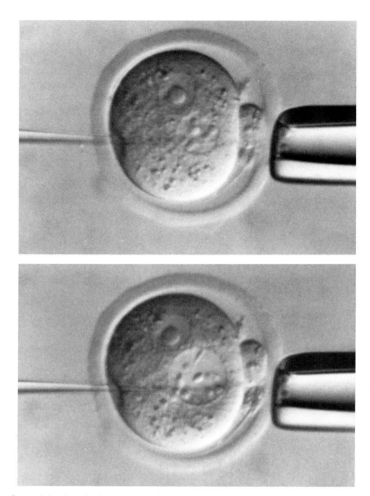

FIG. 3.1. Gene injection in the mouse. A mouse zygote is stabilized with a holding pipette while the gene injection needle is introduced into the male pronucleus. In the lower photo, swelling of the pronucleus as the DNA solution is expelled is evident. (Courtesy of R.L. Brinster, University of Pennsylvania School of Veterinary Medicine.)

the injection procedure, such as delayed withdrawal of the needle, did not result in any significant differences. Several important aspects of the gene injection procedure are illustrated in Fig. 3.2.

In general, the smallest needle that can be used without clogging is desirable. The clogging of the gene injection needle is a frequent problem. Several filled needles should be kept on hand so that work can proceed when a clogged needle must be replaced. Another problem is that nucleolar material

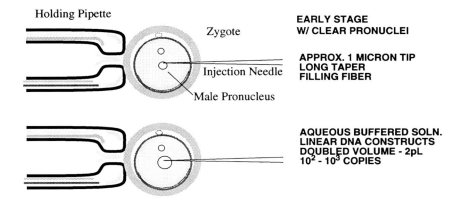

FIG. 3.2. Important factors in gene injection (see refs. 18,19).

can adhere to the needle and will be withdrawn when the needle is removed. In general, pronuclear injection is a straightforward and simple technique. Skill at gene injection, as with all micromanipulative methods, can be obtained only with patience and practice. Some basic aspects of pronuclear injection will be discussed in Chapter 10.

A particularly important aspect of the generation of transgenic mice is the transfer of embryos to surrogate mothers. Early-stage embryos are normally transferred to the fimbria of the oviduct, whereas later-stage morulae or blastocysts are inserted through the uterine wall. One problem with fimbrial transfers is that the bursa membrane, which must be penetrated by the transfer pipette, is heavily vascularized. Bursa dissection often results in substantial bleeding, which may obscure the area and contaminate the oviduct. Pintado and coworkers (20) published an abstract on the use of topical epinephrine (adrenaline) as a hemostatic agent during murine embryo transfer. Epinephrine at a dose of 0.1 μg/mL reduced bleeding, thereby allowing better visibility during the transfer procedure. This dose did not have an adverse effect on embryonic survival.

Transgene Integration

At syngamy, as the genetic material from the two pronuclei combine, the foreign fragments can be incorporated into the new embryonic genome, as illustrated in Fig. 3.3. Integration may sometimes occur later during embryonic cleavage. This delayed integration, which occurs perhaps 30% of the time, results in a genome that is mosaic for the transgene (21). Integration is apparently a random event. Often the fusion constructs link together to form tandem repeats. This results in the integration of multiple copies of the

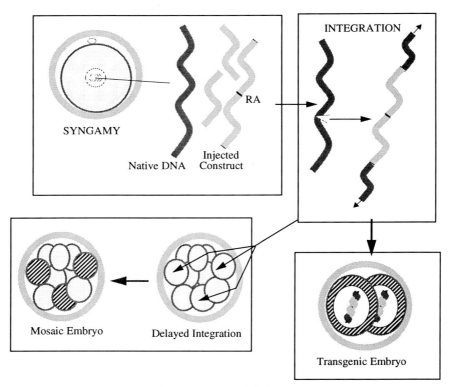

FIG. 3.3. Integration of injected DNA constructs. Constructs often spontaneously fuse to form repeated arrays *(RA)*. At syngamy, constructs can be inserted into naturally occurring breaks in the endogenous DNA, resulting in a transgenic embryo. Integration can be delayed until several cleavage cycles have occurred. This results in a mosaic embryo.

transgene. Unfortunately, this random integration can result in substantial perturbations of the native DNA. Covarrubias et al. (22,23) described the insertion site in several strains of transgenic mice, illustrated in Fig. 3.4. In two of these strains, perturbation of the native DNA during transgene integration resulted in unique recessive lethal mutations. In two other strains, equally substantial DNA rearrangement at the insertion site did not result in any overt phenotypic effect. Transgene expression often varies greatly among different lines of the identical construct (24). Obviously, the chromosomal location and position of the new gene in relation to adjacent genes and regulatory elements is important to expression (21). Once a transgene is integrated into the genome, it becomes like any other gene and can be passed on to offspring. However, there have been cases of transgenes that exhibited altered expression patterns (including failure of expression) in progeny (25).

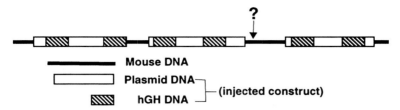

FIG. 3.4. The insertion site of a human growth hormone construct which represents a lethal mutation. Several copies of the construct have integrated interspersed with endogenous mouse DNA sequences which have been disrupted and rearranged. (Adapted from Covarrubias L et al. Early postimplantation embryo lethality due to DNA rearrangements in a transgenic mouse strain. *Proc Natl Acad Sci USA* 1986;83:6020–6024.)

Fusion Constructs

The key to the success and flexibility of the transgenic technique lies in the genetic constructs that are used for injection. As our understanding of the molecular biology of gene regulation has advanced (in no small part owing to transgenic experiments themselves), regulatory DNA sequences have been identified that control gene expression. It was found that these *cis*-acting elements could be isolated and linked to foreign genes to control their expression. Basicly, fusion constructs are created to direct transgene expression to particular tissues or the desired developmental stage. The promoter sequence associated with the elastase gene has been used to direct the expression of transgenes to the pancreas in a highly specific manner (26,27). By using the promoter sequence from the $\alpha_2(1)$-collagen gene, expression of a marker gene was obtained in the appropriate tissues at the correct developmental stage (28).

Regulatory sequences can also put the attached transgene under the control of a desired physiologic or external stimulus. The product of the metallothionein gene is involved with the control of heavy-metal toxicity. Expression of this gene is inducible by heavy metals and glucocorticoid hormones. By fusing the promoter sequence of this gene to a desired transgene and performing gene injection in mice, transgene expression was found to be inducible in the resulting animals by endogenous zinc (25). Interestingly, glucocorticoids did not have an effect on expression. Other promoters have been shown to be inducible by hormones (29,30). Obviously, gene expression is an exceedingly complex system and any attempt at regulation must take the background of random insertion into consideration. The correct positioning of *cis*-acting elements relative to the transgene can be a complex task (21). There have been several cases of incorrect and unexpected expression patterns using fusion constructs (31,32).

TRANSGENIC MOUSE EXPERIMENTS

Hundreds of experiments have been done using transgenic mice to elucidate questions in developmental biology, oncology, immunology, gene regulation, and genetic disease. Several excellent reviews have been published (21,33,34). This section will highlight a few important papers.

In perhaps the most famous transgenic experiment, illustrated in Fig. 3.5, the construct consisted of the metallothioneine promoter (MT) fused to the gene for rat growth hormone (35). Transgenic mice created with this construct exhibited accelerated and increased growth. Several animals were found to be producing enormous amounts of growth hormone. The authors suggested that this high level of gene product, which, in one case, was 10- to 100-fold higher than that of bacterial or mammalian cell culture systems, might indicate that transgenic animals could be used for the commercial production of valuable proteins. This concept of *molecular farming* is currently being developed by several groups. It will be discussed in a later section.

Recently, Yun and coworkers (36) published a fascinating extension of the transgenic experiments with the MT–growth hormone construct. Female mice that are transgenic for an MT–human growth hormone fusion gene are

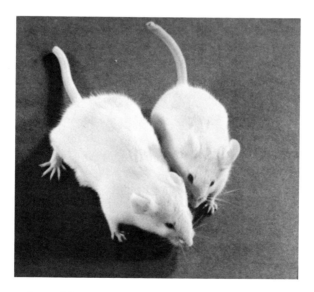

FIG. 3.5. Increased growth in a transgenic mouse produced from gene injection with a mouse metallothionein–rat growth hormone construct (35). The mouse on the *left* is transgenic and weighs 44 g, compared with a nontransgenic sibling on the *right,* weighing 29 g. (Courtesy of R. L. Brinster, University of Pennsylvania School of Veterinary Medicine.)

sterile. Mouse lines that are heterozygous for the transgene are easily acquired by breeding male transgenics with normal females. By surgically transferring the ovaries of transgenic females to normal fertile females and breeding the resulting mice with transgenic male mice, individuals that were homozygous for the transgenic locus were obtained. These mice exhibit a doubled concentration of serum human growth hormone and attain a greater body weight, compared with heterozygous animals. Apparently both copies of the transgene are expressed independently in the homozygous animals.

The transfer of a functional β-globin gene to mice harboring a genetic lesion for this gene resulted in a "cure" for the hemolytic anemia usually associated with the deletion (37). This represented a successful mouse model for the correction of the human hereditary disease β-thalassemia. Isola and Gordon (38) showed that a transgene could be used to confer drug resistance. A mutant gene for dyhydrofolate reductase was used to create transgenic mice. The product of this gene had been shown to be resistant to methotrexate (MTX) toxicity. Mice that expressed the transgene, exhibited greater tolerance to MTX and survived significantly longer than control animals.

By fabricating a construct combining a human heavy chain (variable, diversity, and joining domains—*IgH*) minilocus with a human μ (constant) chain, transgenic mice were created that rearranged the *IgH* locus in their lymphoid tissues and produce human monoclonal antibodies (39). Splenic hybridomas were obtained from these mice, which produced 2 mg of human IgM per liter. This technique might allow the routine production of a range of complete monoclonal antibodies of entirely human origin from transgenic mice strains expressing human light and heavy chain miniloci. Transgenic experiments have also helped elucidate several aspects of the immune system response, particularly self-tolerance (reviewed in 34)

Active developmental domains were probed in transgenic mice by using a construct based on the concept that a weak promoter would permit transgene expression to be determined by the chromosomal insertion site (40). Theoretically, expression of the transgene would be promoted in highly active chromosomal domains during development. The *HSV-tk* promoter was fused to an in situ marker gene and used to create transgenic fetuses that were analyzed during a key developmental period (day 11 of gestation). Histochemical analysis revealed a high degree of variation in the expression pattern for tissue and spatial specificity. The expression patterns were shown to be heritable (40). This technique will be helpful in analyzing mammalian developmental genetics (reviewed in 41).

Another dramatic experiment on mammalian development involved highly specific tissue ablation using the elastase promoter (42). As previously discussed, this promoter is specific in directing expression to the acinar cells of the pancreas. In an ingenious design, it was fused to the gene for the α-polypeptide of diphtheria toxin. The active toxin consists of the α-chain, combined with a β-chain which allows cell binding and endocytosis. Thus, the action of the isolated α-polypeptide, an efficient protein synthesis inhibitor, would be restricted within each cell that expressed the transgene. Expression of this construct in transgenic mice resulted in almost total ablation of pancreatic tissue. Pups were born with no pancreatic tissue or with only rudimentary or necrotic tissue (42). This approach could be of great value by using specific promoters to study cell lineages and relationships between cell types during development.

Transgenic mice have been a natural choice for the study of oncogenes and the inception and progression of neoplasia. A variety of oncogenes have been linked to novel promoters, resulting in directed neoplastic development (43,44). The ability to induce hyperplasia has made possible a careful analysis of cancer progression, such as the importance and timing of angiogenesis in tumor development (45).

Recently, a preliminary report was published concerning the use of a variation of the gene injection technique to successfully insert very large DNA molecules into the murine genome (46). Intact yeast artificial chromosome segments of 350 kilobases (kb) and longer were isolated and injected into the pronuclei of mouse zygotes. Hybridization experiments have shown that these segments were incorporated into the genome of the resulting mice. These mice were termed *transomic* by the investigators. The further development of this transomic technique could have wide-ranging application in the study of gene regulation and expression.

MOLECULAR FARMING

Theoretically, by using regulatory fusion constructs, transgene product synthesis can be directed to the proper site or to a novel site. One concept currently under intense research is the direction of transgene expression to the mammary gland in large domestic animals. In this way, genes for valuable human proteins, such as clotting factors and interferon, could be expressed in the mammary tissue and subsequently harvested from the milk of transgenic animals. At present, transgenic mice and sheep have been created that exhibit this expression pattern by using a promoter sequence from β-lactoglobulin (47,48). Transgenic sheep were created with a fusion construct consisting of the coding sequence of human clotting factor IX combined with sequences from the sheep β-lactoglobulin (β-lac) gene. Milk from these animals contained active human factor IX, which could be isolated and purified. However, the concentration was quite low; only 0.001% of the normal concentration of β-lac in sheep milk. A second group of transgenic sheep was created with human α1-antitrypsin as the transgene. Expression was better here, although still several hundred times less than that of the native gene product. It is hoped that new constructs can be devised that successfully address these expression problems.

Other workers have concentrated on transgenic milk modification through the whey acidic protein (*WAP*) gene (49,50). The promoter sequence from the mouse *WAP* gene was fused with the gene for human tissue plasminogen activator (*tPA*), a vital protein involved with the clotting mechanism. Transgenic mice created with this construct exhibited good expression of the *tPA* gene in the lactating mammary gland, resulting in up to 0.1 mg of tPA per milliliter of mouse milk. In fact, milk from these mice

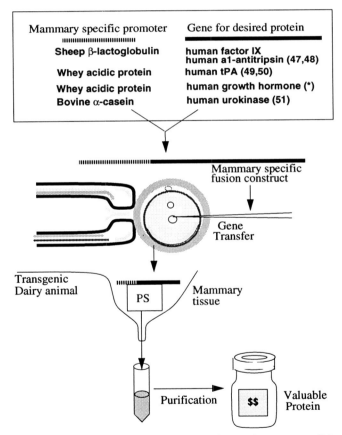

FIG. 3.6. Molecular farming. Several successful experiments have accomplished combining mammary specific promoters with genes for valuable proteins to create a mammary specific construct as indicated in the *upper* section (*, B. G. Brackett, personal communication). Constructs are used to obtain transgenic dairy animals through gene transfer. Expression is directed to the mammary tissue, where synthesis of the desired protein takes place *(PS)*. The protein is excreted into the milk and can be isolated and purified for use.

was able to break up a blood clot in a laboratory dish! Brackett and coworkers (Brackett BG, personal communication) also used the *WAP* promoter to derive mammary-specific expression of the human growth hormone gene in mice. Recently, Meade and Longberg (51) reported high-level expression of the human urokinase gene under the control of a bovine α-casein promoter sequence in transgenic mice.

Molecular farming experiments are summarized in Fig. 3.6. The potential to produce valuable proteins through molecular farming appears to be limited only by our ability to develop more efficient transgenic expression systems. However, ethical and legal questions will have to be addressed as well. No doubt, practical molecular farming will become a reality in the near future.

THE IMPROVEMENT OF LARGE DOMESTIC SPECIES

The transfer of genes providing an improved phenotype would seem to be an ideal tool for use in the development of superior farm animals. Several experiments have been conducted in this area, but advances have been slow. Practical embryology of large-animal species is much more difficult than that of the mouse. Obtaining large-animal zygotes in the quantities required for the gene injection technique is not a trivial task. The in vitro culture of the resulting embryos is also problematic. Nevertheless, transgenic sheep, pigs, and cows have been produced with altered phenotypes (14–16). Massey (52) reported on work conducted at Granada Genetics, a large commercial cattle facility. The results of two recent experiments in the production of transgenic cattle indicate that the efficiency of production is quite low. Following the collection of almost 4,000 bovine pronuclear embryos, only 1,704 were considered suitable for injection. This experiment resulted in the establishment of 79 pregnancies of which only 1 of 16 calves born was transgenic. A second experiment using over 2,000 in vitro-matured–in vitro-fertilized embryos gave similar results, with greater losses during the culture stage. This low efficiency necessitates the large-scale production available only at establishments of this type.

Gene Injection in Large Animals

One specific problem with the application of gene injection lies in the fact that large-animal zygotes, such as those of the cow, goat, and pig, have a dense lipid-rich cytoplasm that prevents visualization of the pronuclei. Two strategies have been successfully applied for solving this problem. Zygotes are subjected to centrifugation, which stratifies the occluding material, allowing the pronuclei to be observed. Wall and coworkers (53) used a protocol of $15,000 \times g$ for 3 minutes for pronuclear visualization in pig zygotes. Centrifugation at 20,000×g for 3 minutes was considered optimum in another study on bovine zygotes (54). Vital DNA stains, such as Hoechst 33258 and diamidinophenylindole (DAPI), have also been used to visualize pronuclei during injection (55,56).

In 1985, the first report of transgenic rabbits, sheep, and pigs was published (14). The construct consisted of the mouse metallothioneine promoter fused with the gene for human growth hormone (*MT-hGH*). Integration frequency was only about 12% for the rabbits and pigs and very low (1.3%) in the sheep. Expression was somewhat better, occurring in 25% of the transgenic rabbits and over half of the transgenic pigs. Varying amounts of hGH were detectable in the animals, with three pigs and one rabbit exhibiting high levels, even in the absence of any endogenous heavy-metal stimulation. No effect on growth was reported. Later work with *MT-GH* constructs in transgenic sheep and pigs did not provide encouragement for this particular route of genetic alteration (57,58). Animals exhibited a range of highly negative side effects, such as muscle weakness and reproductive dysfunction. Apparently, the ubiquitous expression pattern of the *MT* promoter resulted in an abnormal growth hormone profile, causing these effects. However, the transgenic pigs in this experiment did exhibit decreased backfat, indicating that the hormone was, to some extent, promoting more efficient growth metabolism.

McGrane et al. (59) reported a new construct, developed in transgenic mice, in which bovine growth hormone was put under the control of the rat phosphoenolpyruvate carboxykinase (*PEPCK*) promoter. With this promoter, transgenic growth hormone levels are directly linked to metabolism, as the *PEPCK* gene normally responds to carbohydrate and protein intake. In the mouse experiments, gene expression could be regulated by dietary carbohydrate and protein levels. Transgenic pigs have now been created with this construct (60). Approximately 6% of pigs derived from gene transfer were transgenic in these experiments, and germline transmission was evident in at least one case. Overall efficiency in producing expression-positive animals was approximately 0.5%. The transgenic animals exhibited enhanced feed efficiency and dramatically reduced body fat; a 41% reduction compared with control animals. The overall health of the transgenic pigs was superior to that in previous reports using the *MT-GH* construct. However, the same negative symptoms (apparently associated with elevated serum growth hormone in general) were present to a lesser degree and at a later stage in growth. The *PEPCK* promoter is active only from the time of birth in contrast to the *MT* promoter, which is active during gestation. Reproductive dysfunction, joint pathology, and increased stress-related problems were observed in adult transgenic pigs.

The concept of milk alteration for the purpose of molecular farming has been discussed. A related idea is the use of transgenic technology to simply modify milk composition. Animal milk is an important foodstuff for most of the planet, especially in developing countries. The ability to improve the protein content of milk would be highly desirable. In pursuing this goal, Simmons et al. (61) created transgenic mice that expressed a sheep β-lactoglobulin gene and exhibited high levels of this protein in their milk. This approach could be used to alter milk composition in improving nutritive value or in optimizing for particular food science protocols (reviewed in 62).

Despite the problems involved, there would seem to be a multitude of valuable goals that could be reached through the application of transgenic technology in livestock and dairy animal improvement. No doubt the future holds great promise in this direction.

Problems with Gene Injection

Gene injection is currently far from an ideal technique. Serious drawbacks lie in the ambiguity and genetic damage of random integration and in the overall inefficiency of the technique. It is true that biopsy and genetic analysis could be done on gene-injected embryos to increase overall efficiency by identifying positive integration before transfer (63). No doubt this technique will be used in the most critical large-animal procedures. Ninomiya and coworkers (64) reported preliminary experiments in which the polymerase chain reaction (PCR) was used to select embryos for positive integration. Putative transgenic mouse morulae were bisected; one half was set aside for culture and the other half was used for the analysis. Within 7 hours, the PCR analysis was conducted, and positive embryos were identified for transfer. Approximately 36% of analyzed morulae were positive for the transgene. When PCR-negative morulae were transferred, none of the seven resulting mice were transgenic. When PCR-positive embryos were used, one of two animals born was transgenic.

Ideally, new constructs or techniques need to be devised that allow efficient directed integration without perturbation of the genomic DNA. Viral integration occurs in a stable and nondestructive fashion. Possibly the use of novel retroviral control sequences or new artificially synthesized regulatory sequences will provide the answer. Despite its problems, currently, gene injection remains the most workable and successful technique available for animal genetic engineering.

Alternative Methods for Creating Transgenics

Two main alternatives to gene injection have been proposed: retroviral gene transfer and stem cell-mediated gene transfer. Jaenisch (65,66) showed that preimplantation embryos could be infected with a virus, with subsequent integration of the viral sequence into their genome. This observation suggested a method by which an altered virus could act as a vector for embryonic gene transfer. This method does not require the use of micromanipulation and is actually quite ingenious. It relies on the creation of genetically engineered retroviruses that not only carry the coding sequence for the new gene, but have also been rendered incapable of causing further infection. This technique has been used successfully and has the advantage of stable single-copy integration (67,68). However, the size of the gene to be transferred is limited to 10 kb, which would be too small for many genes (69). Also, the presence of viral long-terminal repeat (LTR) sequences can have a detrimental effect on expression (66). However, there have been reports of successful gene transfer and expression using the retroviral method (70). One hopes that future refinements of this technique will result in improved performance.

The second alternative to gene injection is stem cell-mediated transfer. Embryonic stem cells represent one of the most exciting aspects of mammalian genetics. Early work, done by Brinster in the mouse (71), showed that foreign cells, such as teratocarcinoma cells that are introduced into a developing blastocyst, become incorporated into the embryonic tissues and take part in the formation of the new individual. In fact, this work, performed contemporaneously with the retroviral injection work of Jaenisch, may represent the first instance of the creation of genetically altered animals. As discussed in the previous chapter, cell lines have been developed that are derived from the inner cell mass (ICM) of a developing blastocyst (72,73). These cells are maintained in culture in an undifferentiated state and can be manipulated by a wide range of cell culture techniques. However, they are pluripotential and can be introduced into the blastocoele of an embryo and become incorporated into the ICM (74). Thus, a chimera is created, with some cell lineages derived from the stem cells. There are a variety of ways of introducing new DNA into cultured cells, including retroviral infection, electroporation, and chemical transfer methods (75–78). These methods have been used to transform stem cells in culture to create cell lines that contain new genes. These transgenic stem cells are then transferred to a developing blastocyst to create a chimeric individual; mosaic for the new transgene (78). As long as some germ cells contain the new gene, selective breeding can produce nonmosaic transgenic offspring. Stem cell-mediated gene transfer is illustrated in Fig. 3.7. As mentioned in the previous chapter, Robertson (79) described methods for increasing the efficiency of germ cell colonization by using stem cells with an *XY* genotype. The XY cells were particularly successful when the host blastocysts were derived from mouse lines having mutations affecting fertility. In one experiment that used this technique, five of seven fertile males obtained were germline chimeras (79).

The real power of stem cell transfer lies in the cell culture stage. The exact genetic makeup of the cells can be determined, and selection techniques can be applied to obtain the most appropriate transgenic makeup before

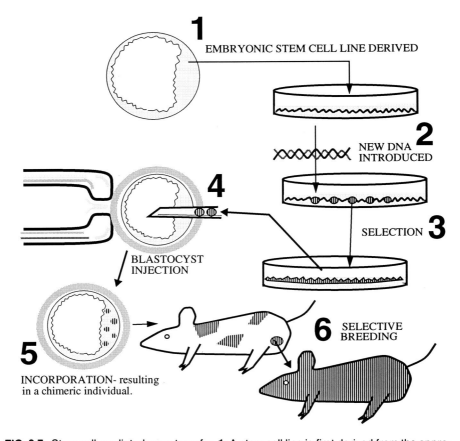

FIG. 3.7. Stem cell-mediated gene transfer. **1:** A stem cell line is first derived from the appropriate embryonic tissue. **2:** New DNA is introduced into the cells by several methods. **3:** Positive transgenic cells are identified and selected by several methods to obtain pure transgenic cell lines with desired characters. **4:** Transgenic cells are injected into the blastocoele of an embryo. **5:** Injected cells become incorporated into the embryo, resulting in a chimeric offspring. **6:** As long as some germ cells are derived from the transgenic lineage, selective breeding can be used to obtain nonchimeric transgenic animals.

transfer. In fact, gene–gene replacement by homologous recombination has been accomplished with this method. This would be the ideal scenario for the treatment of genetic lesions or the improvement of native gene products, since the original gene is, in effect, replaced by the inserted transgene. By use of this method, working with a mouse model, the genetic defect associated with Lesch–Nyhan disorder was reversed through the transfer of a functional hypoxanthine phosphoribosyltransferase (*hprt*) gene, which replaced the defective gene (80,81). Actually, the HPRT-deficient mice were originally created using another important homologous recombination concept: the inactivation of a native gene (77). By replacing it with a disrupted transgene, the native gene is inactivated. Gene inactivation can be used to mimic a particular existing genetic lesion, as in the HPRT-negative mice or to study the role of a gene in development (reviewed in 82). In a recent dramatic experiment, DeChiara et al. (83) reported the inactivation of the insulin-like growth factor II gene through stem cell-mediated gene targeting. Progeny of mice that were germlike chimeras for the inactivated gene exhibited overtly reduced growth (60% of that of their littermates with functional *IGF-II* genes), as illustrated in Fig. 3.8.

Gene targeting relies on the ability to screen the cells for particular traits, such as resistance to antibiotics, that can be derived only from recombination. The vectors for gene transfer usually include the *neo*[r] gene, which provides resistance to neomycin (84). Positive integration is identified by the ability of cells to grow in the presence of a related drug, G418. In early experiments examining various recombination screening strategies, it was found that the frequency of homologous recombination was actually quite high (85). In some cases, such as the *hprt* gene-inactivation experiments, positive targeting can be selected directly (once positive integration is verified by *neo*[r] selection). This gene is present in a single copy (X chromosome) in male cells, so cells in which the *hprt* gene has been inactivated can be selected for by growth in the presence of a cytotoxic guanine analogue (78).

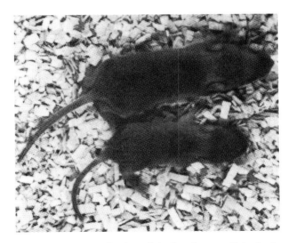

FIG. 3.8. Mouse produced by the inactivation of the insulin growth factor type-II *(IGF-II)* gene. These animals are littermates and are offspring of a chimeric animal derived from stem cells in which the *IGF-II* gene was inactivated by gene targeting. The *upper* animal is of the wild type and the lower animal is heterozygous for the inactivated gene. (Reprinted with permission from DeChiara TM, et al. A growth-deficiency phenotype in heterozygous mice carrying an insulin-like growth factor II gene disrupted by targeting. *Nature* 1990;345:78–80. Copyright © 1990 Macmillan Magazines Ltd.)

Two types of basic-targeting vectors have been described: sequence-replacement vectors and sequence-insertion vectors (77). These are illustrated in Fig. 3.9. In both cases, part of the coding sequence of the targeted gene is disrupted by the *neo*[r] gene. The insertion of sequence-replacement vectors results in a replacement of the normal sequence with the vector sequence. Sequence-insertion vectors are designed so that the two ends of the vector molecule are homologous with adjacent sequences of the endogenous gene. Recombination results in an insertion of the vector into the native sequence with a duplication of some sequences.

For targeting of host genes that are not directly selectable, the positive–negative selection strategy is used as illustrated in Fig. 3.10 (86). This strategy uses a sequence-replacement vector in which a copy of the *neo*[r] gene is inserted into a noncoding exon region and a copy of a positive selectable gene (*HSV-tk*) is inserted adjacent to the homologous sequences. The *HSV-tk* gene is selected for by growth in ganciclovir, a cytotoxic nucleoside analogue that is toxic to HSV-tk–positive cells. When this vector inserts randomly, the entire sequence is integrated and the resulting cells contain functional *neo*[r] and *HSV-tk* genes. When homologous recombination takes place, however, the *HSV-tk* sequences are lost as recombination between the

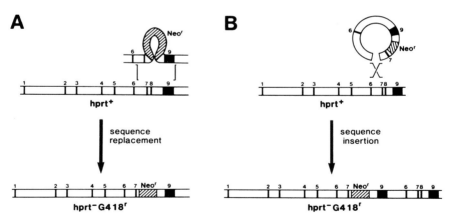

FIG. 3.9. Gene targeting by sequence replacement and sequence insertion vectors. **A:** The *hprt* gene is targeted with a sequence replacement vector that consists of homologous *hprt* sequences with the *neo*[r] gene inserted into the eighth exon. Recombination results in a replacement of some of the endogenous sequences by vector sequences. **B:** The *hprt* gene is targeted by a sequence replacement vector such that adjacent homologous sequences form the ends of the linearized vector. Recombination with this vector causes the entire vector to be inserted into the endogenous gene sequence, with a resulting duplication of the end segments. In both cases the *hprt* gene is disrupted and the *neo*[r] is inserted into the genome for selection procedures (see text for more details). (From Capecchi MR. The new mouse genetics: altering the genome by gene targeting. *Trends Genet* 1989;5:70–76, with permission.)

A **Gene Targeting**

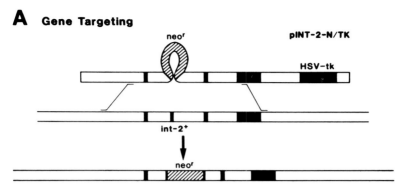

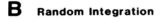

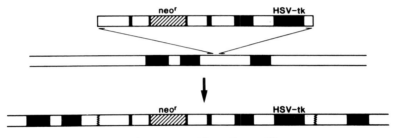

B **Random Integration**

FIG. 3.10. Gene targeting of the *int-2* gene using the positive–negative selection protocol. The sequence replacement vector consists of homologous sequences of the *int-2* gene with the *neo*[r] gene inserted into one of the exons and the *HSV-tk* gene placed in a terminal nonhomologous fashion. **A:** When the vector inserts in a targeted fashion, the *HSV-tk* gene is lost owing to the lack of homology with endogenous sequences. **B:** When the vector inserts randomly, through the ends of the entire linear molecule, the *HSV-tk* gene is retained. The presence of the *neo*[r] and *HSV-tk* genes can be identified by selection techniques as described in the text, and in this way positive homologous recombinants can be identified. (From Capecchi MR. The new mouse genetics: altering the genome by gene targeting. *Trends Genet* 1989;5:70–76, with permission.)

endogenous and vector sequences occurs. This results in cells that have only the *neo*[r] gene incorporated. Selection for cells that grow in the presence of G418 and ganciclovir can, therefore, be used to identify and select positive homologous recombinants.

Stem cell-mediated gene transfer is obviously much more complicated than gene injection. It involves not only difficult micromanipulation techniques, but also the creation and manipulation of the stem cell lines, as well as selective breeding. To date, such lines have been created only in the mouse. The creation of embryonic stem cell lines from large domestic animals is a current goal of many laboratories worldwide. Recently, porcine ICM and embryonic disk cell lines were described (87). The cells exhibited differentiation patterns in culture, which would indicate that they are pluripotential. A second report discussed the establishment of similar cell lines from sheep embryos (88). Two laboratories recently provided preliminary reports on the establishment of stem cell-like lines derived from bovine ICM cells (89,90). The ability of these cells to participate in chimera formation is currently under evaluation. Embryonic stem cell lines will be of tremendous importance not only to genetic engineering, but also to the development of optimum-cloning methods for large animals as will be discussed in the next part of this chapter.

Recently, a report was published concerning a new method for creating transgenic mice (91). Mouse sperm was incubated with a solution of a transgene construct. When this sperm was used to fertilize mouse eggs, the resulting embryos developed into mice that exhibited high levels of transgene integration and expression. Unfortunately, this work has not been reproduced, despite efforts by several top laboratories (92). The authors of the original work continue to claim that the technique is functional in their hands and report on preliminary success with pig embryos (93,94). Gagne et al. (95) recently presented preliminary work using sperm as a vector for genetic transformation in the bovine. Bovine sperm was exposed to a radiolabeled DNA construct solution under a variety of conditions involving electroporation. The fraction of DNA retained by the sperm following several washes ranged from 9% to 15% for the electroporation treatments and was 6.5% following simple incubation without any electrical stimulus. When the acrosome was removed from sperm in these treatments, the percentage of retained label was reduced. Following electroporation with an unlabeled construct, sperm was used to fertilize in vitro matured bovine eggs. The fertilization rate was 83% and development to the morula stage was 24%. The development of a practical technique for sperm-mediated gene transfer would greatly simplify the transgenic methodology.

HUMAN GERMLINE ALTERATION

Because of the problems involved with the various gene-transfer strategies, as outlined earlier, it would seem that attempting to alter the human germline with the current methodology would be highly ill-advised. The random and destructive nature of integration following pronuclear injection would disqualify this technique until improved constructs are developed. The mosaic nature of transgenic organisms developed through stem cell- or retroviral-mediated transfer would also be unacceptable in a human germline treatment scenario. Transgenic animal experiments have shown great promise in the development of somatic gene therapies and for the future of potential germline strategies. The goals of negating the vast array of human genetic lesions and improving the treatment of other major health problems, such as cancer, through germline modification are worthy of much effort. One hopes that the problems with current technologies will be solved and successful germline strategies developed. Human germline therapy strategies will be briefly discussed in Chapter 11.

GENOME EXTENSION

Since the discovery of the relative plasticity of early mammalian embryos, animal scientists have proposed a variety of methods that take advantage of this plasticity in extending the genome of valuable embryos. Large domestic species have been developed over hundreds of years of selective breeding to produce animals that exhibit optimum efficiency and productivity. The individual that produces the most milk or meat per unit of input is obviously of great value. The gametes and embryos of superior animals have become expensive commodities around the world. Therefore, the extension of these valuable genomes through embryological methods is an important goal.

Early Research

Since the work of Roux during the late 1800s, with frog embryos, it was known that separated blastomeres could exhibit some degree of embryonic development (96). Nicholas and Hall (97) repeated this experiment for the first time with mammals in the rat. This concept was taken to its logical conclusion by Seidel (98), who obtained live offspring in the rabbit from half embryos derived from single two-cell stage blastomeres. The work of Tarkowski, Mintz, Gardner, and others, discussed in the previous chapter, further elucidated the nature of mammalian embryo potency and provided an arsenal of techniques for genome manipulation. Several workers attempted to transfer the experimental rodent techniques to large-animal embryology, without great success (99,100). Finally, Willadsen (101) took the lessons of the earlier research and created a practical method with which multicell embryos of large animals could be simply divided to produce multiple identical offspring. A key factor in the success of these experiments was the development of a culture method for the micromanipulated embryos. The embryos that were divided for artificial twinning had very large gaps created in their zona pellucidae. Willadsen realized that upon transfer to the recipient's oviduct, blastomeres could be lost through these gaps, while immune cells or toxins from the oviduct could enter and destroy the developing embryo. The requirement of the early embryo for an intact zona pellucida had been well documented. A further complication was that the in vitro culture of large-animal embryos through the preimplantation period is highly problematic, if not impossible. This problem was solved by the ingenious solution of embedding the micromanipulated embryos in a block of agar gel for protection during a preimplantation culture period in the oviduct of a temporary recipient animal. This gel effectively sealed the opening in the zona pellucida, allowing development to proceed. The method of agar embedding is illustrated in Fig. 3.11. Cracks in some of the agar blocks demonstrated the importance of protecting the embryos in this fashion, as leukocytes invaded through the compromised gel coating, destroying the developing embryos as illustrated in Fig. 3.12. Rabbits were originally used as temporary recipients; however, culture was somewhat compromised, especially with porcine embryos. Sheep were used with greater success and remain the animal of choice for this purpose. After the desired culture period elapsed, the agar chips were flushed from the temporary recipient and dissected with fine hypodermic needles to release the embryos. The blastocyst-stage embryos were then transferred to the recipient mother for gestation to term. With this method, Willadsen (102) showed that blastomeres constituting "half" (individual two-cells, two four-

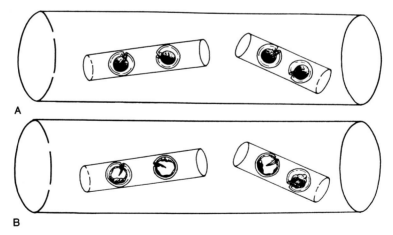

FIG. 3.11. Micromanipulated sheep embryos embedded in agar blocks. The embryos are placed in a warm agar solution, drawn up into a 150-μm–diameter pipette and then expelled after a brief cooling period to form the small agar cylinders. These are, in turn, drawn up from an agar solution into a 0.5- to 0.8-mm pipette to create the larger cylinder, which is placed into the oviduct of a temporary recipient animal **(A)**. Following the preimplantation culture period in the the agar, cylinders are flushed from the recipients tract and examined for development **(B)**. The position of the smaller cylinders with their enclosed embryos is noted before transfer so that identification can be made upon flushing. (Reprinted with permission from Willadsen SM. Micromanipulation of embryos of the large domestic species. In: Adams CE, ed. *Mammalian egg transfer.* 1982:185–210. Copyright CRC Press, Inc., Boca Raton, FL.)

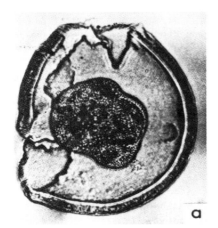 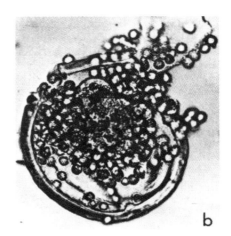

FIG. 3.12. A demonstration of the importance of the agar-embedding procedure. These are sheep embryos, developed from single blastomeres, that were cultured in agar blocks in the oviduct of a temporary recipient animal (rabbit). **A:** This morula was protected by the agar block during the culture period. **B:** Here, there was a crack in the agar block that allowed leukocytes to invade and destroy the developing embryo. (Reprinted with permission from Willadsen SM. Micromanipulation of embryos of the large domestic animal species. In: Adams CE, ed. *Mammalian egg transfer.* 1982:185–210. Copyright CRC Press, Inc., Boca Raton, FL.)

cell stage blastomeres) or even "quarter" embryos (two eight-cell stage blastomeres) could develop to term. Identical animals were produced by this method in cattle, pigs, and horses. Initial work was also undertaken to split bovine embryos at the later stages normally used for nonsurgical commercial embryo transfer (day 5 and 6 morulae) (103).

Genome Extension: Commercial Twinning and Cloning

The concept of artificial "twinning" has developed over the years in two directions. One thrust has been to make the technique of embryo division much more simplistic—allowing the procedure to be carried out "in the back of a pick-up truck" during routine bovine embryo transfer. Other workers have labored to obtain the greatest possible extension of each individual genome through embryo cloning. This uses a different approach to capitalize on the latent totipotency of early embryonic cells.

Routine Embryo Splitting

To a large extent, large-animal husbandry, particularly in the bovine, relies on the application of embryo transfer. Superior animals are superovulated and inseminated to produce many embryos, which are easily recovered from the reproductive tract and transferred to multiple recipients. This is an efficient methodology for the development of superior herds and, moreover, embryos can be cryopreserved for storage and transport to distant locations. As stated in the previous section, early experiments showed that these late-stage embryos could simply be divided into two demiembryos. In the early 1980s, several groups reported on successful bovine and ovine demiembryo transfer (104–107). Later workers reported successful use of embryo splitting in goats, horses, pigs, and rabbits (108–110). Demiembryos can be successfully cryopreserved, and offspring have been produced from the transfer of frozen demiembryos (111). Also, bovine morulae have been split into quarter embryos, the transfer of which resulted in the birth of two identical calves (112).

Basically, morulae-stage embryos are stabilized with a holding pipette while a glass needle or blade is used to free the embryo from the zona and then the morula is simply bisected into two halves, as illustrated in Fig. 3.13 (113,114). The two demiembryos are then placed in empty zona pellucidae for transfer. Over the years, efforts have been made to simplify the embryo-splitting procedure. One method, developed by Rorie and coworkers (115), involves the use of a common razor blade (Fig. 3.14) as the cutting instrument. Embryos were placed on a glass slide, the surface of which had been roughened by an abrasive treatment. This rough surface helped stabilize embryos during the procedure. For greater control, the razor blade was clamped in a pair of hemostats. Late-morula stage bovine embryos were place on the prepared slide in a drop of culture medium. During observation with an inverted microscope, the razor blade was lowered onto the embryo, effectively bisecting it. Variations include the use of blade fragments mounted onto various holders and sharp pins for the bisecting instrument. Herr and coworkers (116) recently described a procedure that uses an ultrasharp ground microblade mounted to a single micromanipulator. The embryo to be split, with an intact zona pellucida, is stabilized by electrostatic attraction to the plastic surface of a tissue culture dish while in a drop of protein-free medium. The blade is lowered, bisecting the embryo, and serum, containing medium, is then added to free the demiembryos from attachment to the dish. This technique was also used in obtaining embryonic biopsies for sexing (117). This will be discussed in a later section.

The pregnancy rate for demiembryos varies between 45% and 65%, compared with a standard embryo-transfer rate of 50% to 75% (Godke RA, personal communication). So, the use of embryo splitting can permit pregnancy rates that are, in effect, above 100% of the number of embryos selected for splitting. Considering the value of prime embryos from genetically superior animals, this is not a trivial goal. Gray and coworkers (118) reported on a major study of commercial bovine embryo splitting. A total of 994 embryos from 435 cows were selected for bisection. The transfer of

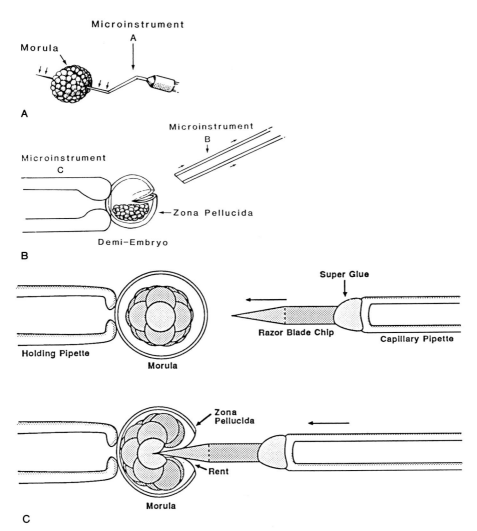

FIG. 3.13. Two methods for the bisecting of late-stage bovine embryos using microma-nipulation. **A:** This technique was developed at Louisiana State University. A glass micro-needle *(A)* is used to bisect a zona-free morula. **B:** A demimorula-transfer pipette *(B)* is used to replace the demiembryo into a zona pellucida stabilized on a holding pipette *(C)*. (Courtesy of Dr. RA Godke. Reproduced from Lambeth VA, Looney CR, Voelkel SA, et al. Microsurgery on bovine embryos at the morula stage to produce monozygotic twin calves. *Theriogenology* 1983;20:85. With permission Butterworth-Heinemann, a division of Reed Publishing (USA) Inc.) **C:** In this method, developed at Colorado State University, a microtool is fabricated from a small section of razor blade glued to a glass micropipette. This tool is simply forced against a morula, effectively bisecting it. The demiembryos would be placed in empty zona as shown in **B**. (Courtesy of Dr. RA Godke. Adapted with permission from Williams TJ, et al. Bisecting bovine embryos: methods, applications, and success rates. In: Proceedings of Annual Conference Artificial Insemination and Embryologic Transfer in Beef Cattle. Denver, Colo; 1983:45–51.)

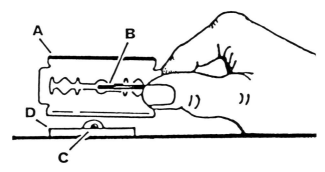

FIG. 3.14. A simplified method for bisecting a bovine morula, without using a micromanipulator, developed at Louisiana State University. A common razor blade *(A)* is held securely with a pair of hemostats *(B)*. An embryo is placed on a preroughened slide *(D)* in a drop of culture medium *(C)*. The blade is lowered onto the embryo for bisection. (From Rorie RW, et al. A new method of splitting embryos without the use of a commercial micromanipulation unit. *Theriogenology* 1985;23:224. Copyright Butterworth-Heinemann, a division of Reed Publishing (USA), Inc.)

1,988 demiembryos resulted in 997 pregnancies, with pregnancies obtained from 72.4% of the embryos selected. These results were considered excellent and highly acceptable to the commercial cattle industry. Embryo splitting will, no doubt, continue to play an important role in maximizing the efficiency and utility of routine embryo transfer.

Embryo Cloning

The simple separation of blastomeres (or later-stage splitting) to create multiple embryos has a limited scope. Single eight-cell–stage blastomeres exhibit a greatly reduced developmental potential. This is due to the simple lack of cytoplasmic material required by the embryo for proper blastocyst formation. The ICM is apparently derived from "inside cell," which are surrounded by other cells at the time of blastulation. Since blastulation occurs based on an absolute schedule, irrespective of cell number, those demiembryos with greatly reduced cell number may begin blastulation with no inside cells. This results in the formation of a trophoblastic vesicle devoid of an ICM (119). Thus, the number of monozygotic offspring that can be obtained from the simple division of an embryo is definitely limited. The largest number of identical animals produced in this way was four (102).

The limitations present in the embryo-splitting methodology were addressed through the development of embryo cloning. Cloning is based on the technique of nuclear transfer. Briggs and King (120) reported on the first nuclear transfer in the frog, *Rana pipiens.* Nuclei from blastula-stage cells were transferred to the cytoplasm of enucleated oocytes. Elsdale et al. (121) reported on the use of a modified enucleation technique for the repetition of this experiment with the embryos of *Xenopus laevis.* Gurdon (122) then attempted transfer with somatic gut cells from tadpoles as the nuclear donors and was successful. Transfer of nuclei from adult cells resulted in limited embryonic development, but not to term. Gurdon also discussed the serial transplantation of nuclei. Blastulas derived from transferred nuclei were then used as donor material for a second round of nuclear transfer. As discussed in the previous chapter, workers developed techniques in the mouse for moving intact genomes through the transfer of nuclei or pronuclei (123). In 1985, Robl and First (124) discussed preliminary work on applying the murine nuclear-transfer technique to porcine embryos. As with gene injection, the lipid-rich pig embryos required centrifugation for visualizing the pronuclei. Basically, the technique was identical with that of the earlier murine experiments. Nuclei were removed as intact karyoplasts, using beveled glass micropipettes with the embryos in a cytoskeletal relaxant cocktail. A similar procedure is illustrated in Fig. 3.15. Electrofusion was used to fuse the nuclear karyoplasts to enucleated embryos. Developmental data were not reported for these experiments. In later work, pigs were produced following the transfer of nuclear clone embryos derived from four-cell–stage donor embryos (125).

In 1986, Willadsen (126) reported on successful nuclear transplant cloning in sheep. Blastomeres from 8- and 16-cell sheep embryos were used as the genome source. Blastomeres were transferred under the zona pellucida of enucleated eggs and fused, using Sendai virus or electrofusion to produce multiple clonal embryos. Electrofusion seemed to be a much

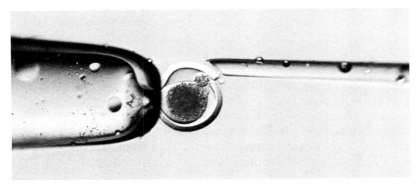

FIG. 3.15. Nuclear transplantation in the bovine. An enucleated egg is stabilized with a holding pipette on the *left.* On the *right,* a transfer pipette has deposited the genome donor cell under the zona pellucida. Fusion between the two cells will be initiated by electrofusion to form a new nuclear-transplant embryo. (Courtesy of Dr. C. L. Keefer, American Breeders Service, DeForrest, Wis.)

more efficient technique, with 90% cell fusion within 1 hour, compared with 50% fusion after 4 hours for the Sendai virus-treated group. When eight-cell blastomeres were used, transfer of the resulting embryos produced three lambs, including two clonal twins. These were the first large-animal clones ever produced.

Smith and Wilmut (127) reported on recent advances in sheep embryo cloning. Lambs were born following the transfer of embryos derived from the fusion (electrofusion) of 16-cell or ICM-stage cells from one sheep variety with the unfertilized, enucleated eggs of another variety. In these experiments, pretreatment with a brief alternating current pulse before the fusion pulse and posttreatment with cytochalasin B were shown to improve the electrofusion results. The positive results obtained from 120- to 150-cell–stage ICM donor cells provided strong evidence that a transcriptionally activated genome can be reprogrammed and bring about the term development of nuclear transfer embryos. This provides some optimism that stem cells will be suitable for use as clonal genomes in the future.

Prather and coworkers (128,129) reported the birth of calves following nuclear transfer in bovine embryos. Recipient oocytes were obtained following either standard oviductal flushing or through the in vitro maturation of ovarian oocytes. Freshly ovulated oocytes were significantly superior. Blastomeres from the 2- to 32-cell stage were used as the source of the donor genome. The success of electrofusion was significantly reduced when later-stage (smaller) cells were used. Several pregnancies were established following the transfer of the resulting embryos, and two calves were delivered.

In 1989, Willadsen (130) reported the birth of the first genetically identical bovine calves produced by nuclear-transfer cloning. In this work, multiple calves were produced from donor material up to the 64-cell stage. Also, by using the concept of serial transfer, in which the clonal embryo is then itself used as a source of donor cells, calves were produced from second- and third-generation material, and apparently normal blastocysts were produced from sixth-generation donor cells. Preliminary work also seems to indicate that in vitro matured oocytes can be used as a source of recipient cells. This would provide not only a more efficacious supply— since these oocytes can easily be obtained from slaughterhouse ovaries—but apparently the timing of the nuclear transfer protocols is simplified by the synchronized maturation possible with these oocytes. The overall pregnancy rates of nuclear-transfer embryos have been reduced with higher abortion rates as well.

Willadsen and coworkers (131) recently discussed the results of a 1-year project on commercial bovine embryo cloning. Embryos from high-quality pure-bred cattle at the 8- to 64-cell stage were used as donor material. Nuclear transplant embryos were transferred to 302 recipients, producing 128 (42.4%) pregnancies, of which 100 (31.1%) survived to term. This number included five sets of quadruplet-clones and ten sets of triplet-clones. When embryo quality was taken into consideration, the transfer of high-quality embryos resulted in a calving rate of nearly 50%; a respectable number, comparable with normal bovine embryo transfer results. There were some abnormalities seen in a few of the clonal animals, including limb and cardiac malformations. Abnormally high birth weight being the most frequent problem. Interestingly, many of the animals exhibiting malformations or increased birth weight had clonal siblings that were completely normal. The majority of the animals were healthy and fertile, and several went on to be sold for commercial agricultural production. Two sets of bovine clones from this work are illustrated in Fig. 3.16.

Yong and coworkers (132) described successful nuclear-transplant cloning in goats. Five goats (including one set of clonal twins) were born following the transfer of embryos derived from 4- to 32-cell–stage donor cells. Nuclear-transplant embryos were apparently transferred shortly after the procedure into recipient animals. An overview of offspring produced by nuclear-transplant cloning is provided by Fig. 3.17.

The interest in nuclear transfer in large domestic species is in providing the largest possible extension of a desired genome. Also important, will be the ability to create clonal lines. With use of serial cloning, large numbers of good quality identical embryos could be developed. Most of these embryos would be cryopreserved, while some were transferred to obtain offspring. These clones would be carefully analyzed to determine their agricultural potential. The most promising clones could then be further developed with the frozen material. Several calves have been born from embryos derived from a frozen donor embryo, including four identical calves from a 32-cell cryopreserved embryo. Another concept is the use of embryonic stem cells

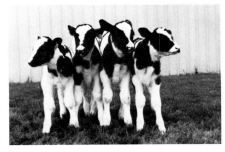 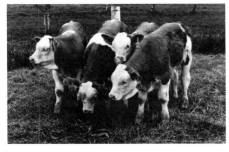

A   B

FIG. 3.16. Two sets of bovine clones. **A:** Four Holstein clones were produced from the transfer of nuclear-transplant–derived blastocysts that had been cryopreserved. **B:** Four Simmental clones were produced from second-generation nuclear transplant embryos. (Courtesy of Dr. S. M. Willadsen, Alta Genetics, Calgary, Canada.)

Nuclear Transplant Cloning

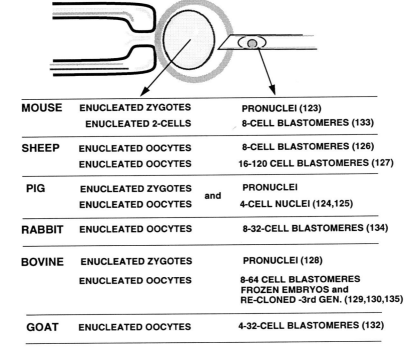

MOUSE	ENUCLEATED ZYGOTES		PRONUCLEI (123)
	ENUCLEATED 2-CELLS		8-CELL BLASTOMERES (133)
SHEEP	ENUCLEATED OOCYTES		8-CELL BLASTOMERES (126)
	ENUCLEATED OOCYTES		16-120 CELL BLASTOMERES (127)
PIG	ENUCLEATED ZYGOTES	**and**	PRONUCLEI
	ENUCLEATED OOCYTES		4-CELL NUCLEI (124,125)
RABBIT	ENUCLEATED OOCYTES		8-32-CELL BLASTOMERES (134)
BOVINE	ENUCLEATED ZYGOTES		PRONUCLEI (128)
	ENUCLEATED OOCYTES		8-64 CELL BLASTOMERES FROZEN EMBRYOS and RE-CLONED -3rd GEN. (129,130,135)
GOAT	ENUCLEATED OOCYTES		4-32-CELL BLASTOMERES (132)

as the genomic source in creating clones. Not only would this provide an unlimited supply of a particular genome, but the genome could be genetically modified by the techniques discussed in the previous section on genetic engineering. Multiple clonal lines could be created, harboring a variety of complementary genetic traits. If this technique is possible, animal improvement would move into a new era, in which phenotypes would be limited only by the imagination and skill of the animal scientist.

Other Uses of Micromanipulation in Animal Husbandry

Sexing of Offspring

In the dairy industry, female animals are obviously the desired offspring. Male animals would be sought for beef production or breeding purposes.

Several methods have been proposed for the sexing of preimplantation embryos. Also, the sorting of X- and Y-bearing sperm has been proposed; with preliminary experiments in rabbits showing some success (136). Embryos could be sexed by the examination of an embryonic biopsy, derived either from simple splitting or the isolation of a few individual blastomeres. Methods for analysis include karyotyping, the detection of male-specific antigens, and direct DNA analysis by PCR (137–139).

Herr and Reed (115) reported on the use of a splitting protocol (discussed in the foregoing section on routine embryo splitting) for obtaining bovine embryo biopsies for analysis. The PCR analysis method was used to identify Y chromosome-specific DNA sequences (140). Sexing could be accomplished within a few hours. In preliminary experiments, a 53.3% pregnancy rate was obtained following the transfer of biopsied embryos.

Microsurgical Fertilization

In general, the genetically superior animals used in animal husbandry are quite fertile. Therefore, techniques for improving reproductive performances are not required. However, in some cases, such as in obtaining the maximum extension of valuable semen, the use of micromanipulation in promoting sperm–egg fusion could have agricultural utility, and some research has been done in this area (reviewed in 141 and 142). This subject will be thoroughly covered in Chapter 5.

REFERENCES

1. Brackett BG, Baranska W, Sawicki W, Koprowski H. Uptake of heterologous genome by mammalian spermatozoa and its transfer to ova through fertilization. *Proc Natl Acad Sci USA* 1971;68:353–357.
2. Jaenisch R, Mintz B. Simian virus 40 DNA sequences in DNA of healthy adult mice derived from preimplantation blastocysts injected with viral DNA. *Proc Natl Acad Sci USA* 1974;71:1250–1254.
3. Jaenisch R. Infection of mouse blastocysts with SV40 DNA: normal development of the infected blastomeres and persistence or SV40 DNA sequences in the adult animals. *Cold Spring Harbor Symp Quant Biol* 1974;39:375–380.
4. Mertz JE, Gurdon JB. Purified DNAs are transcribed after microinjection into *Xenopus* oocytes. *Proc Natl Acad Sci USA* 1977;74:1502–1506.
5. Brown DD, Gurdon JB. High fidelity transcription of 5S DNA injected into *Xenopus* oocytes. *Proc Natl Acad Sci USA* 1977;74:2064–2068.
6. Brinster RL, Chen HY, Trumbauer ME, Avarbock MR. Translation of globin messenger RNA by the mouse ovum. *Nature* 1980;283:499–501.
7. Brinster RL, Chen HY, Trumbauer ME. Mouse oocytes transcribe injected *Xenopus* 5S RNA gene. *Science* 1981;211:396–398.
8. Gordon J, Scangos G, Plotkin D, Barbosa J, Ruddle F. Genetic transformation of mouse embryos by microinjection of purified DNA. *Proc Natl Acad Sci USA* 1980;77:7380–7384.

9. Wagner EF, Stewart TA, Mintz B. The human β-globin gene and a functional thymidine kinase gene in developing mice. *Proc Natl Acad Sci USA* 1981;78:5016–5020.
10. Wagner T, Hoppe PC, Jollick JD, Scholl DR, Hodinka RL, Gault JB. Microinjection of a rabbit β-globin gene into zygotes and its subsequent expression in adult mice and their offspring. *Proc Natl Acad Sci USA* 1981;78:6376–6380.
11. Constantini F, Lacy L. Introduction of a rabbit β globin gene into the mouse germ line. *Nature* 1981;294:92–94.
12. Brinster RL, Chen HY, Trumbauer M, Senear AW, Warren R, Palmiter RD. Somatic expression of herpes thymidine kinase in mice following injection of a fusion gene into eggs. *Cell* 1981;27:223–231.
13. Gordon J, Ruddle FH. Germ line transmission in transgenic mice. In: Burger MB, Weber R, eds. *Embryonic development,* part B: *cellular aspects.* New York: Alan R. Liss;1982.
14. Hammer RE, Pursel VG, Rexroad CE, et al. Production of transgenic rabbits, sheep and pigs by microinjection. *Nature* 1985;315:680–683.
15. Bierry KA, Bondioli KR, DeMayo FJ. Gene transfer by pronuclear injection in the bovine. *Theriogenology* 1988;29:224.
16. Church RB. Embryo manipulation and gene transfer in domestic animals. *Biotechnology* 1987;5:13–19.
17. Seidel GE. Mammalian oocytes and preimplantation embryos as methodological components. *Biol Reprod* 1983;28:36–49.
18. Brinster RL, Chen HY, Trumbauer ME, Yagle MK, Palmiter RD. Factors affecting the efficiency of introducing foreign DNA into mice by microinjecting eggs. *Proc Natl Acad Sci USA* 1985;82:4438–4442.
19. Walton JR, Murray JD, Marshall JT, Nancarrow CD. Zygote viability in gene transfer experiments. *Biol Reprod* 1987;37:957–967.
20. Pintado B, Wall RJ, Pursel VG, Martin S. Attempts to improve efficiency of embryo transfer in transgenic mouse experiments. *J Reprod Fertil* 1990;41(Suppl):221.
21. Palmiter RD, Brinster RL. Germ line transformation of mice. *Annu Rev Genet* 1986;20:465–499.
22. Covarrubias L, Nishida Y, Mintz B. Early developmental mutations due to DNA rearrangements in transgenic mouse embryos. *Cold Spring Harbor Symp Quant Biol* 1985;50:447–452.
23. Covarrubias L, Nishida Y, Mintz B. Early postimplantation embryo lethality due to DNA rearrangements in a transgenic mouse strain. *Proc Natl Acad Sci USA* 1986;83:6020–6024.
24. Chada K, Magram J, Raphael K, Radice G, Lacy E, Constantini F. Specific expression of a foreign β-globin gene in erythroid cells of transgenic mice. *Nature* 1985;314:377–380.
25. Palmiter RD, Chen HY, Brinster RL. Differential regulation of metallothionein-thymidine kinase fusion genes in transgenic mice and their offspring. *Cell* 1982;29:701–710.
26. Swift GH, Hammer RE, MacDonald RJ, Brinster RL. Tissue specific expression of the rat pancreatic elastase 1 gene in transgenic mice. *Cell* 1984;38:639–646.
27. Ornitz DM, Palmiter RD, Hammer RE, Brinster RL, Swift G, MacDonald RJ. Specific expression of an elastase–human growth hormone fusion gene in pancreatic acinar cells of transgenic mice. *Nature* 1985;313:600–603.
28. Khillan J, Schmidt A, Overbeek PA, de Crombrugghe B, Westhphal H. Developmental and tissue specific expression directed by the α_2 type I collagen promoter in transgenic mice. *Proc Natl Acad Sci USA* 1986;83:725–729.
29. Le Meur M, Gerlinger P, Benoist C, Mathis D. Correcting an immune-response deficiency by creating E_α transgenic mice. *Nature* 1985;316:38–42.
30. Leder A, Pattengale PK, Kuo A, Stewart TA, Leder P. Consequences of widespread deregulation of the c-*myc* gene in transgenic mice: multiple neoplasms and normal development. *Cell* 1986;45:485–495.
31. Wanger EF, Stewart TA, Mintz B. The human β-globin gene and a functional thymidine kinase gene in developing mice. *Proc Natl Acad Sci USA* 1981;78:6376–6380.
32. Swanson LW, Simmons DM, Arriza J, Hammer R, Brinster RL. Novel developmental specificity in the nervous system of transgenic animals expressing growth hormone fusion genes. *Nature* 1985;317:363–366.
33. Gordon J. Transgenic animals. *Int Rev Cytol* 1989;115:171–229.

34. Hanahan D. Transgenic mice as probes into complex systems. *Science* 1989;246: 1265–1275.
35. Palmiter RD, Brinster RL, Hammer RE, et al. Dramatic growth of mice that develop from eggs microinjected with metallothionein–growth hormone fusion genes. *Nature* 1982;300:611–615.
36. Yun JS, Li Y, Wright DC, Portanova RP, Wagner TE. Expression of the human growth-hormone transgene in heterozygous and homozygous mice. *J Reprod Fertil* 1990; 41(Suppl):230.
37. Constantini F, Chada K, Magram J. Correction of murine β thalassemia by gene transfer into the germ line. *Science* 1986;233:1192–1194.
38. Isola LM, Gordon JW. Systemic resistance to methotrexate in transgenic mice carrying a mutant dihydrofolate reductase gene. *Proc Natl Acad Sci USA* 1986;83:9621–9625.
39. Bruggemann M, Caskey HM, Teale C, et al. A repertoire of monoclonal antibodies with human heavy chains from transgenic mice. *Proc Natl Acad Sci USA* 1989;86:6709–6713.
40. Allen ND, Cran DG, Barton SC, Hettle S, Reik W, Surani MAH. Transgenes as probes for active chromosomal domains in mouse development. *Nature* 1988;333:852–855.
41. Kothary RK, Allen ND, Surani MAH. Transgenes as molecular probes of mammalian developmental genetics. In: Mclean M, ed. *Oxford survey on eukaryotic genes.* Oxford: Oxford University Press;1989:145–178.
42. Palmiter RD, Behringer RR, Quaife CJ, Maxwell F, Maxwell IH, Brinster RL. Cell lineage ablation in transgenic mice by cell-specific expression of a toxin gene. *Cell* 1987; 50:435–443.
43. Messing A, Chen HY, Palmiter R, Brinster RL. Peripheral neuropathies, hepatocellular carcinomas and islet cell adenomas in transgenic mice. *Nature* 1985;316:461–463.
44. Mahon KA, Chepelinsky AB, Khillan JS, Overbeek DA, Piatigorsky J, Westhphal H. Oncogenesis of the lens in transgenic mice. *Science* 1987;235:1622–1628.
45. Folkman J, Watson K, Ingber D, Hanahan D. Induction of angiogenesis during the transition from hyperplasia to neoplasia. *Nature* 1989;339:58–61.
46. Bennett J, Gearhart J. Introduction of large DNA molecules (> 100 kb) into the germ line of transomic mice. *J Reprod Fertil* 1990;41(Suppl):219.
47. Clark AJ, Bessos H, Bishop JO, et al. Expression of human anti-hemophilic factor IX in the milk of transgenic sheep. *Biotechnology* 1989;7:487–492.
48. Wilmut I, Archibald S, Harris M, et al. Methods of gene transfer and their potential use to modify milk composition. *Theriogenology* 1990;33:113–121.
49. Gordon K, Lee E, Vitale JA, Smith AE, Westphal H, Hennighausen L. Production of human tissue plasminogen activator in transgenic mice. *Biotechnology* 1987;5: 1183–1187.
50. Pittius CW, Hennighausen L, Lee E, et al. A milk protein promoter directs the expression of human tissue plasminogen activating factor cDNA to the mammary gland of transgenic mice. *Proc Natl Acad Sci USA* 1988;85:5874–5878.
51. Meade H, Lonberg N. Bovine alpha casein gene sequences direct high level expression of active human urokinase in mouse milk. *J Reprod Fertil* 1990;41(Suppl):215.
52. Massey JM. Animal production industry in the year 2000. *J Reprod Fertil* 1990; 41(Suppl):199–208.
53. Wall RJ, Pursel VG, Hammer RE, Brinster RL. Development of porcine ova that were centrifuged to permit visualization of pronuclei and nuclei. *Biol Reprod* 1985;32:645–651.
54. Saeki K, Kato H, Hosoi Y, Miyake M, Utsumi K, Iritani A. Detection of pronuclei of in vitro fertilized bovine eggs after centrifugation and their subsequent development in culture. In: *Proceedings Sixth World Congress Human Reproduction;* Tokyo;1988:abstr. 834.
55. Minhas BS, Capehart JS, Bowen MJ, et al. Visualization of pronuclei in living bovine zygotes. *Biol Reprod* 1984;30:687–691.
56. Miyake M, Iritani A. Live staining of nuclear structure in mammalian fertilized eggs. *Jpn J Anim Reprod* 1984;30:37.
57. Pursel VG, Rexroad CE, Bolt DJ, et al. Progress on gene transfer in farm animals *Vet Immunol Immunopathol* 1987;17:303–312.
58. Pursel VG, Hammer RE, Bolt DJ, Palmiter RD, Brinster RL. Integration, expression, and germ-line transmission of growth-related genes in pigs. *J Reprod Fertil* 1990; 41(Suppl):77–87.

59. McGrane MM, de Vente J, Yun J, et al. Tissue-specific expression and dietary regulation of a chimeric phosphoenolpyruvate carboxykinase/bovine growth hormone gene in transgenic mice. *J Biol Chem* 1988;263:1443–1451.
60. Wieghart M, Hoover JL, McGrane MM, et al. Production of transgenic pigs harboring a rat phosphoenolpyruvate carboxykinase–bovine growth hormone gene. *J Reprod Fertil* 1990;41(Suppl):89–96.
61. Simons JP, McClenaghan M, Clark AJ. Alteration of the quality of milk by expression of sheep β-lactoglobulin in transgenic milk. *Nature* 1987;328:530–532.
62. Wilmut I, Archibald AL, Harris S, et al. Modification of milk composition. *J Reprod Fertil* 1990;41(Suppl):135–146.
63. Handyside AH, Penketh RJA, Winston RML, et al. Biopsy of human preimplantation embryos and sexing by DNA amplification. *Nature* 1989;347–349.
64. Ninomiya T, Hoshi M, Mizuno A, Nagao M, Yuki A. Selection of transgenic preimplantation embryos by PCR. *J Reprod Fertil* 1990;41(Suppl):222.
65. Jaenisch R, Fan H, Croker B. Infection of preimplantation mouse embryos and of newborn mice with leukemia virus: tissue distribution of viral DNA and leukemogenesis in the adult animal. *Proc Natl Acad Sci USA* 1975;72:4008–4012.
66. Jaenisch R. Germ line integration and mendelian transmission of the exogenous Moloney leukemia virus. *Proc Natl Acad Sci USA* 1976;73:1260–1264.
67. Jahner D, Haase K, Mulligan R, Jaenisch R. Insertion of the bacterial *gpt* gene into the germ line of mice by retroviral infection. *Proc Natl Acad Sci USA* 1985;82:6927–6931.
68. van der Putten H, Botteri FM, Miller AD, et al. Efficient insertion of genes into the mouse germ line via retroviral vectors. *Proc Natl Acad Sci USA* 1985;82:6148–6152.
69. Shimotohno K, Temin HM. Formation of infectious progeny virus after insertion of herpes simplex thymidine kinase gene into DNA of an avian retrovirus. *Cell* 1981; 26:67–77.
70. Soriano P, Cane RD, Mulligan RC, Jaenisch R. Tissue specific and ectopic expression of genes introduced into transgenic mice by retroviruses. *Science* 1986;1409–1413.
71. Brinster RL. The effect of cells transferred into the mouse blastocyst on subsequent development. *J Exp Med* 1974;140:1049–1056.
72. Evans MJ, Kaufman MH. Establishment in culture of pluriopotent cells from mouse embryos. *Nature* 1981;292:154–156.
73. Martin GR. Isolation of a pluripotential cell line from early mouse embryos culture in medium conditioned with teratocarcinoma cells. *Proc Natl Acad Sci USA* 1981;78: 7634–7639.
74. Bradley A, Evans M, Kaufman MH, Robertson E. Formation of germ-line chimeras from embryo-derived teratocarcinoma cell lines. *Nature* 1984;309:255–256.
75. Stewart CL, Vaneck M, Wagner EF. Expression of foreign genes from retroviral vectors in mouse teratocarcinoma chimaeras. *EMBO J* 1985;4:3701–3709.
76. Robertson EJ, Bradley A, Kuehn M, Evans M. Germ line transmission of gene sequences introduced into cultured pluripotential cells by a retroviral vector. *Nature* 1986; 323:445–448.
77. Thomas KR, Capecchi MR. Site directed mutagenesis by gene targeting in mouse embryo-derived stem cells. *Cell* 1988;51:503–512.
78. Lovell-Badge RH, Bygrave AE, Bradley A, Robertson E, Evans MJ, Cheah KSE. Transformation of embryonic stem cells with the human type II collagen gene and its expression in chimeric mice. *Cold Spring Harbor Symp Quant Biol* 1985;50:707–711.
79. Robertson EJ. Pluripotential stem cell lines as a route into the mouse germ line. *Trends Genet* 1986;2:9–14.
80. Doetschman T, Gregg RG, Maeda N, et al. Targeted correction of a mutant HPRT gene in mouse embryonic stem cells. *Nature* 1987;330:576–578.
81. Thompson S, Clarke AR, Pow AM, Hooper ML, Melton DW. Germ line transmission and expression of a corrected *HPRT* gene produced by gene targeting in embryonic stem cells. *Cell* 1989;56:313–321.
82. Capecchi MR. The new mouse genetics: altering the genome by gene targeting. *Trends Genet* 1989;5:70–76.
83. DeChiara TM, Efstratiadis A, Robertson EJ. A growth-deficiency phenotype in heterozygous mice carrying an insulin-like growth factor II gene disrupted by targeting. *Nature* 1990;345:78–80.

84. Folger KR, Thomas KR, Capecchi MR. Analysis of homologous recombination in cultured mammalian cells. *Cold Spring Harbor Symp Quant Biol* 1984;49:123–138.

85. Thomas KR, Folger KR, Capecchi MR. High frequency targeting of genes to specific sites in the mammalian genome. *Cell* 1986;44:419–428.

86. Mansour SL, Thomas KR, Capecchi MR. Disruption of the proto-oncogene *int-2* in mouse embryo-derived stem cells: a general strategy for targeting mutations to non-selectable genes. *Nature* 1988;336:348–352.

87. Notarianni E, Laurie S, Moor RM, Evans MJ. Maintenance and differentiation in culture of pluripotential embryonic cell lines from pig blastocysts. *J Reprod Fertil* 1990; 41(Suppl):51–56.

88. Notarianni E, Galli C, Larie S, Moor RM, Evans MJ. Derivation of pluripotent, embryonic cell lines from the pig and sheep. *J Reprod Fertil* 1991;43(Suppl):255–260.

89. Streichenko N, Saito S, Niemann H. Toward the establishment of bovine embryonic stem cells. *Theriogenology* 1991;35:274.

90. Stringfellow DA, Gray BW, Toivio-Kinnucan M, et al. A continuous cell line established from a preimplantation bovine embryo. *Theriogenology* 1991;35:275.

91. Lavitrano M, Camaioni A, Fazio VM, Dolch S, Farace MG, Spadafora C. Sperm cells as vectors for introducing DNA into eggs: genetic transformation of mice. *Cell* 1989; 57:717–723.

92. Brinster RL, Sandgren EP, Behringer RR, Palmiter RD. No simple solution for making transgenic mice [Letter]. *Cell* 1990;59:239–240.

93. Lavitrano M, Camaioni A, Fazio VM, Dolci S, Farace MG, Spadafora C. No simple solution for making transgenic mice [Letter]. *Cell* 1990;59:240.

94. Gandolfi F, Lavitrano M, Camaioni A, Spadafora C, Siracusa G, Lauria A. The use of sperm-mediated gene transfer for the generation of transgenic pigs. *J Reprod Fertil Abstr Ser* 1989;4:16.

95. Gagne M, Pothier F, Sirard M. Effect on in-vitro fertilization of electroporation of bovine spermatozoa with a foreign gene. *J Reprod Fertil* 1990;41(Suppl):212.

96. Roux W. Contributions to the developmental mechanics of the embryo (originally published, 1888). In: Willier BH, Oppenheimer JM, eds. *Foundations of experimental embryology.* New York: Hafner Press;1964:3–37.

97. Nicholas JS, Hall BV. Experiments on developing rats. *J Exp Zool* 1942;90:441–459.

98. Seidel F. Die Entwicklugspotenzen einen isolierton Blastomere des Zweizellenstadiums im Saugetierei. *Naturwissenschaften* 1952;39:355–356.

99. Moore NW, Polge C, Rowson LEA. The survival of single blastomeres of pig eggs transferred to recipient gilts. *Aust J Biol Sci* 1969;22:979.

100. Trounson AO, Moore NW. Attempts to produce identical offspring in sheep by mechanical division of the ovum. *Aust J Biol Sci* 1974;27:505.

101. Willadsen SM. A method of culture of micromanipulated sheep embryos and its use to produce monozygotic twins. *Nature* 1979;277:298–300.

102. Willadsen SM. Micromanipulation of embryos of the large domestic species. In: Adams CE, ed. *Mammalian egg transfer.* Boca Raton: CRC Press;1982:185–210.

103. Willadsen SM, Lehn-Jensen H, Fehily CB, Newcomb R. The production of monozygotic twins of preselected parentage by micromanipulation of nonsurgically collected cow embryos. *Theriogenology* 1981;15:23.

104. Ozil J-P, Heyman Y, Renard J-P. Production of monozygotic twins by micromanipulation and cervical transfer in the cow. *Vet Rec* 1982;110:126–127.

105. Lambeth VA, Looney CR, Voelkel SA, Hill KG, Jackson DA, Godke RA. Micromanipulation of bovine morulae to produce identical twin offspring. In: *Proceedings Second World Congress on Embryo Transfer in Mammals.* 1982:55.

106. Williams TJ, Elsden RP, Seidel GE Jr. Identical twin bovine pregnancies derived from bisected embryos. *Theriogenology* 1982;17:14.

107. Willadsen SM, Godke RA. A simple procedure for the production of identical sheep twins. *Vet Rec* 1984;114:240–243.

108. Tsunoda Y, Wakasu M, Yasui T, Sugie T. Micromanipulation and freezing of goat embryos. *Proc World Congr Animal Reprod Artif Insem* 1984;2:249.

109. Slade NP, Williams TJ, Squires EL, Seidel GE Jr. Production of identical twin pregnancies by microsurgical bisection of equine embryos. *Proc World Congr Animal Reprod Artif Insem* 1984;2:241.

110. Rorie RW, Voelkel SA, McFarland CW, Southern LL, Godke RA. Micromanipulation of day-6 porcine embryos to produce split-embryo piglets. *Theriogenology* 1985;23:225.
111. Lehn-Jensen H, Willadsen SM. Deep-freezing of cow "half" and "quarter" embryos. *Theriogenology* 1983;19:49–54.
112. Voelkel SA, Viker SD, Johnson CA, Hill KG, Humes PE, Godke RA. Multiple embryo transplant offspring produced from quartering a bovine embryo at the morulae stage. *Vet Rec* 1985;117:528–530.
113. Williams TJ, Elsden RP, Seidel GE Jr. Bisecting bovine embryos: methods, applications, and success rates. In: *Proceedings Annual Conference Artificial Insemination Embryologic Transfer in Beef Cattle*. Denver, Colo;1983:45–51.
114. Lambeth VA, Looney CR, Voelkel SA, et al. Microsurgery on bovine embryos at the morula stage to produce monozygotic twin calves. *Theriogenology* 1983;20:85.
115. Rorie RW, MacFarland CW, Voelkel SA, Godke RA. A new method of splitting cattle embryos using a simple razor blade technique. *La Cattleman* 1986;19:5–6.
116. Herr CM, Holt NA, Pietrzak U, Old K, Reed KC. Increased number of pregnancies per collected embryo by bisection of blastocyst stage ovine embryos. *Theriogenology* 1990;33:244.
117. Herr CM, Reed KC. Micromanipulation of bovine embryos for sex determination. *Theriogenology* 1991;35:45–54.
118. Gray KR, Bondioli KR, Betts CL. The commercial application of embryo splitting in beef cattle. *Theriogenology* 1991;35:37–44.
119. Tarkowski AK, Wroblewska J. Development of blastomeres of mouse eggs isolated at the 4- and 8-cell stage. *J Embryol Exp Morphol* 1967;18:155–180.
120. Briggs R, King TJ. Transplantation of living nuclei from blastula cells into enucleated frogs' eggs. *Proc Natl Acad Sci USA* 1952;38:455–463.
121. Elsdale TR, Gurdon JB, Fischberg M. A description of the technique for nuclear transplantation in *Xenopus laevis*. *J Embryol Exp Morphol* 1960;8:437–444.
122. Gurdon JB. Adult frogs derived from the nuclei of single somatic cells. *Dev Biol* 1962;4:256–273.
123. McGrath J, Solter D. Nuclear transplantation in the mouse embryo by microsurgery and cell fusion. *Science* 1983;220:1300–1302.
124. Robl JM, First NL. Manipulation of gametes and embryos in the pig. *J Reprod Fertil* 1985;33:101–114.
125. Prather RS, Sims MM, First NL. Nuclear transplantation in early pig embryos. *Biol Reprod* 1989;41:414–418.
126. Willadsen SM. Nuclear transplantation in sheep embryos. *Nature* 1986;320:63–65.
127. Smith LC, Wilmut I. Influence of nuclear and cytoplasmic activity on the development in vivo of sheep embryos after nuclear transplantation. *Biol Reprod* 1989;40:1027–1036.
128. Robl JM, Prather R, Barnes FL, et al. Nuclear transplantation in bovine embryos. *J Anim Sci* 1987;64:642–647.
129. Prather RS, Barnes FL, Sims MM, Robl JM, Eyestone WH, First NL. Nuclear transplantation in the bovine embryo: assessment of donor nuclei and recipient oocyte. *Biol Reprod* 1987;37:59–66.
130. Willadsen SM. Cloning of sheep and cow embryos. *Genome* 1989;31:956–962.
131. Willadsen SM, Janzen RE, McAlister RJ, Shea BF, Hamilton G, McDermand D. The viability of late morulae and blastocysts produced by nuclear transplantation in cattle. *Theriogenology* 1991;35:161–170.
132. Yong Z, Jianchen W, Jufen Q, Zhiming H. Nuclear transfer in goats. *Theriogenology* 1991;35:299.
133. Tsunoda Y, Yasui T, Shioda Y, Nakamura K, Uchida T, Sugie T. Full term development of mouse blastomere nuclei transplanted into enucleated two-cell embryos. *J Exp Zool* 1987;242:147–151
134. Collas P, Robl JM. Factors affecting the efficiency of nuclear transplantation in the rabbit embryo. *Biol Reprod* 1990;43:877–884.
135. Stice SL, Keefer CL, Maki-Laurila M, Phillips PE. Producing multiple generations of bovine nuclear transplant embryos. *Theriogenology* 1991;35:273.
136. Johnson LA, Flook JP, Hawk HW. Sex preselection in rabbits: live births from X and Y sperm separated by DNA and cell sorting. *Biol Reprod* 1989;41:199–203.

137. King WA. Sexing embryos by cytological methods. *Theriogenology* 1984;21:7–17.
138. Anderson GB. Identification of embryonic sex by detection of the H-Y antigen. *Theriogenology* 1987;27:81–97.
139. Bondioli KR, Ellis SB, Prior JH, Williams MW, Harpold MM. The use of male-specific chomosomal DNA fragments to determine the sex of bovine preimplantation embryos. *Theriogenology* 1989;31:95–104.
140. Herr CM, Holt NA, Matthaei KI, Reed KC. Sex of progeny from bovine embryos sexed with a rapid Y-chromosome-detection assay. *Theriogenology* 1990;33:247.
141. Keefer CL. New techniques for assisted fertilization. *Theriogenology* 1990;33:101–112.
142. Iritani A. Micromanipulation of gametes for in vitro assisted fertilization. *Mol Reprod Dev* 1991;28:199–207.

4

Fertilization and Early Embryonic Development in the Human

Beth E. Talansky

Successful mammalian fertilization results from the fine coordination of two very complex reproductive systems. The individual steps involved in this process, ranging from early germ cell maturation to gamete release, seem to have been designed with the common goal of facilitating efficient sperm-egg interaction. However, the integration of two such complicated reproductive systems is subject to perturbation at many levels. The complexity of mammalian gamete interaction is compounded by the use of micromanipulation to assist fertilization. Each approach to microsurgical fertilization interrupts the natural sequence of events that normally precedes fusion. For example, in some methods, sperm interaction with the cumulus cells and zona pellucida is either partially or fully circumvented. Other more invasive types of micromanipulation procedures bypass all oocyte investments, including the plasma membrane.

Normally, spermatozoa gain their full fertilizing ability as a result of interaction with the oocyte barriers. Events such as acrosome reaction induction and, in some species, oocyte activation, are dependent on sperm contact with the zona and the oolemma. To appreciate the ramifications of micromanipulation on these gamete interactions, a comprehensive understanding of mammalian fertilization is necessary. The discussion that follows will present a description of the steps leading to fertilization and formation of the early embryo. In order to clarify the manner in which the male and female reproductive systems are integrated, a separate description of male and female germ cell development will first be presented. This section will be followed by a discussion of gamete interaction and the important mechanisms by which the sperm and oocyte physiologically coordinate into a single entity. In keeping with the scope of this textbook, most of the discussion will directly relate to human gamete physiology. However, when necessary, descriptions of other relevant mammalian models, such as the mouse, will be presented.

MALE GERM CELL DEVELOPMENT

Development of the Spermatozoon

The production of spermatozoa in the seminiferous tubules of the mammalian testis is broadly termed spermatogenesis. Three events comprise spermatogenesis: spermatocytogenesis, meiosis, and spermiogenesis (1). *Spermatocytogenesis* is the continual mitotic replenishment of stem cells that continues throughout the adult life of the male. The committed stem cells, spermatogonia, are produced cyclically. These cells proliferate and differentiate into primary spermatocytes, which undergo meiotic divisions and eventually give rise to four haploid spermatids. Finally, during spermiogenesis, the spermatids acquire the form of mature spermatozoa, characteristic of the particular species. This process includes the acquisition of organelles necessary for motility, and molecular structures necessary for oocyte recognition, binding, penetration, and fusion. This typically involves the compression of the spherical form of the spermatid and its rounded nucleus into an elongated structure with a specialized surface, including an enzyme-containing acrosome, in addition to the development of the flagellum.

An important developmental event during sperm differentiation is the formation of the acrosome. It initially arises during the spermatid stage and is derived from vesicles associated with the Golgi apparatus (2). The products of these proacrosomal vesicles fuse to form a larger acrosomal granule (3,4). The acrosomal granule, which is considered a lysosome-like structure, eventually serves as a cap, conforming with the form of the underlying nuclear envelope. The acrosome is actually confined by a singular membrane that is continuous around the nucleus. At its most posterior region, the acrosome is referred to as the *equatorial segment.* The segment of the acrosome that apposes the nucleus is termed the inner acrosomal membrane, whereas the outer portion, in proximity to the sperm plasma membrane, is the outer acrosomal membrane (Fig. 4.1) (5). The importance of the functional differentiation of these two regions is manifest during the acrosome reaction and will be discussed later in this chapter. Figure 4.2 illustrates the main regions of the differentiated mammalian spermatozoon, including the head, midpiece, and tail. Note also the cross-sectional view of the flagellum, with its classic "9+2" arrangement of microtubules. The sperm head, in its posterior region, contains the proximal centriole, which

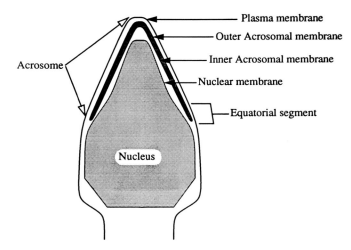

FIG. 4.1. Structure of the head of the human spermatozoon. The inner acrosomal membrane overlies the nucleus, whereas the outer acrosomal membrane apposes the outer plasma membrane.

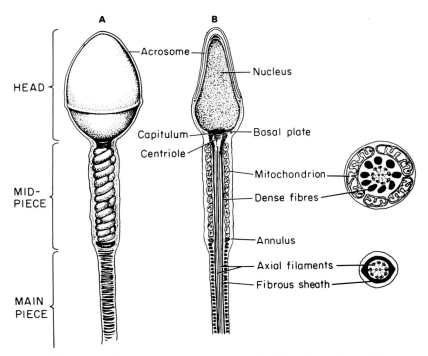

FIG. 4.2. Differentiated human spermatozoon shown in **(A)** surface, **(B)** sagittal, and cross-sectional views. (From Bedford JM, Hoskins DD. The mammalian spermatozoon: morphology, biochemistry, and physiology. In: Lamming GE, ed. *Marshall's physiology of reproduction, Vol 2. Reproduction in the male.* London: Churchill-Livingstone;1990:381, with permission.)

will eventually serve as the centrosome after formation of the male pronucleus.

Epididymal Sperm Maturation

Unlike the spermatozoa of several lower vertebrate species, which are competent to fertilize immediately after their production, most mammalian sperm are incapable of fertilization at the point at which they leave the testis. Important maturational events are initiated and continue during transit through the human epididymis (6). During epididymal maturation, the human sperm cell membrane is altered by the adsorption of epididymal-secreted proteins (7). Modifications of preexisting surface molecules also occur in the epididymis; this has been demonstrated by the observed alteration of lectin-binding sites on the surface of rabbit (8) and rat (9) spermatozoa. During human epididymal maturation, oxidation of protein-bound thiols serves to stabilize the sperm nucleus and tail structure (7,10). Biochemical changes that occur in the tail of the spermatozoon result in the potential for vigorous motility; this potential progressively develops as spermatozoa travel from caput to cauda epididymis. Whether the extensive changes that occur in the full length of the epididymis are absolutely necessary for fertilization in the human, or are simply beneficial, is unknown. Although fertilization by a spermatozoon that has not been exposed to the epididymis has never been demonstrated, human spermatozoa are capable of fertilization after only a brief exposure to the epididymis. Fertilization has been achieved using human sperm extracted from the midcorpus region of the epididymis after epididymovastomy (11). Spermatozoa obtained from the most proximal caput region of the epididymis have been shown to have fertilizing capability in men with a congenital lack of the vas deferens (12). The degree of motility and the fertilizing capability of sperm obtained by aspiration from the proximal caput in this study were considerably less than would be expected for a normal sperm sample. Nevertheless, the establishment of fertilization and pregnancy using sperm from this region indicates that exposure to the complete epididymal tract may not always be necessary.

Capacitation

After ejaculation, mature mammalian epididymal sperm must undergo further modification, either in the female reproductive tract or in vitro, in order to acquire the ability to fertilize (13,14). This process is termed *capacitation.* The nature of the events that occur during the period of capacitation is poorly understood. However, it is known that in vivo human capacitation involves the elimination of seminal plasma constituents from the surface of the sperm as it migrates through the cervical mucus and uterine secretions (15,16). Capacitation may also occur spontaneously in vitro, without any contribution from the female reproductive tract. The time required for the process varies with species. In the human, periods as short as 1 hour have been shown to be sufficient (17). It is also possible to artificially induce capacitation in vitro, by removing sperm from seminal plasma, and washing and incubating the remaining cells in culture medium. Specifically, capacitation involves, at least in part, the removal or alteration of cell surface components. Glycoproteins that were added to the sperm membrane during epididymal maturation may be modified during capacitation. In the absence of this modification, sperm-egg binding is inhibited. Evidence of this phenomenon is found in studies wherein capacitated spermatozoa were incubated with eggs in the presence of high concentrations of surface-associated glycoproteins isolated from uncapacitated sperm. No sperm-egg binding resulted. These glycoproteins have been termed *decapacitation* factors (18,19). Many other modifications occur during mammalian sperm capacitation, including changes in membrane lipids, redistribution of intramembranous particles, metabolism, and nuclear stabilization (for review see reference 20). The significance of many of these alterations remains to be elucidated.

One clear consequence of capacitation is the development in the sperm of a distinctive pattern of tail movement (21,22). Prior to capacitation, spermatozoa move in an essentially linear fashion. Capacitated spermatozoa exhibit a vigorously rapid sinusoidal movement. This hyperactivated sperm motility has been correlated with the ability of the sperm to cross the zona pellucida and to effect fertilization (23).

FEMALE GERM CELL DEVELOPMENT

Oocyte Maturation

In the ovary, proliferating primordial germ cells give rise to mitotically dividing oogonia, which are eventually induced to enter meiosis, as primary oocytes. Meiotic divisions proceed to prophase I, at which point meiosis is arrested at the diplotene stage. Shortly after birth, the oocyte, which resides in a preovulatory antral follicle, experiences a 2- to 3-week growth phase, during which it undergoes a significant increase in volume. At this time, the oocyte remains in meiotic prophase until a hormonal stimulus, a preovulatory surge of gonadotropins, acts as a trigger to resume meiosis. Four days prior to ovulation, the oocyte is at the germinal vesicle stage of development; it is encased in a dense formation of corona and cumulus cells, and its nucleus is in the form of a germinal vesicle containing a nucleolus. At this point, the cytoplasm of the egg is devoid of organelles (16,24,25). During the hours preceding the luteinizing hormone surge, the germinal vesicle migrates toward the periphery of the oocyte and has condensed perinucleolar chromatin (16). In the mouse, during the migration of the meiotic spindle, the nature of the oocyte plasma membrane undergoes an alteration; a restricted region directly overlying the chromosomes becomes devoid of microvilli and is also distinguished by a dense layer of actin filaments (26,27). The significance of this oocyte surface heterogeneity in mammalian gamete interaction is addressed in Chapter 5.

The oocyte and its surrounding granulosa and cumulus cells form an intimate network of syncytial communication, which is needed to sustain the oocyte in its meiotic arrest. The cumulus cells also project processes through the zona pellucida and toward the ooplasm (16). It is thought that meiotic arrest is maintained by the transfer of cyclic adenosine monophosphate (cAMP) from the follicular cells to the oocyte (28,29). However, it has been suggested that additional substances participate in the inhibition of meiosis (30). These include a polypeptide, oocyte meiosis inhibitor (OMI) (30) and purine nucleosides, such as hypoxanthine (31). Particular roles for these substances have been implicated; for instance, it is possible that a reduction in OMI initiates the peripheral migration of the germinal vesicle and the condensation of chromosomes. Breakdown of the nuclear envelope, however, has been attributed to a decrease in the level of cAMP within the oocyte (16). Channing et al. (31) have demonstrated OMI activity, which is inhibitory to meiosis in porcine oocytes, in the follicular fluid of humans. However, further investigation and characterization of such substances are necessary to clarify their role in meiotic inhibition.

Germinal vesicle breakdown, a main feature surrounding meiotic resumption, can occur as early as 15 hours following a surge in luteinizing hormone. Morphologic changes that accompany this gonadotropin-induced cascade include elongation of the corona cells and a dissociation of the cumulus cells from the oocyte. This dissociation of the gap junction-mediated intercellular communication results in a deprivation of exogenous cAMP to the oocyte. The dissociations between the cumulus cells and the oocyte are accompanied by a marked reduction in cell density surrounding the oocyte, caused by a follicle-stimulating hormone-dependent expansion of the cumulus and corona cell complexes (32,33). At this time, the follicle cells begin to produce increased quantities of glycoprotein matrix, rich in hyaluronic acid. Other features of this stage of meiotic resumption into metaphase I include arrangement of the chromosomes on the metaphase plate of the meiotic spindle and formation of cytoplasmic organelles throughout the cytoplasm. Anaphase I is indicated at the point when the oocyte's chromosomes migrate to the spindle pole. The oocyte enters meiotic Metaphase II at approximately 28 to 34 hours after the luteinizing hormone surge. Extrusion of the first polar body occurs, and the chromosomes that remain in the oocyte become situated on the equatorial plate of the second meiotic spindle (Fig. 4.3). Within a few hours, the oocyte-containing follicle ruptures, and ovulation occurs.

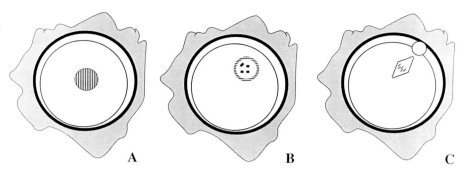

FIG. 4.3. Schematic representation of oocyte maturation. **A:** Oocyte with intact germinal vesicle contained within cumulus complex. **B:** Peripheral migration of the germinal vesicle, breakdown of nuclear envelope. **C:** Arrangement of chromosomes on the metaphase plate of meiotic spindle and extrusion of the first polar body.

The Zona Pellucida

An important part of the developmental program of oocyte growth is the deposition of the zona pellucida. Although the glycoproteins are assembled during this growth phase, the zona does not attain the full ability to be recognized and penetrated until the final stages of oocyte maturation (16). Ultrastructural changes occur in the zona throughout maturation (34), and, during the period from germinal vesicle breakdown until Metaphase I, the oocyte secretes proteoglycan-type molecules into the developing zona pellucida (16). Subsequently, during the next phase of meiotic maturation, that is, between Metaphase I and II, and zona becomes more penetrable by sperm, owing to the presence of proteoglycan-filled pores that develop in its structure.

During the past decade, much information has been generated pertaining to the substructure and function of the mammalian zona pellucida. The zona pellucida is an extracellular glycoprotein matrix that serves several important functions during both fertilization and early embryonic development. The studies, primarily conducted in the mouse model, have elucidated the glycoproteins that compose the zona pellucida and have characterized their functions in mediating species-specific fertilization (35–39). Three glycoproteins that are synthesized and secreted during oocyte growth have been identified in the mouse zona pellucida, designated as ZP-1, ZP-2, and ZP-3 (40–42). With the use of SDS-polyacrylamide gel electrophoresis (SDS–PAGE), the relative molecular masses (M_r) of these components have been identified, respectively, as 200, 120, and 83 kd (35). Each of the three proteins contains both N- and O-linked oligosaccharide chains (40). The overall structure of the zona, however, consists of filaments composed of

ZP-2-ZP-3 dimers cross-linked by ZP-1 (43), the component which thus functions to maintain three-dimensional structure of the zona. ZP-1 is a disulfide-linked homodimer consisting of individual monomers (Fig. 4.4) (35). The reduction of the intermolecular disulfides of ZP-1 can lead to the obliteration of interconnections between the zona filaments and to the overall solubilization of the zona (43,44).

In addition to the descriptions of their molecular structure, additional functions served by two of the glycoproteins of the mouse zona pellucida have been characterized. ZP-2 binds exclusively to acrosome-reacted sperm (45). Thus, it serves as a secondary receptor by which acrosome-reacted spermatozoa maintain their contact with the zona following initial interaction with another of the zona pellucida glycoproteins, ZP-3. As a result of fertilization, ZP-2 undergoes alterations in its structure to become ZP-2$_f$. This modification is the result of protease activity emanating from the oocyte's cortical granule release, which occurs following fertilization (37). As a result of the proteolysis, the ZP-2 molecule is cleaved into fragments that are held together by disulfide bonds. The "new" molecule, ZP-2$_f$, is unable to bind to acrosome-reacted sperm and, therefore, may lead to some of the postfertilization zona modifications, such as zona hardening and inhibition of further sperm binding, which are both involved in the prevention of polyspermic fertilization (45,46).

The third glycoprotein component of the zona pellucida, ZP-3, has been extensively characterized both developmentally and functionally. For instance, it is known that transcription of the ZP-3 gene occurs during a restricted 2- to 3-week period preceding meiotic maturation and ovulation (47,48). It has been demonstrated that during gamete interaction, spermatozoa recognize and bind to ZP-3, the glycoprotein that serves as a sperm

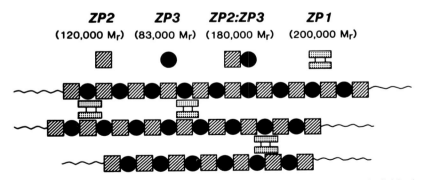

FIG. 4.4. Glycoprotein arrangement of the mouse zona pellucida filaments. Individual elements are illustrated at the *top* of the figure. (Reproduced with permission, from Wassarman PM. Zona pellucida glycoproteins. *Ann Rev Biochem* 1988;57:415–442. © 1988 by Annual Reviews Inc.)

receptor. The receptor activity of ZP-3 is attributed to its O-linked oligosaccharide moiety (43,49,50). Chemical elimination of the oligosaccharide destroys its ability to act as a sperm receptor and, in addition, exposure to the oligosaccharide units precludes sperm binding to ovulated oocytes. ZP-3 has also been identified as an inducer of the acrosome reaction. In contrast with its role as receptor, this function is dependent on the polypeptide, as well as the carbohydrate structure of the molecule (49).

Caused in part by the difficulty in isolating large quantities of zona material, it has been problematic to carry out extensive studies of the molecular structure of the human zona pellucida. However, during the past few years, several investigators have begun to characterize the composition of the human zona pellucida and have identified fertilization-associated changes in its structure as well as the electrophoretic characteristics of its components (51). Three human acidic glycoproteins, likely to be of oligomeric structures, have also been designated as ZP-1, 2, and 3 and have been identified with M_r ranges of 90 to 110, 64 to 78, and 57 to 73 kd. Depending upon whether or not they are assessed under reducing or non-reducing conditions, ZP-1 and ZP-2 co-migrate as either a single band of 92 to 120 kd, or as two distinct bands of lower M_r. ZP-3, however, migrates to the same M_r, regardless of the conditions. In those pools of eggs that had been characterized as fertilized, a dramatic decrease was demonstrated in the labeling of ZP-1. This alteration has been attributed to the cortical granule reaction. The phenomenon is similar to the change that occurs in mouse ZP-2 after fertilization (37) and is also similar to the modifications that occur in the zona structure of the pig oocyte (52); it was therefore suggestive of a structural change in the human zona pellucida that is related to fertilization. In additional studies (53), it was demonstrated that capacitated human spermatozoa could be saturated with heat-solubilized zona pellucidae, thus indicating the existence of human zona pellucida-binding proteins. These binding characteristics were altered when the zonae pellucidae were obtained from fertilized versus unfertilized oocytes. That the human zona glycoproteins served a receptor function was additionally reflected by sperm/zona Western blots, which demonstrated binding of both ZP-3 and ZP-1-2 complexes to spermatozoa.

Cross et al. (54) conducted a series of studies in which human capacitated sperm were assessed for occurrence of the acrosome reaction after coincubation with both intact and disaggregated human zonae. Induction of the acrosome reaction was increased after exposure to intact or digested zonae, as compared with unexposed controls. Although the molecular characteristics of the putative acrosome reaction inducers were not determined, the results suggest that similar to the zonae of other mammalian species, the human zona pellucida has the capacity to induce the acrosome reaction.

Recently, it has been possible to elucidate the substructure of particular moieties of the human zona glycoprotein ZP-3 (55). In an elegant series of experiments, the investigator utilized the antigenic and immunogenic properties of the zona pellucida to compensate for the limited quantity of human zona material. By performing immunizations with small quantities of solubilized human zonae pellucidae to raise mouse polyclonal antibodies, anti-human zona pellucida antibodies were formed. These antibodies were in part used to extend and clarify the previous descriptions of the molecular structure of the human zona and to further assess its role in sperm-egg interaction. Western blot analysis showed strong immunoreactivity against the zona component, which corresponded to ZP-3. In addition, the molecular analysis made it possible to discern the substructure of the glycoproteins in great detail and, therefore, it was determined that ZP-3 is composed of two distinct isomeric chains. In vitro sperm/zona-binding assays were performed to determine whether the antibodies to the human zona could inhibit sperm binding to homologous oocytes. Results indicated that the human zona antibodies were able to interfere with the ability of the sperm to interact with the oocytes; binding to eggs exposed to the zona antibody was significantly reduced, compared with binding to oocytes preincubated in control sera (55). It is suggested that this inhibitory activity of zona antibodies may eventually serve as a model for immunocontraception, which would obviate the need for interference with ovarian function.

Finally, that the genes coding for the mammalian zona pellucida are somewhat conserved among different species has been suggested by results of another recent study in which cross-hybridization of mouse cDNA with human DNA was used to isolate and characterize clones of human ZP-3 (56). It was found that the transcript of human ZP-3 is similar to that of the mouse (57,58), and may also resemble the ZP-3 transcripts of other mammals (58). Despite the conservation in portions of the structures of ZP-3 transcripts, differences in the protein or carbohydrate domains may account for the species specificity of zona-intact fertilization (56).

GAMETE FUSION

Cumulus Cells

The sequence of events, which culminates in sperm-egg fusion, begins with sperm traversal through the series of extracellular matrices that surround the oocyte. The mass of follicle cells that surrounds the ovulated oocyte represents the first obstacle encountered by the sperm en route to the oolemma. Capacitated sperm are able to physically negotiate the cumulus cells (59), which are contained within a hyaluronic acid matrix. Recent evidence suggests that in some mammalian species (e.g., human) spermatozoa that have reached the zona pellucida are acrosome-intact (60). The passage of these spermatozoa may be facilitated in part by the presence of spermatozoa that have undergone premature spontaneous acrosome reactions before reaching the oocyte. The release of hyaluronidase that results from spontaneous acrosome reactions serves to break down the cumulus structure; this may assist the free passage of acrosome-intact sperm. However, White et al. (61) showed that acrosome-intact spermatozoa are capable of penetrating deep into the cumulus cell mass within 3 minutes of insemination. Since little dispersion of cumulus cells occurs in this brief period, this evidence indicates that the effect of spontaneous acrosome reactions in assisting sperm passage may be minimal. It is believed that, although cumulus cells do not participate in direct interaction between sperm and egg, their presence does assist in guiding spermatozoa to the zona pellucida in an orientation that will ensure contact between gametes (62).

Interaction with the Zona Pellucida

Initial Recognition and Binding

Following passage through the cumulus complex, the next oocyte investment encountered by the spermatozoon is the zona pellucida. The initial association formed between the sperm and this zona is a reversible, loose, nonspecific attachment that is no stronger than that between spermatozoa and the zonae of fertilized oocytes (63,64). This is followed by establishment of a tenacious and specific contact, termed *binding* (36). In the mouse, the capacity of the zona pellucida to bind acrosome-intact sperm follows classic saturation kinetics; it reaches a maximum within 10 to 15 minutes of insemination with 10^5 to 10^6 sperm per milliliter (46,65). In light of the widespread use of in vitro fertilization (IVF) technology, additional characteristics are of interest when studying sperm-zona binding in the human. For example, whether or not oocyte maturity is related to the number of sperm that can bind to its zona is not clear. Mahadevan et al. (66) demonstrated that sperm binding was increased in mature oocytes, when compared with atretic or immature ones. Other investigators, however, could not establish an association between egg maturity and sperm-binding ability (16).

The binding of sperm to the zona pellucida is initiated by recognition between the plasma membrane of an acrosome-intact sperm and particular molecules on the zona pellucida, in a manner resembling the ligand–receptor-type interaction that occurs in somatic cells (Fig. 4.5) (67). The approaching acrosome-intact sperm recognizes and binds to tens of thousands of copies of the ZP-3 molecule. The sperm must first recognize a specific region of the ZP-3, which in the mouse and, perhaps, the human, involves the oligosaccharide component of the molecule. Since the sperm is acrosome intact, it is the plasma membrane that is initially exposed to and identified by the zona pellucida.

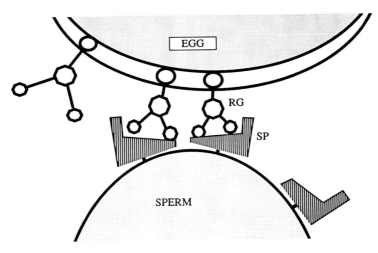

FIG. 4.5. Schematic representation of molecular interaction between sperm receptors on the zona pellucida and "receptors" on the plasma membrane of the acrosome-intact spermatozoon. Specifically, the interaction between the carbohydrate moiety of ZP-3 glycoprotein receptor *(RG)* is shown in association with the sperm protein *(SP)*. (Adapted from Dietl JA, Rauth G. Molecular aspects of mammalian fertilization. *Hum Reprod* 1989;4:869–875, by permission of Oxford University Press.)

It is reasonable to assume that the molecular interaction between the fertilizing spermatozoon and the zona pellucida may also involve sperm proteins that recognize the glycoproteins of the zona pellucida. In mammalian species, including the mouse, rabbit, and guinea pig, several components associated with the sperm plasma membrane have been identified and are considered as possible egg-binding proteins. These include, galactosyltransferase (68), trypsin-like enzymes (69), sialylated residues (70), and a fucose component (71,72). For example, the evidence suggesting that galactosyltransferase mediates gamete recognition is quite convincing. This substance specifically inhibits sperm-egg interaction, in a concentration-dependent manner, and binds to particular N-acetylglucosamine residues on ZP-3 (73). Thus, it is believed that galactosyltransferase may accomplish recognition and binding by forming an enzyme–substrate complex with ZP-3 (74). This association would subsequently lead to the induction of the acrosome reaction (see later). It is possible that this function of galactosyltransferase as an egg-binding protein is operative in human sperm-zona recognition, since a galactosyltransferase has been identified on the surface of the human spermatozoon (73).

Other candidates for proteins involved in mammalian gamete binding include a series of polarized surface proteins that have been described in guinea pig sperm (75,76). These proteins, called PH-20 antigens, migrate from the posterior portion of the sperm head to the inner acrosomal membrane during the course of the acrosome reaction. In addition, monoclonal antibodies directed against these antigens block sperm-zona binding. Although these proteins have not been characterized in human gamete interaction, characteristics, such as their acrosome-dependent modifications, suggest that they may serve an important role in the scheme of gamete recognition and binding.

The Acrosome Reaction

Binding to the zona pellucida is followed by interaction between the sperm and a component of the zona pellucida that will induce the acrosome reaction. The acrosome reaction is an all-important exocytotic event, involving the release of the contents of the acrosome and the exposure of the inner acrosomal membrane. This is necessary for penetration of the zona pellucida and subsequent fusion with the oolemma. In the mouse, it has been demonstrated that both the oligosaccharide and polypeptide portions of the ZP-3 molecule are involved in induction of the acrosome reaction (77,78). Experimental evidence suggests that induction of the acrosome reaction by the ZP-3 molecule involves binding of sperm to multiple O-linked oligosaccharides on individual ZP-3 molecules that are attached by a polypeptide chain. It is possible that this precise scheme applies to the human acrosome reaction, but this remains to be clarified.

The classic scheme of the mammalian acrosome reaction involves multiple fusions between the outer acrosomal membrane and the overlying plasma membrane, followed by fenestration of the acrosome and formation of membrane vesicles. This allows release of the acrosomal contents (Fig. 4.6) (79). It is currently believed that a similar sequence of morphologic changes occurs in the human spermatozoa. In addition, several investigators believe that an alternative series of membrane alterations (80,81) may be associated with a degenerative or unphysiologic acrosome reaction in human spermatozoa (20,61). In this scheme, the vesiculation may involve primarily an invagination of the outer acrosomal membrane. Release of the acrosomal content occurs in the presence of the plasma membrane, and it has been suggested that subtle changes in the consistency of the plasma membrane allow the leeching out of the acrosomal matrix material (Fig. 4.7) (80,81). Although, currently, it is believed that the zona-induced acrosome reaction that occurs in vivo does not involve this unconventional mode of membrane changes, it may occur in those spermatozoa that are induced to acrosome react by artifical methods. In addition, after a micromanipulation procedure, such as subzonal insertion, spermatozoa that are still acrosome-intact, may undergo spontaneous acrosome reactions by this process.

Biochemical changes that accompany the morphologic modifications include sodium and calcium influxes, as well as hydrogen effluxes through

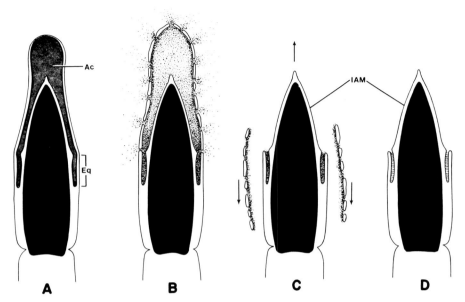

FIG. 4.6. Diagrams of the progressive morphologic changes constituting the typical mammalian acrosome reaction. **A:** Acrosomal cap *(Ac)* is intact. **B:** Fusion of the outer acrosomal membrane and the plasma membrane, leading to the vesiculation of the acrosome. **C:** Progressive loss of membranes and acrosomal contents. **D:** Completion of the acrosome reaction and exposure of the inner acrosomal membrane (IAM). (With permission from Yanagimachi R. Mechanisms of fertilization in mammals. In: Mastroianni I, Biggers JD, eds. *In vitro fertilization and embryo transfer.* New York: Plenum Press; 1981:81–182.)

the plasma membrane. Ion pumps (adenosine 5′-triphosphate-dependent H^+ pumps) facilitate these ionic shifts and lead to changes in intracellular pH that are an integral part of the acrosome reaction (20). In addition, it is believed that phospholipases and phospholipids are involved in the mechanism by which the sperm membranes fuse during the acrosome reaction. The requirement for extracellular calcium in the cascade of events involves specific binding proteins, such as calmodulin, which is located in the region between the plasma and outer acrosomal membranes. This necessity for calcium, for instance, becomes an important factor in the context of microsurgical fertilization, when it is often necessary to artificially induce the acrosome reaction by reagents, such as calcium ionophore.

Secondary Zona Associations and Penetration of the Zona Pellucida

In the mouse model, acrosome-reacted spermatozoa become associated with the secondary sperm receptor, ZP-2 (45). This is a relatively weak inter-

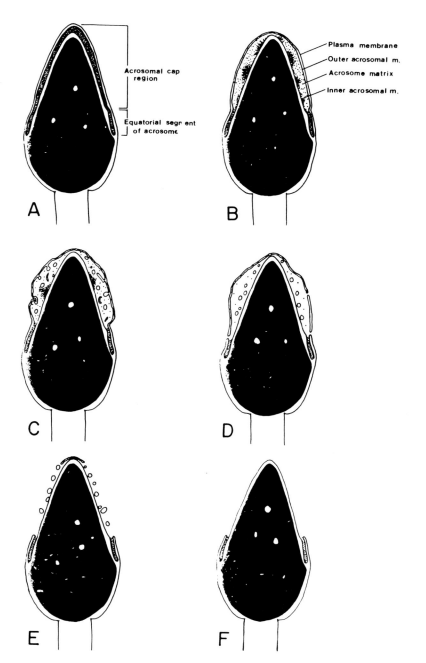

FIG. 4.7. Series of structural changes that may constitute the spontaneous acrosome reaction in human spermatozoa. See text for details of stages **A–F**. Note that unlike the classic acrosome reaction seen in Fig. 4.6, the vesicles shown here in **C–E** may be exclusively composed of outer acrosomal membranes. (From Nagae T, et al. Acrosome reaction in human spermatozoa. *Fertil Steril* 1986;45:701–707, with permission.)

action, which allows the sperm sufficient mobility to begin its course through the zona pellucida. Sperm penetration through the zona pellucida is likely to involve several proteinases. One of the better-characterized enzymes is acrosin, a trypsin-like protease formed from an inactive proenzyme, proacrosin. This enzyme has been isolated in several mammalian species, including the human, and is thought to be associated with the inner acrosomal membrane as well as with several other sperm domains (for review see 82). Once it gains access to the perivitelline space, the sperm can interact and fuse with the vitelline membrane of the oocyte. In the mouse, it is the posterior portion of the sperm plasma membrane that fuses with the oolemma. Microvilli on the surface of the oocyte envelop the sperm, which may no longer be motile at the moment of fusion, and draw it toward the cortex of the egg. In certain mammalian species, fusion will not occur at the microvillus-free region of the oocyte surface (see Chapter 5).

Fusion is followed by oocyte activation. This phase involves depolarization and an intracellular rise in calcium (83), thought to induce completion of the second meiotic division, with the consequent release of a second polar body. In the hamster, failure to extrude the second polar body has been associated with impaired blocks to polyspermy (84). Interestingly, Uchida and Freeman (85) reported that nearly 2% of aborted human fetuses were triploid due to retention of the second polar body. Aside from these activation-induced changes in the oocyte, two mechanisms for preventing supernumerary fertilization are triggered as a result of gamete fusion. The fast block to polyspermy involving the depolarization of the egg membrane is not well characterized in mammals and, in the human, it seems to be minimally effective (86,87).

The second or slow block to polyspermy, operative in the human oocyte, is attributed to alterations in the zona pellucida that occur following fertilization. Cortical granules, membrane-bound organelles containing hydrolytic enzymes such as proteinases and peroxidases (88) located in the cortex of the mammalian egg, undergo an exocytotic event with the oocyte membrane. The fusion of the cortical and egg membranes is propagated as a wave from the point of gamete fusion and is due to release of cytoplasmic calcium stores. As a result, cortical granule contents permeate the perivitelline space and, subsequently, cause modifications in the porous zona pellucida, which are collectively termed the *zona reaction* (Fig. 4.8) (89). The sequelae of the zona reaction involve modifications in both ZP-2 and ZP-3 molecules. After fertilization, ZP-3 can no longer act as a sperm receptor or inducer of the acrosome reaction. In addition, the proteolysis of ZP-2, which occurs after the cortical reaction, renders it incapable of binding to acrosome-reacted sperm (91). Taken together, in addition to their role in the physical "hardening" of the zona pellucida, these modifications are important in physiologically preventing polyspermic fertilization. In the

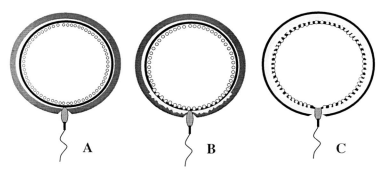

FIG. 4.8. Schematic representation of the cortical reaction as it occurs in the mouse. **A:** Before fertilization, the cortical granules are located in the peripheral region of the oocyte, subjacent to the plasma membrane. **B,C:** After sperm-egg fusion, a wave of fusion between the cortical granules and the plasma membrane is propagated over the egg surface. The cortical granule contents are deposited into the perivitelline space, and ultimately induce the zona reaction. (Adapted from Wassarman PM. Fertilization. In: Yamada KM, ed. Cellular interactions and development: Molecular mechanisms. New York: Wiley-Interscience;1983:1–27. Copyright © 1983 Wiley-Interscience. Reprinted by permission of Wiley-Liss, A division of John Wiley and Sons, Inc.)

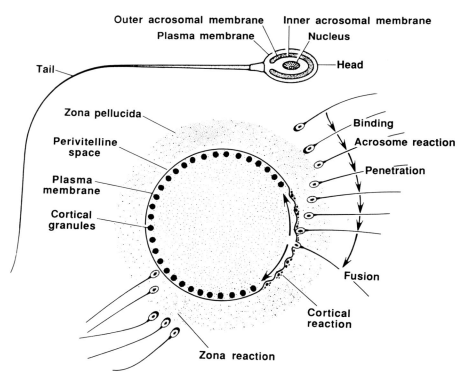

FIG. 4.9. Summary diagram of the sequence of events involved in fertilization in the mouse. (Reprinted with permission from Wassarman PM. The biology and chemistry of fertilization. *Science* 1987;235:553–560. Copyright 1987 by the AAAS.)

human, extensive polyspermic fertilization may result after micromanipulation techniques, such as zona drilling, partial zona dissection, or subzonal insertion, which involve either opening or circumventing the zona pellucida. These observations support the hypothesis that control of supernumerary sperm penetration in the human oocyte is largely under the control of the zona pellucida and not the oocyte plasma membrane.

A chronologic summary of the major events in the mammalian fertilization pathway described thus far is illustrated in Fig. 4.9.

DEVELOPMENT OF EMBRYONIC GENOMIC CONTROL

Pronucleus Formation

The dynamic events that constitute fertilization are not complete with fusion of the sperm and oocyte membranes. Postfusional phenomena, including formation of the maternal pronucleus, decondensation of the sperm, formation of the male pronucleus, and migration and coalescence of the two pronuclei during syngamy, are a complex series of events prerequisite to normal embryonic development.

Within the first few hours after sperm-egg fusion, after the completion of meiotic Anaphase II in the oocyte, a series of morphologic changes occur that lead to formation of the male and female pronuclei. The set of haploid chromosomes that remain following extrusion of the second polar body are dispersed, become surrounded by vesicles that progressively fuse to become a bilaminar envelope and after fusion of the laminae, are encompassed in an irregularly shaped female pronucleus that eventually acquires a spheroid form (92). This process usually requires 12 to 26 hours (93). These events are thought to be analogous to the formation of the mitotic interphase nucleus in a somatic cell (94).

The formation of the male pronucleus, on the other hand, is a more complex process that, in the human, has been recently described in detail. The specific events constituting development of the male pronucleus differ somewhat among organisms. However, common to most species are the degeneration of the nuclear envelope, followed by sperm chromatin decondensation, and transformation of the sperm nucleus into a true male pronuclear structure. In a recent study, Tesarik and Kopecny (95) obtained oocytes that failed to fertilize from an IVF program, removed their zonae, and reinseminated them to assess pronuclear formation. Since the zona pellucida represents the main barrier to sperm penetration in the human oocyte, these oocytes had the capacity to be penetrated by multiple sperm and, therefore, were a good experimental system with which to evaluate the oocytes' ability to support supernumerary sperm fusion. After multiple inseminations, the oocytes were fixed at varying intervals following exposure to sperm and were examined by electron microscopy. The investigators categorized the progressive ultrastructural changes in the sperm nucleus following penetration into the oocyte cytoplasm. Sperm decondensation occurred rapidly, and it was usually complete within 1 hour. The reformation of the nuclear membrane, reorganization of chromatin, and the assembly of nucleolar precursors occurred more gradually. Fully developed male pronuclei were usually observed 12 to 16 hours after sperm penetration; as long as 20 hours was required in some instances. It has also been shown that the development of the male pronucleus in the human is at least partially under ooplasmic control (94). This was demonstrated by the decreasing ability of the oocyte to support transformation of sperm nuclei into pronuclei when increasing numbers of sperm penetrated a single oocyte.

Human male and female pronuclei are morphologically similar, and it is difficult to distinguish between them (96). The male pronucleus normally forms near the point of sperm entry, whereas the female pronucleus is first observed at the ooplasmic pole of the meiotic spindle. From the site of initial formation, the pronuclei migrate to a central position in the cytoplasm, where they will eventually fuse. Male pronuclear movement in mammals is regulated by the formation of the sperm aster (92), which consists of microtubules and associated endoplasmic reticulum. Although the mechanism of pronuclear migration is not known, it may result from microtubule elongation. It is also unknown whether movement of the female pronucleus is governed by the same mechanisms as the migration of the male pronucleus (92).

Human pronuclei enlarge during later states of development. Pronuclei become closely apposed, and they progressively flatten against each other during the period just before syngamy (97). Transmission electron microscopy demonstrates that a very narrow strip of cytoplasm exists between the apposed pronuclei (98,99). Nucleoli are clearly visible within pronuclei; advanced pronuclear stages are characterized by an equatorial alignment of nucleoli (Fig. 4.10). During this final phase of pronuclear movement, there is no increase in the average number of visible pronuclei (97).

Gene Activation in the Human Embryo

The organization of cellular processes in the developing embryo are controlled, in part, by the genetic timetable of differentiation. During the earliest stages of embryogenesis, developmental functions are exclusively under control of the maternal genome. The influence of the maternal genome is manifested by the presence in the cytoplasm of maternal proteins, metabolic products, and RNA. At some point following fertilization, the control of the early embryo is shifted from the maternal to the

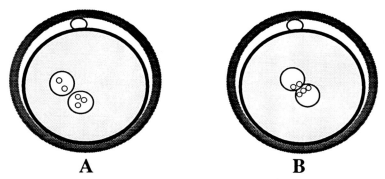

A   **B**

FIG. 4.10. A: Representation of pronuclear zygote with randomly distributed nucleoli. **B:** Zygote at later stage of pronuclear migration. Nucleoli are equatorially aligned. (Adapted from Wright G, et al. Observations on the morphology of pronuclei and nucleoli in human zygotes and implications for cryopreservation. *Hum Reprod* 1990;5:109–115.)

embryonic genome. How and when the control of protein synthesis and gene regulation are assumed by the embryo is of consequence in the application of advanced embryological technology, such as preimplantation diagnosis. Specifically, preimplantation diagnostic technologies involve the use of DNA probes to identify and analyze particular gene sequences (100). Alternatively, products of protein synthesis may be assessed in order to recognize defective or deficient genes. In applying the latter form of diagnosis, one must ascertain that the gene products in question are under the control of the embryonic genome and are not maternal in origin. Thus, the earliest stage at which preimplantation genetic analysis may be performed is a function of the time at which the embryonic genome is activated. Embryonic gene expression has been studied in a variety of mammalian species (reviewed in 101). It is a complex matter, for transition from oocyte to embryonic control is not a perfectly synchronized process in which one system is turned off immediately before the next is activated. In fact, the genetic information present in the unfertilized egg persists during early embryonic development and may transiently coexist with products formed under the regulation of the embryo (102).

Animal Studies

In the mouse, the embryonic genome is inactive until the two-cell stage, at least within the limit of detection (103,104). Qualitative changes in protein content occur late in the one-cell stage, but these changes occur independently of novel RNA synthesis. After inhibition of transcription with inhibitors, such as α-amanitin, investigators evaluated the presence of polypeptides and demonstrated that during the first cell cycle following fertilization, or until the early two-cell stage, almost no novel RNA syntheses occurs (105,106). It has also been shown that protein synthesis in the fertilized oocyte is unaffected by enucleation and, accordingly, is independent of new transcriptional activity (107). The profile of the mouse embryo dramatically changes, however, during the two-cell stage of development. This has been established by studies in which an increase in RNA synthesis was verified following increased uptake of labeled precursors (108–111). Such increases in transcriptional activity have been shown to be concomitant with a change from maternally to embryonically encoded transcripts. The degradation of maternally derived RNA in the two-cell mouse embryo has been shown by the reduction in total RNA content (112), polyadenylated RNA (111,113), and in the number of ribosomes (113). In addition, expression of the paternal genome in two-cell mouse embryos has also been assessed. It has been demonstrated that two-cell mouse embryos heterozygous at the β_2-microglobulin locus can express the paternally derived form of this protein (114). The existence of other gene products, such as surface antigens, have provided evidence that paternally derived gene products are manifest by at least the four- to eight-cell stage (115). Interspecies differences in the onset of embryonic genomic control have been elucidated. In some species, for instance, activation of the embryonic genome is delayed, compared with that of the mouse; maternal regulation of the genome persists until the four-cell stage in the pig embryo (116), until the late eight-cell stage in the cow embryo (117), and until the morula stage in the rabbit (118).

The Human Embryo

Where does the human embryo fit in this mammalian scheme? The phenomenon of gene expression in the human embryo has been approached by autoradiographic, ultrastructural, and biochemical analyses. Studies of human embryos conducted by Tesarik and coworkers (119,120), in which the incorporation of radiolabeled uridine was studied, demonstrated that new RNA synthesis is initiated at the four-cell stage of development. Until this point, the embryo is under the control of the maternal genome. At the four-cell stage, however, RNA synthesis is largely extranucleolar, since the uptake of labeled uridine into blastomere nuclei of four-cell embryos was quite low (119). These observations were correlated with the pattern of nucleogenesis in the early human embryo by parallel ultrastructural and autoradiographic studies (120) that revealed a lack of true DNA-containing nucleolar structures at the four-cell stage. The investigators noted striking structural changes in the nucleolar mass that occurred at the six- to eight-cell stage concurrently with an increase in the amount of embryonic DNA.

Here, it was seen that morphologic changes in the nucleolar structure were associated with increased incorporation of labeled DNA precursors. It was suggested that at the six- to eight-cell stages, embryonic DNA begins to infiltrate the homogeneous fibrillar nucleolus-like bodies. Ultrastructural studies indicated that the initiation of ribosomal RNA synthesis that follows is marked by the change in the nucleolar mass, as it initially becomes permeated with dense fibrils and granules.

In more recent studies, Tesarik et al. (121,122) extended their previous characterizations of the functional and structural modifications by conducting more precise ultrastructural studies of the localization of DNA in the developing nucleolus, thereby providing more specific descriptions of early transcriptional activities in the early human embryo. Interestingly, electron microscopy combined with autoradiographic studies revealed different transcriptional patterns within blastomeres of the same cleavage-stage embryo. Specifically, the investigators showed that, whereas all blastomeres of a four-cell human embryo demonstrate a lack of nucleolar RNA synthetic activity, the blastomeres of an eight-cell embryo are heterogeneous; some reflect a similar low level of transcriptional activity, whereas others have a high level of extranucleolar and nucleolar RNA synthesis (122). In describing this heterogeneity, they categorized the variable blastomeres into those with an early-cleavage transcriptional pattern and those with a progressed-cleavage transcriptional pattern. These patterns of transcriptional activity were correlated with the nucleolar morphology of the blastomeres. That is, those blastomeres with a low level of RNA synthesis were also lacking differentiated nucleolar structure. On the other hand, the progressed-cleavage–stage blastomeres exhibited well-developed nucleoli, with dense fibrillar and granular components. To fully understand the developmental significance of the two types of blastomeres, additional ultrastructural comparisons were made (122). The phenotypic changes associated with elevated transcriptional activity include increases in the endoplasmic reticulum tubule/vesicle ratio and in the amount of lysosomes, as well as a decrease in the Golgi apparatus. Since the measurement of the fractional surfaces of total intracellular membranes was the same in both groups, it was suggested that the modifications were not due to changes in the equilibrium between total membrane production, but were caused by a redistribution of the organelle membranes characteristic of enhanced transcription.

The timing of genomic activation in the human embryo was further substantiated by biochemical evidence (123). In one part of this study, oocytes and embryos were labeled with [^{35}S]methionine and subsequently analyzed by gel electrophoresis. There was no difference detected in polypeptide synthesis between unfertilized oocytes and the two-cell stage embryo. However, changes reflected in losses and gains of electrophoretic bands between the four-cell and morula stages indicated progressive altera-

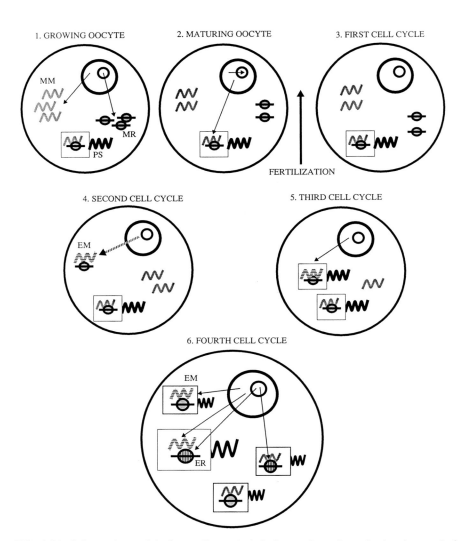

FIG. 4.11. Schematic model of genetic control during early embryonic development. **1:** Growing oocyte in which protein synthesis is entirely under maternal control. *Arrows* indicate that maternal mRNA *(MM)* is produced under the control of the maternal nucleus, and that the nucleolus is controlling the formation of maternal ribosomes *(MR)*. Protein synthesis *(PS)* is indicated by the association of the *MR* and *MM* symbols. **2:** In the maturing oocyte, the nucleolus becomes synthetically inactive and becomes an RNA storage site (see *arrow*). **3,4:** In the two cell cycles following fertilization, protein synthesis is still carried out with the use of maternal mRNA and maternal ribosomes. As indicated by the *dotted arrow,* there may be some embryonic mRNA synthesis *(EM)* during the second cell cycle. **5:** During the third cell cycle, some extranucleolar RNA synthesis occurs (see *arrow*). As indicated by the symbols, at this point, only maternally derived ribosomes are used for protein synthesis. **6:** In the fourth cell cycle after fertilization, the embryonic genome assumes control of protein synthesis using both embryonic ribosomes *(ER)* and the embryonic mRNA. There may be, to a minor extent, some residual activity involving maternal ribosomes and mRNA. (Redrawn from Tesarir J. Developmental control of human preimplantation embryos: a comparative approach. *J In Vitro Fert Embryo Transfer* 1988;5:347–362.)

tions in protein synthesis. It was hypothesized that such modifications in protein synthesis corresponded to those occurring in the two-cell mouse embryo, when maternal expression is reduced and embryonic transcripts are activated. To further clarify these observations, experiments were performed in which embryos were preexposed to α-amanitin, an inhibitor of transcription that will block synthesis of new RNA. In the mouse, α-amanitin has been shown to cause arrest at the two-cell stage and, therefore, blocks embryonic transcription. However, it does not interfere with the decline in maternal expression (105,106). Human embryos that had been exposed to α-amanitin arrested at the four-cell stage of development. Thus, it appeared as though the first two cell cycles in the human embryo are controlled at a posttranscriptional level; the maternal transcripts already present in the embryo were sufficient to support cleavage to four cells. Between the four- and eight-cell stage of cleavage, transcriptional control is assumed by the embryo. Figure 4.11 is a summary of the event surrounding genomic control of the early human embryo. Specifically, the roles of maternal RNA and ribosomes during the period of late follicular maturation until the third cell cycle are illustrated, and the point at which protein synthesis is assumed by the embryo is indicated.

REFERENCES

1. Johnson L. Spermatogenesis (animal species and humans). In: Asch RH, Balmaceda JP, Johnson I, eds. *Gamete physiology.* Norwell, Mass.: Serono Symposia; 1990:3–18.
2. Fawcett DW. Morphogenesis of the mammalian sperm acrosome in new perspective. In: Afzelius BA, ed. *The functional anatomy of the spermatozoon.* Oxford: Pergamon Press; 1975:199–210.
3. Bellve AR. Biogenesis of the mammalian spermatozoon. In: Amann RP, Seidel GE, eds. *Prospects for sexing mammalian sperm.* Boulder: Associated Press; 1982:69–93.
4. Huang TTF, Yanagimachi R. Inner acrosomal membrane of mammalian spermatozoa: its properties and possible functions in fertilization. In: Koehler JK, ed. *Gamete surfaces and their interactions.* New York: Alan R Liss; 1985:249–268.
5. Bedford JM, Hoskins DD. The mammalian spermatozoon: morphology, biochemistry and physiology. In: Lamming GE, ed. *Marshall's physiology of reproduction, vol 2. Reproduction in the male.* London: Churchill-Livingstone; 1990:381.
6. Bedford JM, Calvin HI, Cooper GW. The maturation of spermatozoa in the human epididymis. *J Reprod Fertil* 1973;18(Suppl):199–213.
7. Tezon JG, Ramella E, Cameo MS, Vazquez MH, Blacquier JA. Immunochemical localization of secretory antigens in the human epididymis and their association with spermatozoa. *Biol Reprod* 1985;32:591–597.
8. Nicholson GL, Usui N, Yanagimachi R, Yanagimachi H, Smith JR. Lectin binding sites on the membranes of rabbit spermatozoa. Changes in surface receptors during epididymal maturation and after ejaculation. *J Cell Biol* 1977;74:950–962.
9. Olson GE, Danzo BJ. Surface changes in rat spermatozoa during epididymal transit. *Biol Reprod* 1981;24:431–443.
10. Bedford JM, Calvin HI. Changes in -S-S- linked structures of the sperm tail during epididymal maturation, with comparative observation in submammalian species. *J Exp Zool* 1974;187:181–204.

11. Bedford JM. The bearing of epididymal function in strategies for in vitro fertilization and gamete intrafallopian transfer. In: Jones HW, Schrader C, eds. In vitro fertilization and other assisted reproduction. *Ann NY Acad Sci* 1988;541:284–291.
12. Silber SJ, Ord T, Balmaceda J, Patrizio P, Asch RH. Congenital absence of the vas deferens. The fertilizing capacity of human epididymal sperm. *N Engl J Med* 1990; 323:1788–1792.
13. Austin CR. Observations on the penetration of the sperm into the mammalian egg. *Aust J Sci Res* 1951;4(B):581–596.
14. Chang MC. Fertilizing capacity of spermatozoa deposited into the fallopian tube. *Nature* 1951;168:697–698.
15. Lambert H, Overstreet JW, Morales P, Hanson FW, Yanagimachi R. Sperm capacitation in the human female reproductive tract. *Fertil Steril* 1985;43:325–327.
16. Plachot M, Mandelbaum J. Oocyte maturation, fertilization and embryonic growth in vitro. In: Edwards RG, ed. *Assisted human reproduction.* London: Churchill–Livingstone; 1990:675–694.
17. Plachot M, Junca AM, Mandelbaum J, Cohen J, Salat-Baroux J, Da Lage C. Timing of in-vitro fertilization of cumulus-free and cumulus-enclosed oocytes. *Hum Reprod* 1986;1:237–242.
18. Aunomas S, Mayumi T, Suzuki K, Noguchi T, Iwai M, Okabe M. Studies on sperm capacitation. I. The relationship between a given sperm-coating antigen and a sperm capacitation phenomenon. *J Reprod Fertil* 1973;35:425–432.
19. Reddy JM, Stark RA, Zanveld JD. A high molecular weight antifertility factor from human seminal plasma. *J Reprod Fertil* 1979;57:437–446.
20. Yanagimachi R. Mammalian fertilization. In: Knobil E, Neill JD, eds. *The physiology of reproduction.* New York: Raven Press; 1988:135–185.
21. Yanagimachi R. The movement of golden hamster spermatozoa before and after capacitation. *J Reprod Fertil* 1970;23:193–196.
22. Morales P, Overstreet JW, Katz DF. Changes in human sperm motion during capacitation in vitro. *J Reprod Fertil* 1988;83:119–128.
23. Fraser LR, Quinn PJ. A glycolytic product is obligatory for initiation of sperm acrosome reaction and whiplash motility required for fertilization in the mouse. *J Reprod Fertil* 1981;61:25–35.
24. Szollosi D, Mandelbaum J, Plachot M, Salat-Baroux J, Cohen J. Ultrastructure of the human preovulatory oocyte. *J In Vitro Fert Embryo Transfer* 1986;3:232–242.
25. Bomsel-Helmreich O, Huyen LVN, Durand-Gasselin I, Salat-Baroux J, Antoine JM. Timing of nuclear maturation and cumulus dissociation in human oocytes stimulated with clomiphene citrate, human menopausal gonadotrophin, and human chorionic gonadotrophin. *Fertil Steril* 1987;48:586–595.
26. Nicosia SV, Wolf DP, Inoue M. Cortical granule distribution and cell surface characteristics in mouse eggs. *Dev Biol* 1977;57:56–74.
27. Longo FJ, Chen DY. Development of cortical polarity in mouse eggs: involvement of the meiotic apparatus. *Dev Biol* 1985;107:382–394.
28. Dekel N, Beers WH. Development of the rat oocyte in vitro: inhibition and induction of maturation in the presence or absence of the cumulus oophorus. *Dev Biol* 1980;75: 247–254.
29. Gilula NB, Epstein ML, Beers WH. Cell-to-cell communication and ovulation. A study of the cumulus cell-oocyte complex. *J Cell Biol* 1978;78:58–75.
30. Thibault C, Szollosi D, Gerard M. Mammalian oocyte maturation. *Reprod Nutr Dev* 1987;27:865–896.
31. Channing CP, Liu CQ, Seegar-Jones G, Jones H. Decline of follicular oocyte maturation inhibitor coincident with maturation and achievement of fertilizability of oocytes recovered at midcycle of gonadotrophin-treated women. *Proc Natl Acad Sci USA* 1983; 80:4181–4188.
32. Eppig JJ, Downs SM. The effect of hypoxanthine on mouse oocyte growth and development in vitro: maintenance of meiotic arrest and gonadotrophin-induced oocyte maturation. *Dev Biol* 1987;119:313–321.
33. Eppig J. The relationship between cumulus cell-oocyte coupling, oocyte meiotic maturation and cumulus expansion. *Dev Biol* 1982;89:268–272.

34. Tesarik J, Pilka L, Travnik P. Zona pellucida resistance to sperm penetration before the completion of human oocyte maturation. *J Reprod Fertil* 1988;83:487–495.
35. Bleil JD, Wassarman PM. Structure and function of the zona pellucida: identification and characterization of the proteins of the mouse oocyte's zona pellucida. *Dev Biol* 1980;76:185–202.
36. Bleil JD, Wassarman PM. Mammalian sperm-egg interaction: identification of a glycoprotein in mouse egg zonae pellucidae possessing receptor activity for sperm. *Cell* 1980;20:873–882.
37. Bleil JD, Beall CF, Wassarman PM. Mammalian sperm–egg interaction: fertilization of mouse eggs triggers modification of the major zona pellucida glycoprotein, ZP-2. *Dev Biol* 1981;86:189–197.
38. Bleil JD, Wassarman PM. Sperm-egg interactions in the mouse: sequence of events and induction of the acrosome reaction by a zona pellucida glycoprotein. *Dev Biol* 1983; 95:317–324.
39. Wassarman PM. Zona pellucida glycoproteins. *Annu Rev Biochem* 1988;57:415–442.
40. Bleil JD, Wassarman PM. Synthesis of zona pellucida proteins by denuded and follicle-enclosed mouse oocytes during culture in vitro. *Proc Natl Acad Sci USA* 1980;77: 1029–1033.
41. Greve JM, Salzmann GS, Roller RJ, Wassarman PM. Biosynthesis of the major zona pellucida glycoprotein secreted by oocytes during mammalian oogenesis. *Cell* 1982; 31:749–759.
42. Roller RJ, Kinloch RA, Hiraoka BY, Li SSL, Wassarman PM. Gene expression during mammalian oogenesis and early embryogenesis: quantification of three messenger RNAs abundant in fully grown mouse oocytes. *Development* 1989;106:251–261.
43. Greve JM, Wassarman PM. Mouse egg extracellular coat is a matrix of interconnected filaments possessing a structural repeat. *J Mol Biol* 1985;181:253–264.
44. Moller CC, Bleil JD, Kinloch RA, Wassarman PM. Structural and functional relationships between mouse and hamster zona pellucida glycoproteins. *Dev Biol* 1990;137: 276–286.
45. Bleil JD, Wassarman PM. Autoradiographic visualization of the mouse egg's sperm receptor bound to sperm. *J Cell Biol* 1986;102:1363–1371.
46. Bleil JD, Greve JM, Wassarman PM. Identification of a secondary sperm receptor in the mouse egg zona pellucida: role in maintenance of binding acrosome-reacted sperm. *Dev Biol* 1988;128:376–385.
47. Philpott CC, Ringuette MJ, Dean J. Oocyte-specific expression and developmental regulation of ZP3, the sperm receptor of the mouse zona pellucida. *Dev Biol* 1987;121: 568–575.
48. Liang LF, Chamow SM, Dean J. Oocyte-specific expression of mouse ZP-2: developmental regulation of the zona pellucida genes. *Mol Cell Biol* 1990;10:1507–1515.
49. Wassarman PM, Bleil JD, Florman HM, et al. The mouse egg's receptor for sperm: what is it and how does it work? *Cold Spring Harbor Symp Quant Biol* 1986;50:11–19.
50. Salzmann GS, Greve JM, Roller RJ, Wassarman PM. Biosynthesis of the sperm receptor during oogenesis in the mouse. *EMBO J* 1983;2:1451–1456.
51. Shabanowitz RB, O'Rand MG. Characterization of the human zona pellucida from fertilized and unfertilized eggs. *J Reprod Fertil* 1988;82:151–161.
52. Hedrick JL, Wardrip NJ, Berger T. Differences in the macromolecular composition of the zona pellucida isolated from pig oocytes, eggs and zygotes. *J Exp Zool* 1987;241:257–262.
53. Shabanowitz RB, O'Rand MG. Molecular changes in the human zona pellucida associated with fertilization and human sperm-zona interactions. *Ann NY Acad Sci* 1988; 541:621–632.
54. Cross NL, Morales P, Overstreet JW, Hanson FW. Induction of acrosome reactions by the human zona pellucida. *Biol Reprod* 1988;38:235–244.
55. Shabanowitz RB. Mouse antibodies to human zona pellucida: evidence that human ZP3 is strongly immunogenic and contains two distinct isomer chains. *Biol Reprod* 1990; 43:260–270.
56. Chamberlin ME, Dean J. Human homolog of the mouse sperm receptor. *Proc Natl Acad Sci USA* 1990;87:6014–6018.
57. Ringuette MJ, Sobieski DA, Chamow SM, Dean J. Oocyte-specific gene expression:

molecular characterization of a cDNA coding for ZP-3, the sperm receptor of the mouse zona pellucida. *Proc Natl Acad Sci USA* 1986;83:4341-4345.

58. Ringuette MJ, Chamberlin ME, Baur AW, Sobieski DA, Dean J. Molecular analysis of cDNA coding for ZP-3, a sperm binding protein of the mouse zona pellucida. *Dev Biol* 1988;127:287-295.

59. Cummins JM, Yanagimachi R. Development of ability to penetrate the cumulus oophorus by hamster spermatozoa capacitated in vitro, in relation to the timing of the acrosome reaction. *Gamete Res* 1986;15:187-212.

60. Saling PM. How the egg regulates sperm function during gamete interaction: facts and fantasies. *Biol Reprod* 1991;44:246-251.

61. White DR, Phillips DM, Bedford JM. Factors affecting the acrosome reaction in human spermatozoa. *J Reprod Fertil* 1990;90:71-80.

62. Bleil JD. Sperm receptors of mammalian eggs. In: Wassarman PM, ed. *Elements of mammalian fertilization, vol 1.* Boca Raton: CRC Press; 1991:133-151.

63. Hartmann JF, Gwatkin RBL, Hutchison CF. Early contact interactions between mammalian gametes in vitro: evidence that the vitellus influences adherence between sperm and zona pellucida. *Proc Natl Acad Sci USA* 1972;69:2767-2769.

64. Inoue M, Wolf DP. Fertilization associated changes in the murine zona pellucida: a time sequence study. *Biol Reprod* 1975;13:546-551.

65. Florman HM, Saling PM, Storey BT. Fertilization of mouse eggs in vitro. Time resolution of the reactions preceding penetration of the zona pellucida. *J Androl* 1982;3:373-381.

66. Mahadevan MH, Trounson AO, Wood C, Leeton JF. Effect of oocyte quality and sperm characteristics on the number of spermatozoa bound to the zona pellucida of human oocytes inseminated in vitro. *J In Vitro Fert Embryo Transfer* 1987;4:223-231.

67. Dietl JA, Rauth G. Molecular aspects of mammalian fertilization. *Hum Reprod* 1989;4:869-875.

68. Shur BD, Hall NG. A role for mouse sperm surface galactosyltransferase in sperm binding to the egg zona pellucida. *J Cell Biol* 1982;95:574-579.

69. Saling PM. Involvement of trypsin-like activity in binding of mouse spermatoza to zona pellucida. *Proc Natl Acad Sci USA* 1981;78:6231-6235.

70. Lambert H, Le AV. Possible involvement of a sialylated component of the sperm plasma membrane in sperm-zona interactions in the mouse. *Gamete Res* 1984;10:153-163.

71. O'Rand MG, Irons GP, Porter JP. Monoclonal antibodies to rabbit sperm autoantigens. I. Inhibition of in vitro fertilization and localization on the egg. *Biol Reprod* 1984; 30:721-729.

72. Huang TTF, Yanagimachi R. Inner acrosomal membrane of mammalian spermatozoa: its properties and possible functions in fertilization. *Am J Anat* 1985;174:249-268.

73. Lopez LC, Bayna EM, Litoff D, Shaper NC, Shaper JM, Shur BD. Receptor function of mouse sperm surface galactosyl transferase during fertilization. *J Cell Biol* 1985; 101:1501-1510.

74. Wassarman PM. The biology and chemistry of fertilization. *Science* 1987;235:553-560.

75. Myles DG, Primakoff P. Localized surface antigens of guinea pig sperm migrate to new regions prior to fertilization. *J Cell Biol* 1984;99:1634-1641.

76. Primakoff P, Hyatt M, Myles D. A role for the migrating sperm surface antigen PM-20 in guinea pig sperm binding to the egg zona pellucida. *J Cell Biol* 1985;101:2239-2244.

77. Florman HM, Bechtol KB, Wassarman PM. Enzymatic dissection of the functions of the mouse egg's receptor for sperm. *Dev Biol* 1984;106:243-255.

78. Florman HM, Wassarman PM. O-Linked oligosaccharides of mouse egg ZP3 account for its sperm receptor activity. *Cell* 1985;41:313-324.

79. Barros C, Bedford JM, Franklin LE, Austin CR. Membrane vesiculation as a feature of the mammalian acrosome reaction. *J Cell Biol* 1967;34:C1-C5.

80. Nagae T, Yanagimachi R, Srivastava PN, Yanagimachi H. Acrosome reaction in human spermatozoa. *Fertil Steril* 1986;45:701-707.

81. Stock CE, Fraser LR. The acrosome reaction in human sperm from men of proven fertility. *Hum Reprod* 1987;2(2):109-119.

82. Urch UA. Biochemistry and function of acrosin. In: Wassarman PM, ed. *Elements of mammalian fertilization, vol 1.* Boca Raton: CRC Press;1991:233-248.

83. Cuthbertson KSR, Whittingham DG, Cobbold PM. Free Ca^{2+} increases in exponential phases during mouse oocyte activation. *Nature* 1981;294:754–757.
84. Stewart-Savage J, Bavister BD. Failure of hamster eggs fertilized in vitro to extrude the second polar body correlates with high levels of polyspermy. *Gamete Res* 1987;18: 333–338.
85. Uchida IA, Freeman VCP. Triploidy and chromosomes. *Am J Obstet Gynecol* 1985; 151:65–69.
86. Gordon JW, Grunfeld L, Garrisi GJ, Talansky BE, Richards C, Laufer N. Fertilization of human oocytes by sperm from infertile males after zona pellucida drilling. *Fertil Steril* 1988;50:68–73.
87. Cohen J, Malter H, Wright G, Kort H, Massey J, Mitchell D. Partial zona dissection of human oocytes when failure of zona pellucida penetration is anticipated. *Hum Reprod* 1989;4:435–442.
88. Gulyas BJ. Cortical granules of mammalian eggs. *Int Rev Cytol* 1980;63:357–392.
89. Wolf DP. The mammalian egg's block to polyspermy. In: Mastroianni L Jr, Biggers JD, eds. *Fertilization and embryonic development in vitro.* New York: Plenum Press; 1981:183–197.
90. Wassarman PM. Fertilization. In: Yamada KM, ed. *Cellular interactions and development: molecular mechanisms.* New York: Wiley-Interscience; 1983:1–27.
91. Moller CC, Wassarman PM. Characterization of a proteinase that cleaves zona pellucida glycoprotein ZP2 following activation of mouse eggs. *Dev Biol* 1989;132:103–112.
92. Longo FJ. *Fertilization.* London: Chapman and Hall; 1987.
93. Trounson AO, Mohr LR, Wood C, Leeton JF. Effect of delayed insemination on in vitro fertilization, culture and transfer of human embryos. *J Reprod Fertil* 1982;64:285–294.
94. Tesarik J, Kopecny V. Development of human male pronucleus: ultrastructure and timing. *Gamete Res* 1989;24:135–149.
95. Tesarik J, Kopecny V. Developmental control of the human male pronucleus by ooplasmic factors. *Hum Reprod* 1989;4:962–968.
96. Wiker S, Malter H, Wright G, Cohen J. Recognition of paternal pronuclei in human zygotes. *J In Vitro Fert Embryo Transfer* 1990;7:33–37.
97. Wright G, Wiker S, Elsner C, et al. Observations on the morphology of pronuclei and nucleoli in human zygotes and implications for cryopreservation. *Hum Reprod* 1990; 5:109–115.
98. Soupart P, Strong PA. Ultrastructural observations on human oocytes fertilized in vitro. *Fertil Steril* 1975;25:11–44.
99. Soupart P, Strong PA. Ultrastructural observations on polyspermic penetration of zona pellucida-free human oocytes inseminated in vitro. *Fertil Steril* 1975;26:523–537.
100. Saiki R, Gelfand DH, Stoffel S, et al. Primer-directed enzymatic amplification of DNA with a thermostable DNA polymerase. *Science* 1988;239:487–491.
101. Tesarik J. Developmental control of human preimplantation embryos: a comparative analysis. *J In Vitro Fert Embryo Transfer* 1988;5:347–362.
102. West JD, Green JF. The transition from oocyte-coded to embryo-coded glucose phosphate isomerase in the early mouse embryo. *J Embryol Exp Morphol* 1983;78:127–140.
103. Young RJ, Sweeney K, Bedford JM. Uridine and guanosine incorporation by the mouse one-cell embryo. *J Embryol Exp Morphol* 1978;44:133–148.
104. Johnson MH. The molecular and cellular basis of preimplantation mouse development. *Biol Rev* 1981;56:463–498.
105. Braude PR, Pelham HRB, Flach G, Lobatto R. Post-transcriptional control in the early mouse embryo. *Nature* 1979;282:102–105.
106. Flach G, Johnson MH, Braude PR, Taylor RS, Bolton VN. The transition from maternal to embryonic control in the 2-cell mouse embryo. *EMBO J* 1982;1:681–686.
107. Petzoldt U, Hoppe PC, Illmensee K. Protein synthesis in enucleated fertilised and unfertilised mouse eggs. *Roux Arch Dev Biol* 1980;189:215–219.
108. Woodland HR, Graham CF. RNA synthesis during early development of the mouse. *Nature* 1969;221:327–332.
109. Knowland J, Graham C. RNA synthesis at the two-cell stage of mouse development. *J Embryol Exp Morphol* 1972;27:167–176.

110. Clegg KB, Piko L. Size and specific activity of the UTP pool and overall rates of RNA synthesis in early mouse embryos. *Dev Biol* 1977;58:76–95.
111. Levey IL, Stull GB, Brinster RL. Poly (A) and synthesis of polyadenylated RNA in the preimplantation mouse embryo. *Dev Biol* 1978;64:140–148.
112. Olds PJ, Stern S, Biggers JD. Chemical estimates of the RNA and DNA contents of the early mouse embryo. *J Exp Zool* 1973;186:39–46.
113. Piko L, Clegg KB. Quantitative changes in total RNA, total poly(A), and ribosomes in early mouse embryos. *Dev Biol* 1982;89:362–378.
114. Sawicki J, Magnuson T, Epstein C. Evidence for expression of the paternal genome in the two-cell mouse embryo. *Nature* 1981;294:450–451.
115. Magnuson T, Epstein CJ. Genetic control of very early mammalian development. *Biol Rev* 1981;56:369–408.
116. Tomanek M, Kopecny V, Kanka J. Studies on RNA synthesis in early pig embryos. *Histochem J* 1986;18:138.
117. Camous S, Kopecny V, Flechon JE. Autoradiographic detection of the earliest stage of [³H]uridine incorporation into the cow embryo. *Biol Cell* 1986;58:195–200.
118. Manes C. Nucleic acid synthesis in preimplantation rabbit embryos. II. Delayed synthesis of ribosomal RNA. *J Exp Zool* 1971;176:87–96.
119. Tesarik J, Kopecny V, Plachot M, Mandelbaum J. Activation of nucleolar and extranucleolar RNA synthesis and changes in the ribosomal content of human embryos developing in vitro. *J Reprod Fertil* 1986;78:463–470.
120. Tesarik J, Kopecny V, Plachot M, Mandelbaum J, Da Lage C, Flechon JE. Nucleologenesis in the human embryo developing in vitro: ultrastructural and autoradiographic analysis. *Dev Biol* 1986;115:193–203.
121. Tesarik J, Kopecny V, Plachot M, Mandelbaum J. High-resolution autoradiographic localization of DNA-containing sites and RNA synthesis in developing nucleoli of human preimplantation embryos: a new concept of embryonic nucleologenesis. *Development* 1987;101:777–791.
122. Tesarik J, Kopecny V, Plachot M, Mandelbaum J. Early morphological signs of embryonic genome expression in human preimplantation development as revealed by quantitative electron microscopy. *Dev Biol* 1988;128:15–20.
123. Braude P, Bolton V, Moore S. Human gene expression first occurs between the four- and eight-cell stages of preimplantation development. *Nature* 1988;332:459–462.

5

Microsurgical Fertilization in Mammals

Beth E. Talansky

Mammalian models, used in conjunction with micromanipulation systems, are ideal for conducting fertilization studies. The requirements for maturational events necessary for gamete fusion, such as oocyte activation, capacitation, the acrosome reaction, and interaction between sperm and egg membranes have been brought into a new perspective since fertilization has been examined through micromanipulation. In this chapter, we will discuss the development of micromanipulation procedures to assist fertilization of mammalian gametes. We begin with a description of the early experiments in which sperm or sperm nuclei from one species were microinjected into oocytes of another species. By providing evidence that microinjected spermatazoa were capable of undergoing at least some of the nuclear changes involved in "natural" fertilization events, these early studies set the stage for further and extensive progress in the field of assisted mammalian reproductive technology.

This discussion will concentrate on the three major categories of micromanipulation-assisted fertilization that have been explored in mammalian systems (Fig. 5.1). The first and most invasive form of microsurgical fertilization is the microinjection of sperm into the cytoplasm of the oocyte. This method entails traversal of all outer barriers of the oocyte: the cumulus-corona complex, the zona pellucida (ZP), and the vitelline membrane. A second category of micromanipulation directed at facilitating sperm–egg interaction is the subzonal insertion of sperm. Less invasive than direct microinjection, this procedure involves placement of sperm into the perivitelline space. The third subgroup of microsurgical fertilization technology entails the creation of an artificial gap in the (ZP). Thus, the micromanipulated oocyte is inseminated according to standard in vitro fertilization (IVF) protocols. This form of micromanipulation is broadly termed *zona drilling*.

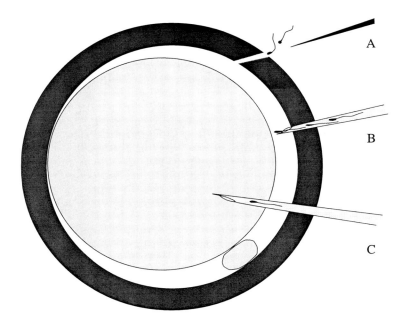

FIG. 5.1. Representation of the three methods of micromanipulation-assisted fertilization. **A:** Zona drilling: methodologies that entail the introduction of an opening in the zona pellucida, thereby allowing sperm direct access to the oolemma. Following micromanipulation, the oocyte is inseminated. **B:** Subzonal insertion: Spermatozoa are aspirated into a hollow microneedle and are deposited directly into the perivitelline space of the oocyte. **C:** Direct sperm microinjection: Sperm contained within a microneedle are microinjected into the cytoplasm of the oocyte.

Classically, a discussion pertaining to the various forms of gamete methodologies to assist fertilization, is constructed so that techniques are presented in order of invasiveness. Here, on the other hand, we follow our discussion of direct sperm microinjection with a description of the least invasive variation of assisted fertilization; zona pellucida drilling. In this way, the development of the procedures will be clear, in a historical perspective. Specifically, it will be clearer to the reader how subzonal insertion was a natural successor to zona drilling methods, in terms of addressing increasingly severe fertilization disorders.

MICROMANIPULATION-ASSISTED
FERTILIZATION TECHNIQUES

Direct Sperm Microinjection

Microinjection entails circumvention of all oocyte barriers, including the plasma membrane. Physiological studies of nonmammalian gametes provided evidence that events such as sperm nuclear decondensation did not require prior interaction between sperm and oocyte membranes. Hiramoto's studies (1) involving sea urchin sperm microinjection and Brun's (2) demonstration that living *Xenopus* spermatozoa were able to decondense in oocytes following injection, suggested that direct interaction between the fertilizing spermatozoon and the oocyte membrane was not a prerequisite to pronuclear formation. Similar microinjection procedures were performed in both mammalian heterospecific (3–5) and homospecific (6–10) systems. Such attempts occasionally resulted in sperm decondensation or the formation of male pronuclei. However, the procedure was often detrimental to the oocyte, if not fatal. This is not surprising, for not only does microinjection involve handling of both sperm and egg, but, since it completely bypasses the oocyte's ability to bind and select sperm, it may interfere with the sequence of events that precede normal embryonic development. These processes must be accomplished by artificial means. Such manipulations may interfere with the normal sequence of embryonic development.

The success of microinjection is dependent on several factors. First, ova of different species vary in their ability to withstand piercing of the oolemma. Whereas mouse and rat oocytes are particularly sensitive to microinjection, hamster oocytes are more receptive to injection of sperm from a variety of species and readily support decondensation of the sperm nucleus (5,11). Another consequence of microinjection methodologies is that the ability of the oocyte to undergo activation and pronuclear formation is partially affected by the sperm treatment utilized to induce capacitation and the acrosome reaction (11). An example is provided by the results of Keefer's rabbit experiments (11) in which significantly higher rates of pronuclear formation were obtained after microinjection of spermatozoa subjected to defined capacitation protocols. Specifically, it was found that preparation of sperm nuclei by salt extraction, for example, had an inhibitory effect on oocyte activation. Also, introduction of intact sperm was associated with higher rates of oocyte activation and pronuclear formation than microinjection of sperm prepared by sonication. These observations led to the suggestion that subtle modifications may occur during capacitation and the acrosome reaction that are prerequisite to the ability of the spermatozoon to undergo postfusional events in the ooplasm. Although some methods of sperm preparation for microinjection may be somewhat effective in inducing capacitation and the acrosome reaction, they could affect sperm structure of function in such a way as to interfere with those modifications needed for interaction with the ooplasm (11).

Improvements in the use of the rabbit model for microinjection has not only led to pronuclear formation, but has also resulted in further embryonic cleavage and the birth of normal, live offspring (12,13). Such progress has indicated the application of sperm microinjection procedures for large domestic species. However, microsurgical fertilization in some large species is complicated by the fact that microinjection alone is not sufficient to induce oocyte activation. In cattle, single sperm were microinjected into oocytes that had been activated by preincubation in calcium ionophore A23187. In some studies, cleavage development was obtained (14,15) and, additionally, transfer of morulae-blastocysts derived from this procedure resulted in the birth of a calf (16). Thus, it has been confirmed that, in some species, microinjection may be a viable method with which to achieve fertilization and embryonic development to term.

There is undoubtedly a subset of gamete defects that might be refractory to less invasive methods of micromanipulation, such as zona drilling or subzonal insertion. However, what is the reality of applying microinjection to clinical IVF? Severe morphologic defects (17), including complete absence of an acrosome, may render sperm incapable of undergoing the prerequisite interactions necessary for fusion and may require application of direct microinjection technology. This hypothesis has been tested by Lazendorf and coworkers (17), who showed that spermatazoa with defects specific to the acrosome and associated structures were able to decondense in the cytoplasm of hamster oocytes. In addition, similar studies have been carried out using spare human oocytes and sperm. In these investigations, it was demonstrated that, to a certain extent, human oocytes were capable of surviving microinjection and 7 of 20 microinjected oocytes were able to support formation of male and female pronuclei (18). Although these data are somewhat encouraging, assisted fertilization by direct sperm microinjection remains a tedious and difficult procedure, requiring great manual dexterity. It will be necessary to establish sperm microinjection as a viable and repeatable technique that poses minimal danger to the oocyte before it can be considered a microsurgical method with which to assist human fertilization on a routine clinical basis.

In addition to potentially disturbing the oocyte, microinjection may also be traumatic to the spermatozoon. The work of Martin et al. (19) provides an illustration of a serious hazard posed by sperm microinjection. This group devised a technique involving microinjection of human spermatozoa into hamster oocytes, initially for the purpose of conducting chromosomal analyses. Sperm were treated either by sonication or incubation in TEST-yolk buffer to induce capacitation and to reduce motility and facilitate their capture for micromanipulation. Analyses of resulting chromosomal complements reflected a significantly increased damage rate (91%), including multiple breaks and rearrangements in the sperm that had been subjected to sonication. On the other hand, chromosomal damage was greatly reduced in the sperm karyotypes derived from the TEST-yolk buffer pretreatment group (39%). These results suggest that, although they might be effective methods for promoting capacitation and ease of micromanipulation, protocols, such as sonication, might be destructive to the chromosomal structure of the spermatozoon. Since it involves more extensive sperm contact and preparatory treatment than other types of gamete micromanipulation, the risks might preclude the use of microinjection as a viable tool for assisting fertilization.

Zona Pellucida Drilling (Zona Micromanipulation)

Although the early studies suggested that gametes from a variety of species might be compatible with microinjection, the first successful demonstration of microsurgical fertilization in mammals was provided by Gordon and Talansky (20). Zona drilling is a procedure designed to circumvent the complications posed by disorders, such as reduced sperm counts, that minimize the likelihood of normal gamete interaction. In contrast with the microinjection of sperm, zona drilling is a relatively atraumatic form of micromanipulation, since it does not involve interruption of the oocyte plasma membrane or direct handling of spermatozoa, but entails only creation of a small opening in the zona pellucida.

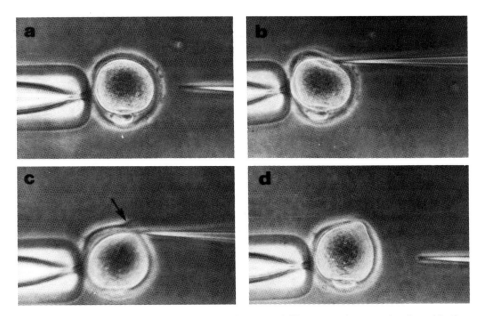

FIG. 5.2. The successive steps involved in the zona-drilling procedure, as developed in the murine model. **A:** Oocyte is secured by suction onto a holding pipet. **B:** Microneedle containing acid Tyrode's solution is brought into tangential contact with the zona pellucida. **C:** A small volume of Tyrode's solution is expelled from the microneedle to create a minute opening in the zona. **D:** After manipulation is completed, the microneedle is withdrawn. Note the area where a restricted portion of the zona pellucida has been removed. (From Gordon JW, Talansky BE. Assisted fertilization by zona drilling: a mouse model for correction of oligospermia. *J Exp Zool* 1986;239:347–354, with permission. Copyright © 1988. Reprinted with permission Wiley-Liss, a division of John Wiley and Sons, Inc.)

In the original zona-drilling procedure developed in a mouse model, the oocyte was secured by suction on a holding pipet and a microneedle loaded with acid Tyrode's solution was brought into contact with a restricted region of the zona pellucida (Fig. 5.2) (20). A minute volume of solution was gently released from the microneedle just until the point at which the zona was breached. In some cases, when the procedure was done more aggressively, the opening in the zona became obvious, as the underlying oocyte protruded from the site of manipulation. Routine insemination followed the procedure. In the mouse model, the creation of an artificial gap in the zona was associated with increased rates of fertilization at both normal and reduced sperm concentrations. Initial pronuclear formation was observed about 45 minutes earlier in manipulated groups than in controls. In addition, zona drilling resulted in rates of supernumerary sperm penetration that did not differ from the incidence of polyspermy in zona-intact controls. Mouse zygotes that resulted from assisted fertilization by zona drilling, when transferred to the oviducts of pseudopregnant

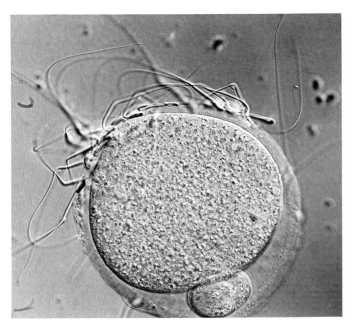

FIG. 5.3. A zona-drilled mouse oocyte 35 minutes after insemination. Note that the spermatozoa are accumulated near the region of micromanipulation where the underlying plasma membrane is exposed. (From Talansky BE, Gordon JW. Cleavage characteristics of mouse embryos inseminated and cultured after zona drilling. *Gamete Res* 1988;21:277–278, with permission. Copyright © 1988. Reprinted with permission Wiley-Liss, a division of John Wiley and Sons, Inc.)

foster female mice, gave rise to normal live young. The zona-drilling procedure exposed sperm to a region of direct access to the oocyte (Fig. 5.3), while allowing the intact portion of the zona pellucida to retain its function in the block to polyspermic fertilization and in support of early embryonic development.

To develop zona drilling as a tool for clinical IVF, additional animal studies were undertaken. Since replacement of pronuclear-stage zona-drilled embryos did not permit direct observation of embryonic development, cleavage to the blastocyst stage was observed in vitro following micromanipulation (21). The result of these investigations demonstrated that, frequently, after the creation of a relatively large hole in the zona pellucida, the embryo tended to protrude through the gap as development progressed. This sometimes resulted in embryonic development both inside and outside the zona, or in the loss of intact blastomeres (Fig. 5.4). When a portion of the blastocyst protruded through the small gap in the zona, the resulting constriction frequently caused the formation of twin blastocysts (Fig. 5.5)

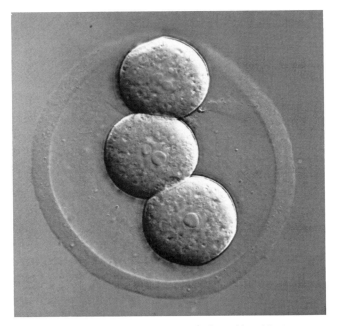

FIG. 5.4. Mouse embryo derived from zona drilling. One of four blastomeres was lost through the opening in the zona *(top)*. Note the linear configuration of blastomeres, which contrasts with the tetrahedral formation typically seen in four-cell embryos. (From Talansky BE, Gordon JW. Cleavage characteristics of mouse embryos inseminated and cultured after zona drilling. *Gamete Res* 1988;21:277–278. Copyright © 1988. Reprinted with permission Wiley-Liss, a division of John Wiley and Sons, Inc.)

(21,22). Also, hatching routinely occurred 1 day earlier than usual in micromanipulated embryos (22).

Removal of a portion of the zona pellucida is undoubtedly effective in exposing sperm directly to the oocyte. That the sperm actually utilize the artificially created gap to gain access to the egg has been demonstrated by several techniques. It is known that, in the mouse, premature induction of the acrosome reaction prevents fertilization of zona-intact oocytes (23). With this in mind, Gordon and Talansky (20) induced the acrosome reaction in populations of mouse sperm with dibutyrlcyclic guanosine monophosphate (dBcGMP), and demonstrated that these acrosomeless sperm were able to penetrate zona-drilled, but not zona-intact oocytes. Conover and Gwatkin (24) exposed oocytes to an antibody to the zona glycoprotein ZP-3, and showed that in the absence of micromanipulation, penetration occurred in only a single oocyte. The fertilization rates were significantly elevated to 65%, however, when antibody-treated eggs were zona-drilled. Recently, it was shown that a method of zona drilling greatly increased the rate of fertilization in a strain of random-bred mice that is normally refractory to sperm penetration in vitro (25). These results all indicate that spermatozoa are indeed traversing the opening in the zona pellucida following micromanipulation.

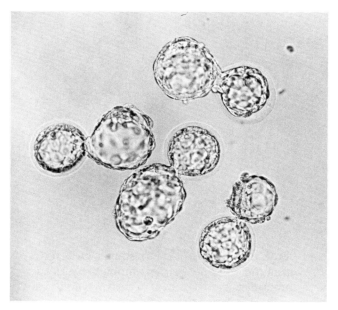

FIG. 5.5. Twin mouse blastocysts formed as a result of partial extrusion of the embryo through the site of zona drilling.

Since the outcome of the initial studies were encouraging, micromanipulation-assisted fertilization was applied to clinical IVF (26). Although fertilization was frequently achieved, embryonic cleavage was often abnormal, and no pregnancies resulted after embryo transfer. The human zona pellucida appeared to differ from the mouse zona in its response to acid Tyrode's solution. Even though the outer layer of the human zona was easily dissolved by the acidic solution, the inner, more resistant layer required longer exposure to be completely breached.

A method introduced by Cohen et al. (27) for introducing a gap in the mammalian zona pellucida resulted in the first human pregnancy from microsurgical fertilization. Partial zona dissection (PZD) is a mechanical technique that does not entail the use of acid Tyrode's solution, which was obviously detrimental to the human oocyte (26,28). Sucrose solution is used to shrink the oocyte so that a single glass microneedle can be introduced into the perivitelline space without damaging the oocyte. The microneedle is threaded through one side of the zona pellucida at the 1-o'clock position and out through the side of the zona at the 11-o'clock position. The oocyte is released from the holding pipet, which is then used to massage the portion of the zona that is incorporated between the points at which it is pierced by the microneedle. After repeated massage by the holding pipet, the oocyte drops off, and the result is a clear slit in the zona where the microneedle was threaded (Fig. 5.6). The actual size of the slit is a function of the position along the microneedle at which the zona is threaded; the wider portion of the needle will produce a larger gap in the zona. After this procedure, the oocyte is removed from the sucrose solution, reexposed to medium of normal osmolarity, and is inseminated. This method, employs fewer and more simply designed microtools than other methods that were subsequently attempted for producing an effective gap in the zona. The clinical use of partial zona dissection has been highly successful. To date, well over 50 births have resulted from this method of microsurgical fertilization, and many pregnancies are ongoing.

Several other variations on the zona drilling procedure have been attempted during the past few years. As mentioned earlier, local digestion of the human zona with acid Tyrode's solution was found to be harmful to the oocyte (28,29), despite that it was a safe and effective treatment in the mouse model. Alternative enzymatic methods for opening the human zona pellucida were also attempted; however, due to the persistent action of the enzyme, such treatments were not effective for use with human oocytes (29). In addition, several other investigators sought alternative mechanical methods for opening the zona pellucida. Among the procedures attempted in animal and human models were zona cutting and cracking (tearing) (30,31). For example, zona cutting, which was adapted from the enucleation technique of Tsunoda et al. (32), involved the use of a single bevelled needle to mechanically create a slit in the zona. While this method was associated

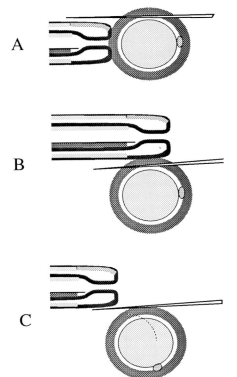

FIG. 5.6. Schematic illustration of the partial zona dissection procedure. **A:** The microneedle is threaded through the zona pellucida. **B:** The oocyte is released from the holding pipet, which is then used to massage the portion of zona incorporated by the microneedle. **C:** The rubbing motion is complete and the oocyte is released from the microneedle. A clear slit in the zona results (see text).

with enhanced fertilization, successful embryonic development, and the production of live offspring, it was less effective in promoting fertilization when compared with zona drilling with acid Tyrode's solution. Zona cracking, on the other hand, is a technique that involves a more complex arrangement of microtools than the other methods of zona manipulation. Two glass microhooks are used to pierce the zona and produce a localized tear (Fig. 5.7). To expedite this safe manipulation of the oocyte, a hyperosmolar sucrose solution is used to widen the perivitelline space. A novel variation of zona drilling is the use of lasers (Laufer N, personal communication) to standardize the type of gap created in the zona pellucida. An argon fluoride excimer laser guided through a glass pipet was used to introduce holes in the zonae of mouse oocytes. Ultrastructural analysis demonstrated the creation of uniform, round holes with clearly defined edges. Insemination of oocytes subjected to this type of zona-drilling procedure were fertilized at rates similar to intact controls. However, it was observed that the rate of blastocyst hatching was significantly increased in the laser-drilled group, compared with untreated controls (73% versus 17%).

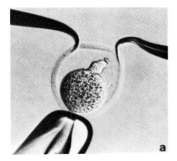

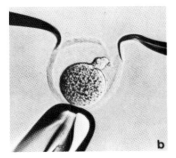

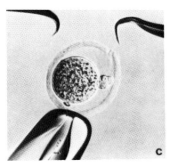

FIG. 5.7. Three stages of the zona cracking (tearing) procedure using two glass microhooks. **A:** Microhooks are used to pierce the zona pellucida. **B:** The zona is stretched by the microhooks and the tear is widened. **C:** Microhooks are removed leaving a narrow fissure at the point of the tear. (From Odawara Y, Lopata A. A zona opening procedure for improving in vitro fertilization at low sperm concentrations: a mouse model. *Fertil Steril* 1989;51:699–704. Reproduced with permission of the publisher, The American Fertility Society.)

The investigators suggest that the laser may, therefore, be a useful tool for performing assisted-hatching procedures and, perhaps, may be useful at enhancing fertilization at very low sperm concentrations.

What types of fertilization disorders may be alleviated by zona micromanipulation procedures such as zona drilling or partial zona dissection? Initially, zona drilling was devised to assist fertilization in cases in which sperm are available only in reduced numbers. In instances of oligospermia, insemination of zona-intact oocytes frequently results in low rates of fertilization (33). Animal models have exemplified the usefulness of micromanipulation. After zona drilling was performed, insemination with sperm counts as low as ten sperm per egg were associated with fertilization rates that were significantly higher than zona-intact controls. Similar results were obtained in mouse studies involving other forms of zona breaching, such as zona cracking (31). As discussed earlier, the motility that is acquired and enhanced during sperm maturation is important for penetration through outer egg investments. It has been shown, however, that motility may not be necessary for traversal of the plasma membrane. In 1982, Cohen et al. (34) noted that human spermatozoa that lacked progressive motility were able to penetrate zona-free hamster oocytes. These observations were substantiated by Aitken and coworkers (35), who indicated that sperm from a patient with Kartagener's syndrome, a disease characterized by immotile cilia, were able to penetrate zona-free hamster oocytes. These were interesting observations, in spite of the fact that hamster egg penetration by human sperm is not representative of physiologic gamete interaction. Thus, it has been established that sperm with nonprogressive, abnormal, or limited motility may be relatively inefficient in traversing only the outermost barriers of the oocyte.

Several investigators have applied the use of zona drilling to "rescue" the fertility of mice that carry, for instance, some genetic defect that renders them incapable of fertilizing a zona-intact oocyte. For example, zona drilling was used to overcome the infertility in male mice that were heterozygous for two t haplotypes ($T^{tw5/w71}$)(36). Spermatozoa from such mice, which transmit the t haplotype, have severely reduced motility and a consequent inability to penetrate intact zonae pellucidae. Additional animal models have demonstrated the application of zona manipulation for sperm in which abnormal morphology was associated with an inability to penetrate intact zonae. Gordon et al. (37) generated a line of transgenic mice in which male homozygotes were sterile. Ultrastructural studies showed severe flagellar defects in the sperm of affected males, and it was hypothesized that this condition led to motility disorders that rendered the sperm incapable of penetrating the outer egg investments. These sperm were incapable of penetrating an intact zona pellucida and could fertilize eggs only after zona drilling was performed. Although there is no direct human analogy for this model, it demonstrates that motility defects resulting in infertility can be overcome with zona drilling.

Other types of morphologic anomalies, such as severe teratozoospermia, have been clinically treated by application of zona manipulation (38). In addition to the aforementioned sperm factors, micromanipulation may be useful when the zona pellucida is impenetrable, even by "normal" sperm. The glycoproteins comprising the zona pellucida serve as sperm receptors, and, if masked in some way, will cause the zona to be refractile to sperm binding and penetration. In the human, antibodies to sperm can be present in the follicle and may result in infertility due to interference with fertilization (39). Additionally, properties of the zona pellucida are altered with time in culture and exposure to serum (40,41). The zona hardening that results from in vitro culture can inhibit sperm penetration. In both of these instances, it may be possible to bypass the zona barrier with microsurgical fertilization.

Subzonal Sperm Insertion

We have now defined the two ends of the spectrum of gamete micromanipulation technologies. Actually, of these forms of microsurgical fertilization, only zona drilling, the less invasive of the techniques has represented a realistic and successful approach to treating human infertility. A third category of gamete micromanipulation is one of intermediate invasiveness of the oocyte, compared with microinjection and zona drilling. Subzonal insertion (SZI) of sperm is a procedure in which the zona pellucida is not merely opened, but is functionally and physically bypassed. Sperm are aspirated into a hollow microneedle and are deposited into the perivitelline space of the oocyte (Fig. 5.8). Like zona drilling methods, subzonal insertion has been attempted in both animal and human models. However, because it involves placement of preselected sperm directly into the perivitelline space, subzonal insertion poses a greater challenge to the oolemma than zona drilling. Both the "quality and quantity" of sperm placed in the perivitelline space may be determined by the individual performing micromanipulation. As we have discussed, only sperm that have undergone capacitation and the acrosome reaction will be capable of fusing with the eggs' plasmalemma. Since the zona pellucida is no longer involved in the selection process, it may be necessary to use artificial induction of the acrosome reaction to ensure that the "selected" sperm will be capable of fertilization. Thus, in terms of sperm management, subzonal insertion may be tedious. Spermatozoa of certain mammalian species are fragile and easily prone to mechanically induced damage. Therefore, several animal models have been investigated to create a suitable prototype for subzonal insertion. These studies included the development of efficient methods by which to prepare and subzonally insert spermatozoa.

Much progress has been made in refining the use of perivitelline sperm insertion in the mouse model. In 1986, Barg et al. (7) attempted to introduce immobilized, yet acrosome-reacted sperm into the perivitelline space of oocytes. Results indicated that sperm rendered immotile by several methods (e.g., cold exposure, treatment with calcium ionophore, mechanical immobilization) after subzonal insertion, were unable to fuse with the oocyte and form pronuclei. These results raised the possibility that the methods used to immobilize and/or acrosome react the sperm might have disrupted the integrity of the spermatozoon membrane and, thereby, rendered it incapable of fertilization. In fact, it was subsequently shown that

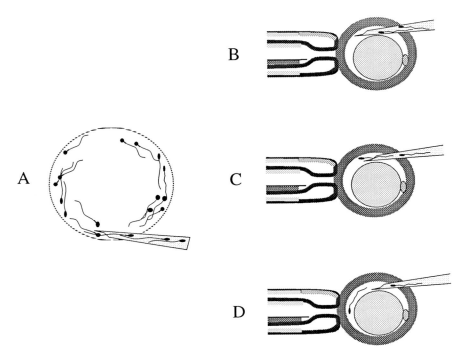

FIG. 5.8. Successive steps of the subzonal insertion procedure. **A:** Aspiration of sperm from a microdrop. Note that sperm are taken from the periphery of the drop where the most motile cells accumulate. **B:** The microneedle is brought through the zona at the 1-o'clock position and is gently introduced into the perivitelline space. **C,D:** Sperm are slowly released from the microneedle, in a minimum of medium. Subsequently, the needle is carefully withdrawn through the initial point of entry (not shown).

even acrosome-reacted spermatozoa require a functional ion pump ($Na^+K^+ATPase$) to fuse with the vitelline membrane of the oocyte (23). Accordingly, it is possible that aggressive contact between sperm and a microneedle can disrupt a membrane function that is associated with motility and the ability of the sperm to undergo normal fusion with the egg. Other groups who attempted subzonal insertion, using motile spermatozoa that were not artificially induced to undergo the acrosome reaction, showed that such sperm could penetrate the oocytes, albeit at a low rate (42). Yamada and coworkers (43), before performing subzonal insertion, used a protocol in which mouse spermatozoa were subjected to a cyclic nucleotide treatment (23), which induced the acrosome reaction without affecting motility. This treatment led to higher rates of fertilization than were previously attained in the mouse model. Finally, full embryonic development and live birth was achieved in a mouse subzonal insertion study by Mann

(44), who placed mouse sperm, which had been capacitated under "normal" conditions, in a viscous solution of methyl cellulose. This treatment served to slow the motility of the spermatozoa and facilitate their capture into the microneedle. It is likely that exposure to the methyl cellulose protected vulnerable mouse spermatozoa from the mechanical and functional damage caused by aspiration into the microneedle that was described by other investigators. Others have tried to combine the use of methyl cellulose with various methods of acrosome reaction induction to improve the results of subzonal insertion by generating more uniform populations of acrosome-reacted sperm (45).

Subzonal insertion has been further modified for use in other mammalian species. For example, in the rabbit, efficient microinjection of sperm into an enlarged perivitelline space has been facilitated by exposing the oocyte to hyperosmotic solutions, such as those used in the partial zona dissection procedure (46). Interestingly, fertilization occurred in the absence of acrosome-reacting agents. Thus, to develop the most suitable animal model for clinical subzonal insertion, it is important to remember that conditions that are ideal for gamete fusion differ significantly among the mammalian species that have been studied. The requirements for single versus multiple sperm insertion within an individual species, such as the mouse, may also differ. Furthermore, the ideal methods for acrosome reaction induction may also vary according to species.

The need to identify treatments specifically applicable to the induction of capacitation and the acrosome reaction in human spermatozoa was investigated in a heterospecific model. Since hamster oocytes are receptive to human sperm penetration, they provide another system with which to evaluate the effects of protocols to which human sperm will be subjected during micromanipulation (47). It is important to bear in mind that this use of hamster oocytes does not replace the use of animal models in which physiologic gamete interaction may be achieved. However, it has shown to be instructive for assessing various pretreatment protocols of human sperm to be used for microsurgical fertilization (for review see 48). The induction of the acrosome reaction before subzonal insertion significantly increased the rate of human sperm penetration of hamster oocytes (49). In this study, sperm that were induced to acrosome-react with calcium ionophore penetrated oocytes at a higher rate than untreated sperm. Penetration was further enhanced when sperm were acrosome-reacted by freeze-thaw. The optimal number of inserted sperm was five in both cases; lower penetration rates resulted when fewer sperm were inserted and multiple penetrations were significantly increased when more than five sperm were inserted.

Recently, some of the developmental work on subzonal insertion has come to fruition in the clinical IVF laboratory. Successful application of a method for synchronizing capacitation in which spermatozoa are incubated in medium in which strontium chloride is substituted for calcium has been reported (50,51). This method enabled the investigators to obtain fertilization after a single, motile spermatozoon was placed under the human zona pellucida. Subsequently, others reported a pregnancy after transfer of multiple (seven to ten) sperm under the zona pellucida (52). Special methods of sperm preparation were not employed in this study. Fertilization in human oocytes subzonally inserted with immotile sperm from a male with Kartagener's syndrome has also been reported (53). This result, which contrasts with the inability to achieve fertilization with immobilized mouse sperm (7), emphasizes the distinction between different mammalian systems in the application of subzonal insertion. Perhaps it also indicates that, unlike naturally occurring motility dysfunctions, the type of immotility achieved by artificial means (7) may prevent fertilization by directly compromising the integrity of the spermatozoon. Cohen and coworkers (54) have recently applied subzonal insertion to severe cases of male factor infertility. The data obtained from these clinical trials has clarified several biologic principles and has raised interesting questions pertaining to mammalian fertilization. For example, although both partial zona dissection and subzonal insertion may be effective treatments for cases of extreme teratozoospermia, it has become clear that those embryos derived from subzonal insertion implant at a significantly higher rate than those resulting from the partial zona dissection procedure (54). It is believed that this phenomenon is related to the presence of increased seminal debris in the semen of patients with severe teratozoospermia. Upon insemination of oocytes that have been subjected to partial zona dissection, products from the sperm preparation gain access to the embryo through the gap in the zona pellucida. This might have detrimental effects on the oocyte and, after fertilization, on a developing embryo, and it may eventually interfere with normal implantation. In contrast, subzonal insertion does not involve creation of relatively large openings in the zona that can leave the embryo vulnerable to invasion. Sperm are individually handled and placed into the perivitelline space, with care taken not to introduce extraneous matter. The clinical applications of subzonal insertion, as well as all other currently applied forms of microsurgical fertilization technology, will be dealt with in great detail in Chapter 7.

BIOLOGICAL ASPECTS OF ZONA PELLUCIDA MICROMANIPULATION

The evolution of gamete micromanipulation has not only introduced an important and novel approach to treating fertilization disorders, but has also provided new insight into the biology of fertilization in different mammalian species.

Function of the Differentiated Surface of the Mammalian Oocyte

Zona manipulation has helped to elucidate the biological role of the mammalian egg surface during fertilization. In a recent investigation conducted in our laboratory, partial zona dissection was used in conjunction with IVF to study the function of the heterogeneous surface structure of the mouse and hamster oocyte (25). It is well established that the oocytes of several mammalian species, while extensively covered with microvilli, are characterized by a localized region that is devoid of the microscopic projections (Fig. 5.9) (55,56). The microvillus-free area directly overlies the region of the meiotic spindle and, therefore, is eventually associated with the first polar body (58,59). Previous studies have also established that sperm binding is reduced in the microvillus-free area. The goal of our investigation was to clarify the role of this differentiated surface in mammalian sperm–egg interaction. The effect of introducing gaps over different regions of the egg surface in conjunction with subsequent insemination was evaluated. It was assumed that the gaps produced either near or opposite the first

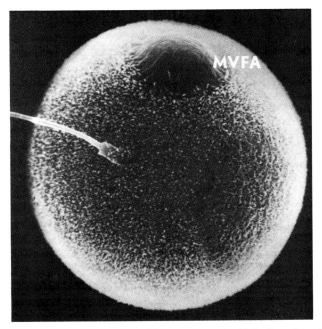

FIG. 5.9. Scanning electron micrograph of hamster oocyte. Note the microvillus-free area *(MVFA)* located away from the region of sperm-egg fusion. (From Yanagimachi R. Mechanisms of fertilization in mammals. In: Mastroianni L, Biggers JD, eds. *Fertilization and embryonic development in vitro.* New York: Plenum Press; 1981:81–182, with permission.)

polar body were accordingly located either close to or away from the microvillus-free region of the oocyte. Two different animal models were deliberately chosen. First, we used a model in which we performed partial zona dissection on mouse oocytes and inseminated them with mouse sperm. This model served several important purposes. Since it involved gametes of the same species, it provided demonstration of real or "physiologic fertilization." Also, we chose mouse strains in which sperm could not penetrate intact zonae in vitro. This ensured us that any contact between egg and sperm was the result of sperm passage through the gap introduced by micromanipulation. The experimental design, therefore, enabled us to direct the site of fusion to predetermined domains on the egg surface. However, to potentially extend our observations to the human, it was also necessary to create an animal model that more closely resembled the human oocyte in terms of size, area of perivitelline space, and thickness of the zona pellucida. For these reasons, the hamster oocyte was chosen. As in the mouse experiments, it was important to avoid sperm penetration at any site other than that produced by micromanipulation; thus, mouse sperm were used for insemination. Relative differences in the sizes of the perivitelline spaces and in the zona thickness in the two oocyte models are illustrated in Fig. 5.10. The mouse zona is thin and surrounds a subzonal space of substantial size, whereas the thicker hamster zona creates a more limited perivitelline area, which restricts free movement of sperm, a configuration that more closely resembles the human oocyte.

The results of the experiments using the mouse gametes are illustrated in Fig. 5.11. Following partial zona dissection opposite the polar body, fertili-

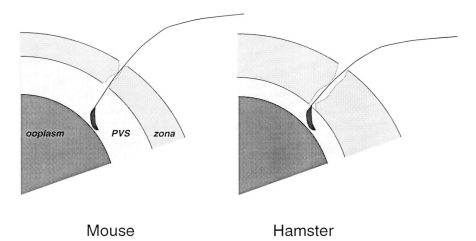

Mouse   Hamster

FIG. 5.10. Comparison of the zonae pellucidae and perivitelline spaces of the mouse and hamster oocytes. The thinner zona of the mouse oocyte is associated with a wider perivitelline space, whereas the thicker hamster zona surrounds a more narrow subzonal area.

MOUSE OOCYTES /
MOUSE SPERMATOZOA

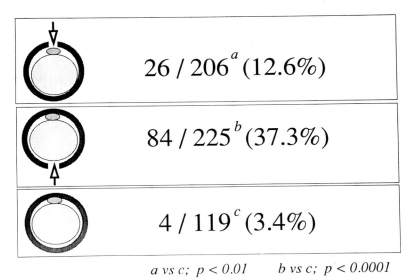

$26 / 206^{a} (12.6\%)$

$84 / 225^{b} (37.3\%)$

$4 / 119^{c} (3.4\%)$

a vs c; p < 0.01   *b vs c; p < 0.0001*

FIG. 5.11. Comparison of fertilization rates in mouse oocytes with mouse spermatozoa after partial zona dissection is performed near and opposite the first polar body. The lower panel provides the fertilization rate of unmanipulated controls.

zation was significantly higher (37.3%) than when the zona was opened near the polar body (12.6%). Similar results were obtained with the hamster–mouse model. A sperm penetration rate of nearly 61% was achieved after zona manipulation was done opposite the first polar body, whereas a significantly lower penetration rate of 34% was attained in the group of oocytes subjected to partial zona dissection near the polar body (Fig. 5.12). Therefore, it seemed that the site of zona manipulation in relation to the first polar body was correlated with the ability of sperm and oocyte to interact. That the sperm were, in fact, fusing with the egg at or near the region predetermined by the site of micromanipulation was demonstrated by the following observations: First, we were relatively certain that sperm did not pass through the breach in the zona, swim around the perivitelline space, and eventually, fuse with another area of the egg. In fact, in the mouse model, after partial zona dissection, most eggs were completely devoid of perivitelline space sperm. This result was true, regardless of where partial zona dissection was performed in relation to the polar body. On the rare occasion that a perivitelline space sperm was present, it appeared with its tail doubled-up upon itself and was never fully extended around the perimeter of the perivitelline space (Fig. 5.13). This observation confirmed that

HAMSTER OOCYTES / MOUSE SPERMATOZOA

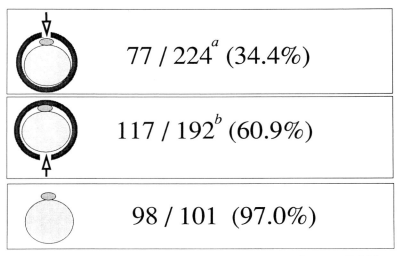

a vs b; $p < 0.001$

FIG. 5.12. Numbers of mouse sperm penetrations in hamster oocytes following partial zona dissection proximate to and opposite the first polar body. The lower panel represents the results of zona-free inseminations.

the spermatozoa were unable to move freely within the subzonal area and that their interactions with the oocyte were likely to occur at the site at which they initially traversed the zona. An additional observation that suggested that the spermatozoa were interacting with the oocyte at the site of zona dissection, was the existence of a unique binding pattern seen in both mouse and hamster oocytes. Frequently, there was an accumulation of sperm near the region in which the zonae were manipulated. The notion that sperm penetration occurred near the site of zona manipulation was further substantiated by the accretion of decondensed sperm heads and/or pronuclei (Fig. 5.14). Furthermore, when the opening in the zona was produced in the vicinity of the polar body, the pronuclei that eventually formed after insemination were located in proximity to one another (Fig. 5.15A). In contrast, partial zona dissection on the side of the oocyte opposite the first polar body was associated with widely separated pronuclei (see Fig. 5.15B). Since the maternal nucleus is always located in the region of the spindle apparatus, it follows that the female pronucleus will develop in the area subjacent to the polar body. Therefore, it is reasonable to assume that

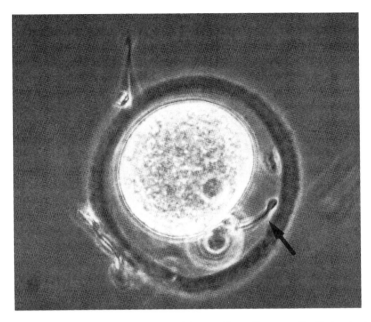

FIG. 5.13. A mouse zygote derived from partial zona dissection near the first polar body. The *arrow* indicates a sperm tail doubled up within the perivitelline space. (From Talansky BE, et al. A preferential site for sperm-egg fusion in mammals. *Mol Reprod Dev* 1991;28:183–188, with permission. Copyright 1991 Wiley-Liss, a division of John Wiley & Sons, Inc.)

the location of the male pronucleus is dependent on the position of zona manipulation and, thus, in our experimental model, is a reflection of where the sperm actually interacts with the oocyte. Whether these results are applicable to human IVF is not clear.

Clinical data generated in our laboratory relating the site of partial zona dissection with respect to the polar body to fertilization outcome has been examined (Cohen J, Alikani M, unpublished results). The results suggest that, in terms of the structure and function of surface topography, the human oocyte may be quite different from the animal models we studied. A significantly higher rate of polyspermy results after partial zona dissection was performed near the polar body (Fig. 5.16). This indicates that, in the human, a functional microvillus-free region may not be present. Currently, the model with which we explain this is based on the fact that the perivitelline area is locally enlarged due to the presence of the polar body. This expanded space acts as a "sink" in which multiple sperm may gather (Fig. 5.17). Since there is no strong block to polyspermy at the level of the human plasma membrane, supernumerary fertilization may result from an accumulation of sperm.

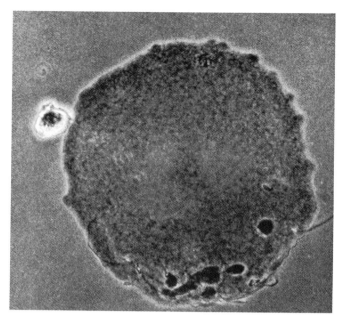

FIG. 5.14. A hamster oocyte that was micromanipulated away from the first polar body (zona was removed for microscopy). The sperm tails remain in close association with the cluster of swelling sperm heads located at the region of micromanipulation. (From Talansky BE, et al. A preferential site for sperm–egg fusion in mammals. *Mol Reprod Dev* 1991;28:183–188, with permission. Copyright 1991 by Wiley-Liss, a division of John Wiley & Sons, Inc.)

The Block to Polyspermy in the Human

Results of several studies have clarified the role served by the zona pellucida in the oocytes' block to polyspermy. Although limited levels of polyspermy were reported in the mouse model with zona drilling (20), these rates increase when such techniques are applied to the human oocyte (26,27). Whether or not the human vitelline membrane maintains a slow or transient function has not yet been defined. However, clinical trials of subzonal insertion show that the rate of polyspermy is elevated when increased numbers of sperm were placed within the perivitelline space (60). This observation suggests that the plasma membrane plays, at most, a minor role in the prevention of polyspermy.

Polyspermy Control by Activation of the Oocyte Plasma Membrane

During the initial phases of clinically applied partial zona dissection, it was noted that the degree of polyspermic fertilization was reduced as the

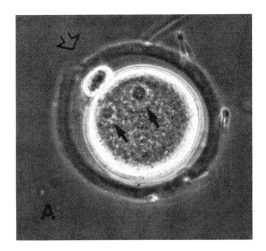

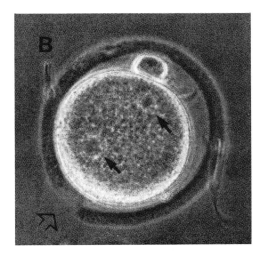

FIG. 5.15. Mouse zygotes resulting from partial zona dissection. *Open arrows* indicate the site of zona manipulation; *closed arrows* indicate pronuclei. **A:** Micromanipulation near the first polar body is associated with closely apposed pronuclei. **B:** Zona micromanipulation opposite the first polar body results in widely spaced pronuclei. (From Talansky BE, et al. A preferential site for sperm-egg fusion in mammals. *Mol Reprod Dev* 1991;28:183–188, with permission. Copyright 1991 by Wiley-Liss, a division of John Wiley & Sons, Inc.)

interval between exposure to sucrose and insemination was increased (61). It was postulated that the sucrose was somehow affecting the sperm receptivity of the plasma membrane. This effect became enhanced with increased time after initial exposure to sucrose. The hypothesis was tested further in a trial of partial zona dissection performed on day-old reinseminated oocytes (61). By varying the periods of exposure to sucrose following micromanipulation, it was demonstrated that polyspermy rates were significantly altered by changing the interval during which oocytes were exposed to sucrose. The investigators suggested that the changes in the cell membrane resembling activation were triggered by sucrose. Whether such changes

HUMAN SPERMATOZOA / HUMAN OOCYTES

	MONOSPERMY	POLYSPERMY	TOTAL
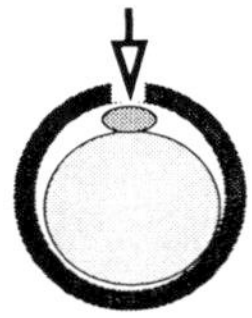	6 / 27 (22%)	7 / 27 (26%)	13 / 27 (48%)
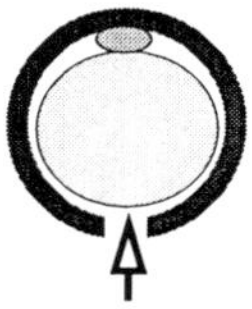	12 / 28 (43%)	0 / 28 (0%)	12 / 28 (43%)

FIG. 5.16. Clinical results of fertilization after partial zona dissection near and opposite the first polar body. Note that the polyspermy rate was significantly increased after zona manipulation in the region of the polar body.

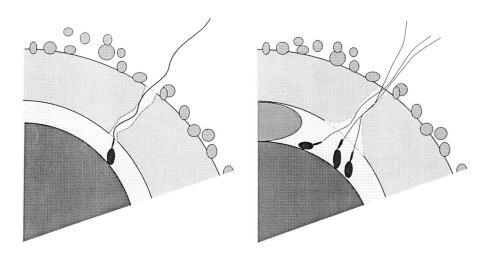

A

PZD near polar body 1

B

FIG. 5.17. The result of partial zona dissection (PZD) near and opposite the first polar body in the human oocyte. **A:** PZD distant from polar body 1. Note that the narrow perivitelline space is associated with a reduced number of sperm. **B:** PZD near polar body 1. The widened perivitelline space near the polar body accommodates multiple spermatozoa.

involve any of the biologic processes associated with physiologic "activation" (62), such as calcium oscillations or metabolic alterations, remains unclear. Whatever the mechanism, however, the receptivity and fusogenic characteristics of the oocyte plasma membrane are subject to effects of the micromanipulation protocol (likely related to sucrose exposure). Technical details such as these appear to have profound consequences for subsequent sperm–egg interaction.

REFERENCES

1. Hiramoto Y. Microinjection of the live spermatozoa into sea urchin eggs. *Exp Cell Res* 1966;27:416–426.
2. Brun RB. Studies on fertilization in *Xenopus laevis*. *Biol Reprod* 1974;11:513–518.
3. Thadani VM. A study of heterospecific sperm–egg interactions in the rat, mouse, and deer mouse using in vitro fertilization and sperm injection. *J Exp Zool* 1980;212:435–453.
4. Naish SJ, Perreault SD, Zirkin BR. DNA synthesis following microinjection of heterologous sperm and somatic cell nuclei into hamster oocytes. *Gamete Res* 1987; 18:109.
5. Perreault SD, Barbee RR, Elstein KH, Zucker RM, Keefer CL. Interspecies differences in the stability of mammalian sperm nuclei assessed in vivo by sperm injection and in vitro by flow cytometry. *Biol Reprod* 1988;39:157–167.
6. Perreault SD, Zirkin BR. Sperm nuclear decondensation in mammals: role of sperm-associated proteinase in vivo. *J Exp Zool* 1982;224:252–257.
7. Barg PE, Wahrman MZ, Talansky BE, Gordon JW. Capacitated, acrosome-reacted, but immotile sperm, when microinjected under the mouse zona pellucida, will not fertilize the oocyte. *J Exp Zool* 1986;237:365–374.
8. Uehara T, Yanagimachi R. Microsurgical injection of spermatozoa into hamster eggs with subsequent transformation of sperm nuclei into male pronuclei. *Biol Reprod* 1976; 15:467–470.
9. Markert CL. Fertilization of mammalian eggs by sperm injection. *J Exp Zool* 1983; 228:195–201.
10. Gomibuchi H, Kayama F, Sato K, Mizuno M. Decondensation of sperm head injected into oocyte under micromanipulation. *Acta Obstet Gynaec Jpn* 1985;37:2639.
11. Keefer CL. Fertilization by sperm injection in the rabbit. *Gamete Res* 1989;22:59–69.
12. Hosoi Y, Miyake M, Utsumi K, Iritani A. Development of rabbit oocytes after microinjection of spermatozoa. In *Proceedings of the 11th International Congress on Animal Reproduction and Artificial Insemination* 1988:abstr 331.
13. Iritani A. Micromanipulation of oocytes and embryos. In *Proceedings 13th World Congress on Fertility and Sterility*. Marrakash, Morocco Oct. 1-5, 1989. England: Parthenon Publishing (in press).
14. Keefer CL, Younis Al, Brackett BG. Cleavage development of bovine oocytes fertilized by sperm injection. *Mol Reprod Dev* 1990;25:281–285.
15. Goto K, Kinoshita A, Takuma Y, Ogawa K. Fertilization by sperm injection in cattle. *Theriogenology* 1990;33:238.
16. Goto K, Kinoshita A, Takuma Y, Ogawa K. Birth of calves after the transfers of oocytes fertilized by sperm injection. *Theriogenology* 1991;35:205.
17. Lanzendorf SE, Maloney M, Ackerman S, Acosta A, Hodgen G. Fertilizing potential of acrosome-defective sperm following microsurgical injection into eggs. *Gamete Res* 1988; 19:329–337.
18. Lanzendorf SE, Maloney MK, Veeck LL, Slusser J, Hodgen GD, Rosenwaks Z. A preclinical evaluation of pronuclear formation by microinjection of human spermatozoa into human oocytes. *Fertil Steril* 1988;49:835–842.
19. Martin RH, Ko E, Rademaker A. Human sperm chromosome complements after microinjection of hamster eggs. *J Reprod Fertil* 1988;84:179–186.

20. Gordon JW, Talansky BE. Assisted fertilization by zona drilling: a mouse model for correction of oligospermia. *J Exp Zool* 1986;239:347–354.
21. Talansky BE, Gordon JW. Cleavage characteristics of mouse embryos inseminated and cultured after zona drilling. *Gamete Res* 1988;21:277–278.
22. Malter HE, Cohen J. Blastocyst formation and hatching in vitro following zona drilling of mouse and human embryos. *Gamete Res* 1989;24:67–80.
23. Talansky BE, Barg PE, Gordon JW. Ion pump ATPase inhibitors block the fertilization of zona-free mouse oocytes by acrosome-reacted spermatozoa. *J Reprod Fertil* 1987;79: 447–455.
24. Conover JC, Gwatkin RBL. Fertilization of zona-drilled mouse oocytes treated with a monoclonal antibody to the zona glycoprotein, ZP3. *J Exp Zool* 1988;247:113–118.
25. Talansky BE, Malter HE, Cohen J. A preferential site for sperm-egg fusion in mammals. *Mol Reprod Dev* 1991;28:183–188.
26. Gordon JW, Grunfeld L, Garrisi GJ, Talansky BE, Richards C, Laufer N. Fertlization of human oocytes by sperm from infertile males after zona pellucida drilling. *Fertil Steril* 1988;50:68–73.
27. Cohen J, Malter H, Wright G, Kort H, Massey J, Mitchell D. Partial zona dissection of human oocytes when failure of zona pellucida penetration is anticipated. *Hum Reprod* 1989;4:435–442.
28. Malter HE, Cohen J. Partial zona dissection of the human oocyte: a nontraumatic method using micromanipulation to assist zona pellucida penetration. *Fertil Steril* 1989;51: 139–148.
29. Garrisi GJ, Talansky BE, Grunfeld L, Sapira V, Gordon JW. Clinical evaluation of three approaches to micromanipulation-assisted fertilization. *Fertil Steril* 1990;54:671–677.
30. Depypere HT, McLaughlin KJ, Seamark RF, Warnes GM, Matthews CD. Comparison of zona cutting and zona drilling as techniques for assisted fertilization in the mouse. *J Reprod Fertil* 1988;84:205–211.
31. Odawara Y, Lopata A. A zona opening procedure for improving in vitro fertilization at low sperm concentrations: a mouse model. *Fertil Steril* 1989;51:699–704.
32. Tsunoda Y, Yasui T, Nakamura K. Effect of cutting the zona pellucida on the pronuclear transplantation in the mouse. *J Exp Zool* 1986;240:119–125.
33. Cohen J, Edwards R, Fehilly C, et al. In vitro fertilization: a treatment for male infertility. *Fertil Steril* 1985;43:422–432.
34. Cohen J, Weber RFA, van der Vijer JCM, Zeilmaker GH. In vitro fertilizing capacity of human spermatozoa with the use of zona-free hamster ova: interassay variation and prognostic value. *Fertil Steril* 1982;37:565–572.
35. Aitken RJ, Wang YF, Liu J, Best F, Richardson DW. The influence of medium composition, osmolarity and albumin content on the acrosome reaction and fertilizing capacity of human spermatozoa. Development of an improved zona-free hamster egg penetration test. *Int J Androl* 1983;6:180–193.
36. Ahmad T, Conover JC, Quigley MM, Collins RL, Thomas AJ Jr, Gwatkin RBL. Failure of spermatozoa from T/t mice to fertilize in vitro is overcome by zona drilling. *Gamete Res* 1989;22:369–373.
37. Gordon JW, Uehlinger J, Dayani N, et al. Analysis of the hotfoot *(ho)* locus by creation of an insertional mutation in a transgenic mouse. *Dev Biol* 1990;137:349–358.
38. Cohen, J, Talansky BE, Malter HM, et al. Microsurgical fertilization and teratozoospermia. *Hum Reprod* 1991;6(1):118–123.
39. Bronson RA, Cooper GW, Rosenfeld DL. Sperm antibodies: their role in infertility. *Fertil Steril* 1984;42:171–183.
40. DeFelici M, Siracusa G. "Spontaneous" hardening of the zona pellucida of mouse oocytes during in vitro culture. *Gamete Res* 1982;6:107–113.
41. DeFelici M, Salustri A, Siracusa G. "Spontaneous" hardening of the zona pellucida of mouse oocytes during in vitro culture. II. The effects of follicular fluid and glycosaminoglycans. *Gamete Res* 1985;12:227–235.
42. Mettler L, Yamada K, Kuranty A, Michelmann HW, Semm K. Microinjection of spermatozoa into oocytes. In: Jones H, Schrader C, eds. In vitro fertilization and other assisted reproduction. *Ann NY Acad Sci* 1988;541:591–600.

43. Yamada K, Stevenson AFG, Mettler L. Fertilization through spermatozoal microinjection: significance of acrosome reaction. *Hum Reprod* 1988;3:657–661.
44. Mann J. Full term development of mouse eggs fertilized by a spermatozoon microinjected under the zona pellucida. *Biol Reprod* 1988;38:1077–1083.
45. Lacham O, Trounson A, Holden C, Mann J, Sathananthan H. Fertilization and development of mouse eggs injected under the zona pellucida with single spermatozoa treated to induce the acrosome reaction. *Gamete Res* 1989;23:233–243.
46. Yang X, Chen J, Chen YQ, Foote RH. Improved developmental potential of rabbit oocytes fertilized by sperm microinjection into the perivitelline space enlarged by hypertonic media. *J Exp Zool* 1990;255:114–119.
47. Yanagimachi R, Yanagimachi H, Rogers BJ. The use of zona-free animal ova as a test system for the assessment of the fertilizing capacity of human spermatozoa. *Biol Reprod* 1976;15:471–476.
48. Iritani A. Micromanipulation of gametes for in vitro assisted fertilization. *Mol Reprod Dev* 1991;28:199–207.
49. Lassalle B, Testart J. Human sperm injection into the perivitelline space (SI-PVS) of hamster oocytes: effect of sperm pretreatment by calcium ionophore A23187 and freeze-thawing on the penetration rate and polyspermy. *Gamete Res* 1988;20:301–311.
50. Mortimer D, Curtis EF, Dravland JE. The use of strontium-substituted media for capacitating human spermatozoa: an improved method for the zona-free hamster egg penetration test. *Fertil Steril* 1986;46:97–103.
51. Laws-King A, Trounson A, Sathananthan H, Kola I. Fertilization of human oocytes by microinjection of a single spermatozoon under the zona pellucida. *Fertil Steril* 1987; 48:637–642.
52. Ng S, Bongso A, Ratnam SS, et al. Pregnancy after transfer of sperm under zona. *Lancet* 1988;2:790.
53. Bongso TA, Sathananthan AH, Wong PC, Ratnam SS, Anandakumar C, Ganatra S. Human fertilization by micro-injection of immotile spermatozoa. *Hum Reprod* 1989; 4:175–179.
54. Cohen J, Alikani M, Malter HE, Adler A, Talansky BE, Rosenwaks Z. Partial zona dissection or subzonal sperm insertion: microsurgical fertilization alternatives based on evaluation of sperm and embryo morphology. *Fertil Steril* 1991;56 (in press).
55. Johnson MH, Eager D, Muggleston-Harris A. Mosaicism in organization of concanavalin A receptors in surface membrane of mouse egg. *Nature* 1975;257:221–322.
56. Longo FJ, Chen DY. Development of cortical polarity in mouse eggs and oocytes. *Dev Biol* 1985;107:382–394.
57. Yanagimachi R. Mechanisms of fertilization in mammals. In: Mastroianni L, Biggers JD, eds. *Fertilization and embryonic development in vitro*. New York: Plenum Press; 1981: 81–182.
58. Maro B, Johnson MH, Pickering SJ, Flach G. Changes in actin distribution during fertilization of the mouse egg. *J Embryol Exp Morphol* 1984;81:211–237.
59. Maro B, Johnson MH, Webb M, Flach G. Mechanism of polar body formation in the mouse oocyte: an interaction between the chromosomes, the cytoskeleton and the plasma membrane. *J Embryol Exp Morphol* 1986;92:11–32.
60. Cohen J, Grifo J, Malter HE, Talansky BE. Gamete and embryo micromanipulation. In: Marrs RP, ed. *The assisted reproductive technologies*. Oxford: Blackwell Scientific Publications (in press).
61. Malter H, Talansky B, Gordon J, Cohen J. Monospermy and polyspermy after partial zona dissection of reinseminated human oocytes. *Gamete Res* 1989;23:377–386.
62. Yanagimachi R. Mammalian fertilization. In: Knobil E, Neill JD, eds. *The physiology of reproduction*. New York: Raven Press; 1988:135–185.

6

A Practical Guide to Microsurgical Fertilization in the Human

Jacques Cohen

PRIMARY AND SECONDARY FACTORS

A successful microsurgical fertilization method is determined not only by primary aspects (i.e., the preparation and handling of microtools), but also by secondary factors (i.e., the immediate environment of the oocyte during micromanipulation). Moreover, the embryos created are, depending on the technique used, physiologically very different from regular embryos owing to the presence of an artificial gap in the zona pellucida. Primary factors, therefore, are limited to the actual duration of the micromanipulation procedure, whereas secondary factors extend until the moment of zona shedding at the blastocyst stage (Table 6.1). The factors described in Table 6.1 are a guide to problem areas one may encounter when setting up microsurgical fertilization.

There are not only a considerable number of microsurgical fertilization techniques to chose from, but there are also a number of technical alternatives within each method. Moreover, there is a wide variety of instrumentation to consider (see Chap. 10). This often unnecessarily intimidates those who are inexperienced with micromanipulation. Basically, there are three microscopic setups for performing micromanipulation: (a) the use of hanging droplets under coverslips, using a regular microscope; (b) the use of medium-filled tops or bottoms of large petri dishes and dissecting microscopes; and (c) the use of medium-filled petri dishes or microdroplets under oil, in combination with an inverted microscope. The first method requires considerable handling experience and, therefore, is not recommended for routine application. The use of a simple dissecting microscope is limited for

TABLE 6.1. *Primary and secondary factors determining
the success of microsurgical fertilization*

Primary factor	Secondary factor
Before micromanipulation	
Tool making (glass manufacturer)/ instruments/cleaness of tools/tool storage	Allocation of quiet, clean, and vibration-free work area within the egg laboratory
During micromanipulation	
Optimal optical system and microscope	Maintenance of appropriate temperature (approx. 37°C)
	Maintenance of pH (7.4)
	Maintenance of sterility
Optimal size and configuration of microtools	Careful handling of sperm and egg; size of the hole in the zona pellucida; number of spermatozoa used; extensive washing of eggs
Duration of each procedure (complexity of technique/ experience of technician)	Accuracy and gentleness of procedure
Following micromanipulation	
	Number of spermatozoa used
	Removal of corona cells after fertilization
	Careful pipetting of zygotes
	Careful transfer of embryos
	Inhibition of intrauterine immune attack
	Inhibition of uterine contractions

clinical purposes, since it would not reveal sufficient detail, especially when inserting individual spermatozoa. Consequently, the use of an inverted microscope is recommended. Although one may apply most micromanipulation techniques by using a variety of optical systems, considerable depth is required to maintain safety. Therefore, we recommend use of the Hoffman or Nomarski systems.

Now that the main setup (an inverted microscope with a three-dimensional optical system) has been chosen, there are still several options left, considering the type of micromanipulators and injection devices, the angle at which microtools approach the cells, and the type of compartment (petri dish or depression slide) used for micromanipulation. The first two aspects are discussed in detail in Chapter 10.

We prefer to use micromanipulators with fine and coarse controls that are not hooked up to the actual microscope stage. In addition, we prefer a mouth-controlled suction system, hooked up by sterile tubing, with a sterile filter, to either the holding pipette during partial zona dissection (PZD) or the sperm insertion needle during subzonal sperm injection (SZI) (see Chap. 10). Control of suction or expulsion of air or fluid by mouth control is more accurate and immediate than most electronically or manually controlled suction devices (1).

Basically, we do not have a preference for the size and shape of the micromanipulation chamber. However, the use of a mineral oil covering for microdroplets has so many advantages, especially when unfertilized eggs are handled outside the incubator for prolonged periods, that any other system would impose clinical limitations. Moreover, preparation of semen and concentration of spermatozoa from men with extreme forms of infertility may yield low volumes of sperm-rich suspensions, often insufficient for either pickup of sperm into an insertion needle or insufficient for insemination in a regular in vitro fertilization (IVF) dish (the open-well method) or tube system. Accordingly, it is practical to use the oil method (droplets of 100 µL or less under a layer of pretreated mineral oil) also for the general IVF procedure or, at least, during insemination when applying microsurgical fertilization.

PREPARATIVE TECHNIQUES

The Oil-Microdroplet Method for Gamete and Embryo Culture

Relatively large amounts of medium are required for the preparation of mineral or paraffin oil. Hence, it is economically and technically more advantageous to use the well-slide technique for the actual micromanipulation procedure. Very small amounts of culture medium and oil are needed for successful application of this technique (approximately 2 µL of medium and 70 µL of oil per slide). Micromanipulation can be easily performed with straight microtools hooked up to the micromanipulator arms, approaching the target cells under a shallow angle of approximately 30° (Fig. 6.1).

The use of mineral or paraffin oil for in vitro culture of gametes and embryos has long been recognized (2,3). Whereas most experimental and veterinarian embryologists use this system, the number of clinical IVF programs who use it is actually very low, possibly because of fear that toxic compounds will be released by the oil. There are two other systems for support of human gametes and early embryos that are usually preferred. The *culture tube* and *organ culture dish* systems are essentially "open" systems in which oocytes and embryos are cultured in a relatively large volume of medium and placed in a humidified atmosphere of 5% CO_2 in air or 5% O_2, 5% CO_2, and 90% N_2 at 37°C.

We have used the oil–microdroplet system for over a decade without any problems, and we recommend its use, provided the preparations and precautions outlined in the following are used. The oil we currently use is Squibb mineral oil (Squibb, Princeton, New Jersey), which is an intestinal lubricant made for human consumption. The "microdroplets under oil"

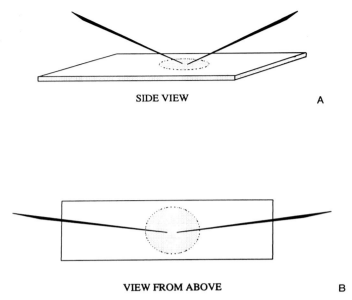

SIDE VIEW   **A**

VIEW FROM ABOVE   **B**

FIG. 6.1. Position of microtools and depression slide. *Black lines* represent the tools. Note that the tools are positioned **(A)** at an angle of 20–30° in the horizontal plane (relative to upper and lower edge of the slide) and **(B)** at an angle of 30–40° in the vertical plane (relative to the microscope stage).

system can either be used in a nonhumidified or humidified atmosphere of 5% CO_2. Although pH and temperature changes are inevitable during gamete manipulations in the other two culture systems, oil, by virtue of its physical properties—a high heat capacity and slow gas diffusion—largely prevents such rapid changes. To maintain an appropriate pH and to initiate a simple extraction process, it is advisable to preequilibrate oil with medium in 5% CO_2 for several days.

One volume of medium (either Earl's balanced salt solution or human tubal fluid) is added to three volumes of mineral oil in a 500-mL sterile plastic Falcon bottle and the mixture is bubbled with 5% CO_2 through a 5 or 10 mL sterile pipette (Falcon) for 10 minutes until the pH indicator obtains the appropriate color. The pipette is hooked up onto sterile tubing, connected by a sterile air filter and a humidification flask filled with sterile water, to a gas mixture of 5% CO_2 in air. The slow gas diffusion of mineral oil is advantageous, since gametes and embryos incubated in bicarbonate-buffered medium under oil can be kept in a relatively constant pH for 10 to 15 minutes when outside the CO_2 incubator.

Exposure of cells to unequilibrated oil should be avoided at all times, since the pH of oil stabilizes only after several hours in a regular CO_2 incubator. Pregassing is also advantageous, since trace elements will diffuse into the aqueous phase. Sterilization of oil may be disadvantageous and is actually unnecessary, since oil cannot be easily innoculated. This characteristic provides another advantage to the microdroplet method. After each work day, the contents of the bottles are regassed and closed. The biphased bottles are kept at room temperature, but dishes needed for the procedures are filled to approximately 75% of their depth the day before the actual procedure. It is advisable to discard the tops of the petri dishes, since oil may seal the narrow gaps between the top and bottom of the dish, reducing exchange of gas. This will lower the diffusion rate of CO_2 and, hence, may increase the pH. Moreover, the tops of the dishes are not really needed because the oil phase provides enough protection against contamination.

Patient culture medium (10% homologous serum solution or 6% human serum albumin) used for fertilization is slowly gassed with a 5% CO_2 mixture (10 mL in 50 mL flask), using a sterile pipette. The protein-enveloped bubbles thus created are advantageous, since these conserve the gas, allowing the embryologist to close and open the bottle several times, without a significant pH change. The bottles are stored overnight at 4°C (for preservation purposes) and droplets are pipetted into the warm preequilibrated oil dishes at least 30 minutes before the egg collection. One can pipette seven to eight 100-μL droplets (for 7 to 14 eggs) in each dish. Normally, we prepare at least two of these dishes. However, for microsurgical fertilization, which involves many washes, at least three are needed. There are two advantages to pipetting medium droplets into an oil layer (rather than pipetting oil over medium droplets). First, a shallow layer of oil will remain between the oocyte and the dish, providing less surface tension, which may reduce flattening of the corona (followed by stretching of the zona pellucida). Second, the chance of medium evaporation is reduced.

It is important to choose an uncoated petri dish like Nunc (Copenhagen, Denmark), since the droplets may otherwise flatten under the weight of oil, reducing the optical resolution. In addition, a small, flattened microdroplet of 10 μL, for instance, including all the spermatozoa of a severely oligospermic patient, could then run together with other empty droplets, limiting the frequency of interaction between the gametes. However, it is not recommended that only one small droplet be pipetted into a large dish, since trace elements left in the oil phase (that is, if there are any left) may accumulate in the aqueous phase.

Culture Media and General Culture Conditions

A multitude of media and media supplements are available for embryology laboratories and, although many trials have been reported, there is still some controversy over the optimum preparation. Unsupplemented media can be frozen or refrigerated as stocks, or in their final solutions. However, freezing and refreezing is not advisable. Sera, serum substitutes, and proteins can be kept frozen, depending on the storage facility, although many specialists prefer to use fresh samples. Regardless of the formula, the most crucial component of culture media is water. Ionic resistance should be measured regularly, preferably with two separate monitoring devices, and cytotoxins could either be assayed directly—with the use of the limulus test—or indirectly with standard quality control assays.

We have used two different culture media for regular IVF cases, as well as micromanipulation procedures. These are Earle's solution and human tubal fluid, although, recently, we mostly perform micromanipulation procedures in phosphate-buffered saline (PBS), supplemented with pyruvate and penicillin (4,5). The results between these media do not seem to be any different, although the use of a non-bicarbonate–buffered system has technical advantages. The ingredients and preparation procedures for these culture media are listed in Tables 6.2 to 6.4.

The final osmolarity used is 285 mOsm. Maternal serum-supplemented Earle's medium or human tubal fluid (HTF) culture medium is used.

TABLE 6.2. *Human tubal fluid culture media*

Stock A solution (stable for approx 2 mo)

59.31 g	NaCl
3.5 g	KCl
0.49 g	$MgSO_4 \cdot 7H_2O$
0.5 g	KH_2PO_4
37 mL	Na lactate
5.0 g	Glucose
3.0 g	$CaCl_2 \cdot 2H_2O$
0.6 g	Penicillin G

Using a 2-L Falcon roller bottle, dissolve one component at a time into 1,000 mL Milli-Q ultra pure water
Vacuum-filter, sterilize, and store in a 1,000-mL bottle at 4°C

Stock B solution (stable for 2–3 days)

Dissolve 5.25 g $NaHCO_3$ in 247.5 mL Milli-Q ultra pure water
Add 2.5 mL phenol red 0.5% solution
Vacuum-filter, sterilize, and store in 200-mL flask

Stock C solution (stable for 2–3 days)

Dissolve 0.37 g Na pyruvate in 100 mL
Vacuum-filter, sterilize, and store in 10-mL tubes

For 1 L of culture medium

Using a 2-L Falcon roller bottle
  Start with 790 mL Milli-Q ultra pure water (or slightly less!)
  Add 100 mL of stock A solution
  Add 100 mL of stock B solution
  Add 10 mL of stock C solution
  Adjust osmolarity to 284–286 mOsm by the addition of H_2O
Vacuum-filter, sterilize, and store in 1,000-mL Nalge bottle at 4°C, and/or aliquot 9.0 mL and 8.5 mL into 50-mL Nunc flasks

---

TABLE 6.3. *Earle's balanced salt solution*

Stock solutions

Dissolve 0.055 g Na pyruvate into 50 mL H_2O
Dissolve 2.1 g Na bicarbonate into 100 mL H_2O
Dissolve 0.550 g phenol red in 50 mL H_2O
Weight out the following:

$CaCl_2 \cdot 2H_2O$	0.2649 g
KCl	0.4000 g
$MgSO_4 \cdot 7h_2O$	0.2000 g
NaCl	6.8000 g
NaH_2PO_4	0.1220 g
Glucose	1.0000 g

Dissolve each of the above to 50 mL H_2O
Add each solution into a 2-L Falcon roller bottle
Add 550 mL of H_2O
Ad 0.25 mL phenol red 1.1% solution
Add Na bicarbonate solution dropwise while swirling medium
Add 10 mL Na pyruvate solution
Adjust osmolarity to 284–286 mOsm by addition of H_2O
(Volume: 960 mL)
Add penicillin G (100 IU/mL)
Vacuum filter, sterilize, and store in a 1,000-mL Nalge bottle at 4°C and/or aliquot 9.0 mL and 8.5 mL into 50-mL flasks

---

Homologous serum supplementation is not used during fertilization if the female partner has antibodies against spermatozoa, severe endometriosis, idiopathic infertility, or when normally colored serum cannot be isolated. In these instances, 6% human serum albumin (HSA; Plasmanate, Cutter Biological, Miles Inc., Elkhart, IN) is used for the first 24 hours of the procedure. After fertilization, 15% homologous serum is used for zygote and embryo culture, although the culture can also be performed in 10% Plasmanate. The embryos selected for replacement are pipetted into a preequilibrated droplet, containing 75% homologous serum or 50% Plasmanate in culture medium (4).

TABLE 6.4. *Dulbecco's phosphate-buffered saline (PBI)[a]*

Compound	gm/500 mL	Concentration in final medium (mM)
NaCl	4.0	136.9
KCl	0.1	2.68
Na_2HPO_4	0.58	8.17
KH_2PO_4	0.1	1.47
$MgCl_2 \cdot 6H_2O$	0.05	0.50
$CaCl_2 \cdot 2H_2O$	0.066	0.90
Glucose	0.5	5.56
Phenol red (1.1% solution)	0.05 mL	0.001%
Na pyruvate	0.0185g/500 mL	

[a]Store at 4°C
PBI + sucrose (0.01 M solution): 56.3 mL PBI, 3.6 mL Plasmanate, 2.04 g sucrose

The general culture conditions and gamete handling procedures we use have been described in several publications over the last decade (4,6–8). Some important details with emphasis on the use of the oil–microdroplet method are presented below.

Oocytes are collected and washed in either an Earle's solution containing low amounts of bicarbonate or in HTF, buffered with HEPES (Table 6.5). During every step of the procedure, the pH (7.4), temperature range (35° to 37°C), and osmolarity (285 mOsm) are kept as constant as possible.

TABLE 6.5. *Flushing media*

Human tubal fluid flush medium

For 2-L Falcon of flush medium

Using a 2 L Falcon roller bottle,
    Start with 1692 mL Milli-Q ultra pure water (or slightly less)
    Add 200 mL of stock A solution
    Add 32 mL of $NaHCO_3$ solution (stock B)
    Add 20 mL of stock C solution
    Add 45.88 mL of HEPES solution (1 M)
    Adjust pH to 7.36–7.38 with 1 N NaOH
    Adjust osmolarity to 284–286 mOsm by the addition of Milli-Q ultra pure water approx.
     7 mL NaOH)
    Take out 150–200 mL to be used for oocyte wash medium
    Add 1.0 mL heparin to the remainder
    Vacuum filter, sterilize, and store in 1,000-mL Nalge bottle at 4°C,
    and/or aliquot 25 mL into 50-mL Nunc flasks

Earles balanced salt solution flush medium—approx. 1.5 L

Stock solutions

Dissolve 0.055 g Na pyruvate into 50 mL Milli-Q ultra pure water
Dissolve 1.25 g Na Bicarbonate into 75 mL Milli-Q ultra pure water
Dissolve 0.550 g phenol red into 50 ml Milli-Q ultra pure water
Weigh out the following:
    $CaCl_2 \cdot 2h_2O$ 0.4636 g
    KCl   0.7000 g
    $MgSO_4 \cdot 7H_2O$ 0.3500 g
    NaCl   11.9000 g
    NaH_2PO_4 0.1952 g
    Glucose   1.7500 g
Dissolve each of the above into 50 mL Milli-Q ultra pure water
Add each solution into a 2-L Falcon roller bottle
Add 1160 mL of Milli-Q ultra pure water
Add 0.35 mL phenol red 1.1% solution
Add Na bicarbonate solution dropwise while swirling medium
Add 16 mL Na pyruvate solution
Adjust osmolarity to 284–286 mOsm by addition of Milli-Q ultra pure water
(Volume: 1552 mL)
Take out 150–200 mL to be used for oocyte wash medium. Add heparin to the remainder at 4 IU/mL
Take out 400 mL of penicillin-free flush medium
Add penicillin G to the remainder at 100 IU/mL
Vacuum filter, sterilize, and store in 1,000-mL Nalge bottle at 4°C, and/or aliquot 25 mL into 50-mL Nunc flasks

Although the effects of pH and osmolarity changes on unfertilized human eggs have not been studied in depth, it has been demonstrated that temperature fluctuations are detrimental. A short exposure to room temperature may lead to changes in the cytoskeletal structure, causing damage to the metaphase plate. Whereas these effects are reversible in the mouse egg, similar changes are apparently not repaired in human oocytes (9). Although this does not necessarily have consequences for the ability of the oocyte to interact with spermatozoa and form pronuclei, normal development of the embryo may be inhibited. This pattern is not necessarily noticed before processes involving gene expression. Since the latter occurs mostly following transition into the eight-cell embryo, IVF specialists may be observing activated oocyte-derived artifacts—rather than embryos—upon the moment of replacement (10). Consequently, it is recommended that precisely controlled warming plates be placed on each microscope (dissecting and inverted) during handling of unfertilized eggs. The use of a covering oil layer during all steps—including cumulus–corona removal and micromanipulation—will provide the embryologist with the ability to monitor and control temperature fluctuations precisely.

Eggs are separated from granulosa cells and blood-stained fluid in a dish filled with flushing medium. Parts of the cumulus that are stained with blood are immediately removed with hypodermic needles. Atretic cumuli are also dissected, until only the corona cells remain. The oocytes contained in debris-free expanded cumuli are pipetted into a washing droplet in the culture dish containing oil and then transferred into another culture droplet. Depending on the size of the dissected cumuli, two to four eggs may be housed in a single droplet. During the egg-collection procedure, the culture dish is placed on a warm plate in the back of the laminair flow area, providing a temperature of 35° to 37°C. The dish is covered with a cover or funnel connected to a humidified 5% CO_2 inlet. The culture dish can be placed in this pseudoincubator area for up to approximately 30 minutes, although such lengthy periods are not recommended. If CO_2 conditions are not optimal, the dish may be left on a warming plate uncovered for 10 to 15 minutes. Longer periods seem not to change the pH indicator immediately. However, the changes in pH will be noticeable only after 1 to 2 hours, owing to the low gas diffusion through the oil layer after the dish has been placed back into the incubator. Such changes may be not only detrimental, but may go by unnoticed.

Oocyte Preparation for Micromanipulation

Immediate enzymatic treatment following egg retrieval may interfere with oocyte maturation and activation. Preparation for micromanipulation is therefore timed between 4 and 8 hours after the egg retrieval, depending on the level of estradiol, follicular response, and continuing expansion of the cumulus. The oocytes are gathered in one or two microdroplets of the first dish. One or two other microdroplets are emptied and replaced with culture medium containing a 0.1% sterilized solution of hyaluronidase. The eggs are pipetted into these droplets and, consequently, because of the small size of the hyaluronidase droplets, the amount of enzyme may be diluted. Therefore, the 0.1% level provides an upper limit.

Two to five milligrams, of the hyaluronidase crystals (sheep testes type III, Sigma, St. Louis, Missouri) are weighted out into 5-mL sterile Falcon tubes, properly sealed, and stored at 4°C. Depending on the amount, the crystals are dissolved in HTF, Earle's solution, or modified phosphate-buffered saline (PBS with pyruvate and penicillin) supplemented with either 10% maternal serum or 6% Plasmanate, sterile filtered, gassed with small bubbles of CO_2, and placed in a dry bath at 37°C. Excess corona cells are removed with hypodermic needles or with a narrow-bore glass pipette connected to a mouth-controlled piece of tubing. Oocytes are washed at least four times in culture medium and gently manipulated with a probe to visualize and select those with a clear first polar body under a dissecting microscope. Up to this point, only a single dish has been used for egg collection, hyaluronidase treatment, and washing. Mature and immature eggs are now separately pipetted into a second oil dish, and the droplets are marked underneath with a sharp needle.

Small droplets of approximately 2 µL 0.1 M sucrose solution (in PBI with 6% Plasmanate) are pipetted in depression or well slides (Clay-Adams 3720, Baxter, New York) and immediately covered with 5% CO_2 preequilibrated warm mineral oil pipetted from the actual egg collection oil dish. One must ensure that the sucrose droplets are not in contact with air, since this may lead to detrimental osmolarity changes. The slides are then stored for 5 to 10 minutes in the incubator or on a warm plate. This holding time is used for connecting the micromanipulator arms to new microtools (see later discussion). The slides are not kept outside the incubator for more than 15 minutes. Depending on the number of eggs, two to four slides are prepared and kept in the incubator. When subzonal insertion is performed, a separate depression slide is prepared with a microdroplet of the final sperm suspension. This slide may be prepared and kept in the incubator for up to 1 hour prior to the procedure. During the procedure, the slide is kept on the microscope stage warming plate without gassing. Although this may increase the pH slightly, it has no inhibitory effects on the spermatozoa.

When the microtools are satisfactorily positioned and angled, the dish is removed from the incubator and a maximum of two or three eggs are carefully pipetted into a well slide. After micromanipulation, sucrose is removed by washing the eggs four times. The eggs are then moved into the final and third oil dish.

All pipetting during micromanipulation is done with prepulled and sterilized borosilicate 8-mm–bored glass pipettes. The pipettes are made from 30-cm–long pieces of cleaned (H_2O rinsing and ultrasound) and heat-sterilized glass. The pieces are pulled over a hot flame, broken in two with a diamond needle, and the tips are polished by moving quickly in and out of the flame. The pipettes are then again heat-sterilized and stored in stainless steel cans or glass cylinders.

Micromanipulated eggs and embryos can be easily damaged during pipetting. The embryologist can avoid most of the damage by pipetting very slowly and by checking each pipette before use. Oil or debris may be stuck to the inside (Fig. 6.2), reducing the lumen of the pipette. This may cause elongation of the zona pellucida, possibly resulting in a change of shape in the egg or embryo. Normally, when the zona is intact, the integrity of the cells will remain unharmed. However, partial release of the egg or loss of blastomeres can occur when the zona has an artificial gap (Fig. 6.3). Oil droplets stuck to the inside of the pipette can be removed by pipetting oil up and down into the pipette.

Preparation of Sperm

Semen analysis is performed at least twice prior to the IVF cycle. This includes morphologic analysis, according to strict criteria (see Chap. 7), and standard semen assessment, including a sperm survival test at 37°C in human tubal fluid and 6% Plasmanate (11). Men with severely abnormal samples and few normally shaped motile spermatozoa should be advised to have karyotyping prior to IVF. Electron microscopy is performed on sperm of men with fewer than 2% normal sperm. Assessment of microbial infection is performed when indicated. Basically, any type of semen abnormality is currently acceptable in our program, provided some spermatozoa are alive (not necessarily motile). Subzonal insertion has been performed on one occasion in a couple for whom the male partner had semen cryopreserved due to malignant disease. None of the spermatozoa (count fewer than 1×10^6/mL) were motile after thawing. All the straws were thawed and spermatozoa were collected through a mini-Percoll column and concentrated in

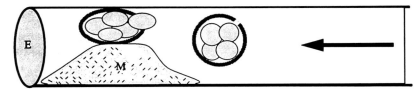

FIG. 6.2. Possible explanation of blastomere or embryonic loss following zona micromanipulation, when the transfer is performed before the formation of intercellular connections (E, end opening of catheter; M, mucus accumulated during cervical passage). A similar phenomenon may be encountered when pipetting through a narrow-bored pipette lined with small oil droplets.

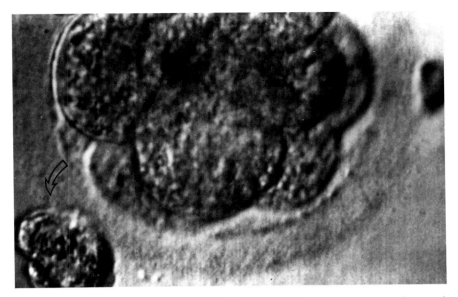

FIG. 6.3. Single blastomere lost through artificial gap several hours following micromanipulation of the zona pellucida with acidic Tyrode's solution for assisted hatching. *Arrow* indicates extruded blastomere. (Courtesy of Ms. Mina Alikani.)

approximately 20 μL of medium. This was pipetted into an oil-covered depression slide. A total of 15 motile spermatozoa were located, and these were all sucked into a beveled subzonal insertion needle. It was technically possible to inject 12 of these spermatozoa into the perivitelline space of eight eggs. Although none of the spermatozoa fertilized, it demonstrates that microsurgical fertilization can be technically accomplished in extreme cases.

The period of abstinence is preferably 3 to 5 days. In instances of autoimmunity, the sample is collected in a mixture of 50% serum and 50% medium. Men with normal semen volumes and more than 5×10^6 spermatozoa per milliliter are usually asked to collect semen in two fractions. Split ejaculates are not necessarily recommended in cases of extreme oligospermia, since suspensions of both fractions are often combined at the end of the preparation, due to lack of motile spermatozoa. Semen is produced before the egg collection and the patient is usually asked to collect once more after 3 to 5 hours. Sperm aggregation and storage of suspensions at room temperature over a period of 5 days before the procedure, as described several years ago, is no longer practiced because of the low survival rates of spermatozoa from patients selected for microsurgical fertilization (12). Highly viscous samples can be prepared either with the use of chymotrypsin or by vigorously pipetting followed by Percoll treatment. Sterile vials of chymotrypsin may be obtained in quantities of 5 mg (13,14). This should be dissolved in several milliliters of culture medium and mixed with the sample at room temperature. Viscous samples will be liquefied after 10 minutes. The sample would be washed four times to remove chymotrypsin completely.

Semen is prepared according to sedimentation, multitube layover, or Percoll techniques by procedures described elsewhere (1,6,15,16). In cases where subzonal sperm insertion was applied and sperm numbers and motility were extremely poor, it was not possible to do standard sedimentation. In such cases very low volumes of culture media were used. Final pellets were resuspended and stored in only 20 to 50 μL, at room temperature, under mineral oil (Squibb). Droplets from these concentrated suspensions were pipetted into tops of large petri dishes or onto depression slides and covered with mineral oil. Although some motile spermatozoa were present throughout the droplets, they were concentrated especially around the periphery, probably owing to increased surface tension. Debris, spermatogenic and inflammatory cells were usually retained in the center of the droplets. In such cases, 12- to 15-μm–wide, beveled glass, sperm injection needles were lowered near the edges of the droplets by the micromanipulator system and motile spermatozoa were aspirated by gentle suction using a mouth-controlled connection tube (Fig. 6.4A).

Alternatively, virtually debris-free sperm samples were obtained using an adapted mini-Percoll gradient (16). Semen samples were centrifuged once, resuspended in 0.5 mL of protein-supplemented culture medium, and layered on a discontinuous gradient of 90, 70, and 50% isotonic Percoll. Isotonic Percoll was made from nine parts of Percoll and one part of (10×) Ham's F10 (Gibco, Grand Island, New York). After 15 minutes of centrifugation of 300 *g,* the 90% fraction was collected and washed twice before use in SZI or PZD procedures.

It is beneficial to combine different preparation methods or repeat the same procedure several times. Consequently, some suspensions may be centrifuged five or more times. This apparently does not inhibit the chances of conception, although it is advisable to limit the centrifugation force as much as possible. Durations and forces of centrifugation used in regular IVF are usually excessive and can be reduced considerably. Swim-ups and sedimentation methods can be repeated several times to yield a more densely concentrated and debris-free suspension of motile spermatozoa. This is important because immotile spermatozoa may produce free radicals or other potentially toxic compounds (17,18). Indeed, the morphology of embryos inseminated with sperm from men with extreme teratozoospermia is often more abnormal than those embryos that were not inseminated, but injected with a few sperm during subzonal insertion. Moreover, it has been suggested that even immotile spermatozoa from fertile men may inhibit the sperm-decondensing ability of normal motile spermatozoa (19).

(view from above)

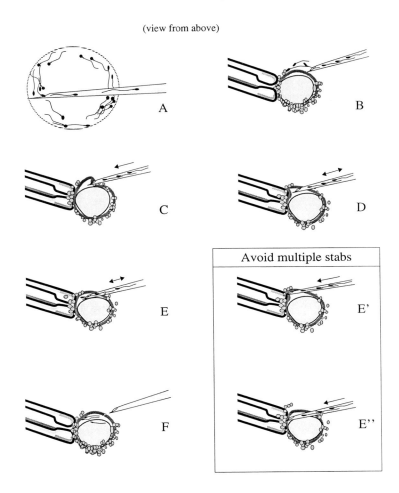

FIG. 6.4. Clinical subzonal sperm insertion step by step. **A:** Spermatozoa are picked up from the edge of a microdroplet, and the beveled needle is lowered next to the oocyte. **B:** Medium and spermatozoa are expelled from the aperture to minimize the amount of fluid in the tip of the needle when inserting it through the zona. The suction on the needle side is now minimal. **C:** The needle is pushed through the 1-o'clock position and the suction on the holding pipette is increased. **D:** The needle is moved from left to right several times (if needed) to reduce the tension of the instrument at the side of piercing. **E:** This will allow free movement of this tool through the perivitelline area. **F:** The spermatozoa are released slowly using minimal pressure.

INSERTION TECHNIQUES

Partial Zona Dissection: Step by Step

Microtools can be positioned in a variety of ways. However, the needle and holding pipette freely move past each other if the microtools are angled in two different planes (see Fig. 6.1). The straight tools are angled in the vertical plane between 30° and 45° parallel to the longitudinal axis of the microscope; this angle is comparable with that of holding a knife and fork, if the microscope stage is considered to be the plate. While keeping this angle relatively constant, the microtools are also angled (10° to 20°) in a horizontal plane parallel to the microscope stage, with the microtool tips facing slightly toward the direction of the binoculars. This double angle has the advantage that the needle passes alongside the holding pipette freely during the insertion procedure (see Fig. 6.1). At this point, the tools are centered through the microscope at the lowest magnification. The microtools are then elevated (only vertically) with the coarse controls of the micromanipulators, and the depression slide with the oocyte is placed on the microscope stage. We usually use a 20× objective and calibrate the Nomarski or Hoffman optics in such a way that the inside of the zona pellucida is clearly visible. The microtools are now lowered one by one, starting with the holding pipette side. Mouth suction is used to remove large pieces of corona radiata, until at least a fraction of the inside of the zona pellucida is visualized at the 12 o'clock position.

The corona cells may be very sticky, and the needle has to be lowered as a second tool to roll the oocyte around on the holding pipette. If the oocyte is not in an appropriate position and cannot be removed or rolled around, one can elevate the holding pipette rapidly through the oil layer while releasing the suction. The oocyte cannot be dragged through the viscous oil layer and, therefore, is released. This oocyte removal maneuver may also be applied after micromanipulation, and the micromanipulated oocyte is always released without apparent damage. This technique is preferred over tedious attempts to remove the oocyte with the tools, since that can be very time-consuming, increasing the period of sucrose exposure.

Oocytes secured by suction and oriented so that the zona pellucida is at least partially visible at the 12-o'clock position are checked for the possible presence of cytoplasmic processes between the membrane and the inside of the zona pellucida. Such processes, although rare in normally matured oocytes, become visible after shrinkage of the oocyte in sucrose. The processes are part of the oocyte and may cause lysis when pierced. After the aperture of the holding pipette is checked (it should be located in such a way that the zona and holding pipette tip are in focus at the same time), the microneedle is focused and gently probed on the 1-o'clock position, to ensure appropriate alignment of the tools (Fig. 6.5A). The needle is intro-

(view from above)

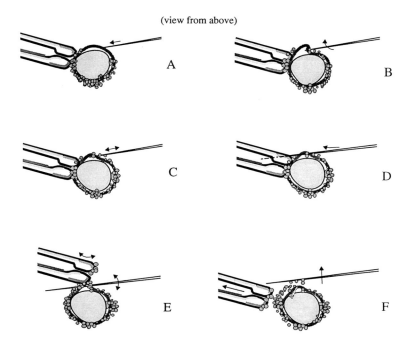

FIG. 6.5. Clinical partial zona dissection step by step. The *arrows* indicate tool movements. **A:** The two tools are focused in the same plane. The area on the top should be relatively free of corona cells. **B:** The 1-o'clock position is gently probed with the microneedle and the needle is inserted superficially while the suction is increased. **C:** The needle is moved upward and from left to right to lower the tension on the needle. **D:** The needle is moved through the 11-o'clock side in one relatively swift move, again while increasing the suction. **E:** The holding device is removed without sucking the zona from the needle and brought over the area contained between the parts of the needle stuck through both sides of the zona. The focus is slightly changed for both tools by altering the up and down controls of the micromanipulators. **F:** The holding pipette is moved below the egg and the needle and the suction is increased to remove the egg from the sticky corona cells.

duced through that side of the zona pellucida while the suction is increased, carefully threaded through the perivitelline space, moved upward to the 12-o'clock position (this is necessary to limit the size of the hole), and brought out through the zona again at approximately the 1-o'clock position (see Fig. 6.5*B–D*). Threading through the zona in two steps is advantageous, since it is important to limit the size of the hole. The suction is now interrupted, and we recommend expelling air slowly, to avoid accidental removal from the needle by suction. The microneedle and suspended oocyte are brought under the holding pipette, which is then used to rub against the portion of zona incorporated by the microneedle until the oocyte "drops off." The tip of the holding pipette and the portion of the zona being "massaged" need to be continuously adjusted during the procedure to ensure proper contact between the tool and the egg. The oocyte rarely drops off completely and usually sticks to the microneedle (see Fig. 6.5*F*). The oocyte can be sucked off by bringing the holding pipette under the oocyte while applying suction.

Partial zona dissection results in the creation of a slit in the zona that usually cannot be visualized owing to the presence of corona cells or the transparency of the zona. It is not advisable to check the presence of the slit by exercising pressure on the zona and checking for expelled cytoplasm. The formation of two or more slits may be disadvantageous for normal hatching. The oocytes are immediately removed from the sucrose droplet and incubated in a fresh droplet.

The insemination is usually timed 30 to 45 minutes after sucrose exposure. This is based on evaluation of a series of experiments using reinseminated day-old oocytes [20]. In these experiments a trend was found toward a reduced fertilization (not significant) and polyspermy (significant) rate as the time between sucrose exposure and insemination in sucrose-free medium increased. These results indicated that changes resembling activation occur following sucrose exposure and that sucrose activation can be used to reduce the risk of polyspermic fertilization in micromanipulation procedures.

The number of spermatozoa needed for insemination of partially zona-dissected oocytes is considerably lower than that used for regular insemination of zona-intact oocytes. Fertilization has been observed in suspensions with fewer than 20,000 motile spermatozoa per milliliter. However, the number of fertilizing spermatozoa varies per patient and may not be accurately assessed on the basis of motility or morphology. To improve the chances of fertilization, two parameters can be varied if a large batch of oocytes is available. First, the size of the artificial gap can be varied by increasing the area of the zona incorporated between the insertion and exit of the microneedle during microsurgery (however, this usually causes polyspermy). Second, droplets with different sperm concentrations may be used. Although monospermic fertilization may occur only in one of the droplets of a particular patient, analyses of all the data from all patients do not provide evidence that an optimal sperm concentration exists that can be applied to all patients.

Subzonal Sperm Insertion: Step by Step

Sperm insertion needles are front loaded with spermatozoa by either applying suction near the edge of the small sperm droplet containing motile spermatozoa (in cases for which layering of Percoll was successful) or by removing spermatozoa from the edges of droplets still contained within the sedimentation dish (when a motile fraction can not be secured) see Fig. 6.4*A*). Occasionally, several needles were filled and stored temporarily in the humidified incubator. However, this method was rapidly abandoned, as prolonged storage of large numbers of spermatozoa in narrow spaces appeared to be detrimental to the motility of some spermatozoa.

Fresh spermatozoa are sucked into the needle after each injection. Needles with apertures that are too small—noticeable after the spermatozoa have to be forced in and out of the opening—are discarded. Large needles, which upon insertion through the zona pierced through two sides, were also discarded (see Fig. 6.4*E'*, *E''*). Blockage of the needle tip with debris, corona cells, and spermatozoa must also be avoided. Therefore, it is important, more so than for partial zona dissection, to clean the oocytes free from corona cells, at least on one side of the Zona (the side to be pierced). Rather than attempting to clean an occluded needle tip, we usually change the needle immediately.

It is particularly important to visualize the perivitelline space in an area in which shrinkage has occurred prior to actual insertion (see Fig. 6.4*B*). The technique that we employ does not use a viscous solution, such as methyl cellulose or oil, to reduce the flow of spermatozoa. However, the flow is mouth-controlled, which, with some practice, can be very finely tuned. Spermatozoa are aspirated in such a way that limited amounts of fluid are aspirated between them. We usually pick up relatively large numbers of spermatozoa (>25), if available. This is necessary, since medium may be sucked into the needle when the tool is lowered into the droplet containing the oocyte. After the area to be pierced is chosen, the medium is expelled slowly, until motile spermatozoa are released (still outside the zona pellucida) from the needle tip, indicating the correct level of expulsion pressure (see Fig. 6.4*B*). The level of suction–expulsion on this tool is now maintained. The sperm insertion needle is tangentially inserted, while increasing the suction on the holding pipette, into the upper region (the 12-o'clock position) of the perivitelline space with the holding pipette at the 9-o'clock position (see Fig. 6.4*C, D*). This can rarely be achieved in one smooth movement. It is recommended to follow the same rules, as described earlier for partial zona dissection, focusing on both tool tips and the zona pellucida simultaneously. Small amounts of medium can be released from the needle tip when it is only partially inserted through the zona. This usually widens the perivitelline space and reduces the gripping force applied to the insertion instrument by the zona. The needle can also be more properly inserted by moving it back and forth over a very short distance several times, without coming back out of the zona. The insertion tool may be pushed alongside the vitellus into the aperture region of the holding pipette, if the instruments are angled as for partial zona dissection. This should be done carefully, since a small secondary hole may be created at the 9-o'clock position (see Fig. 6.4*E''*). Inserted spermatozoa may then be sucked out of the perivitelline space by suction from the holding pipette. A similar phenomenon occurs when the zona is pierced for a second time above the holding pipette between the 10- and 12-o'clock positions. Insertion of spermatozoa may result in increased pressure in the perivitelline space, and the excess of fluid, including spermatozoa, may then be released through the second gap. With experience, the number of inserted spermatozoa can be quite effectively controlled. If needed, spermatozoa can sometimes be removed by prompt suction applied on the insertion pipette. It is important to limit the amount of fluid inserted, since the oocyte's cytoskeleton may be adversely affected. Although we have gathered only limited data, it appears that previous shrinkage in sucrose solution is advantageous for subzonal insertion, limiting the amount of trauma when fluid is injected into the perivitelline space. However, in some cases (when sperm concentrations are very low), the zona may expand considerably, and the oocyte may distort due to the relatively high amounts of fluid injected along with the few spermatozoa in the needle. The insertion needle may be partially withdrawn until it is positioned half in, and half outside, the zona. Excess fluid can then be removed until a sperm cell appears in the opening, when the tool can be moved back into the perivitelline space. This technique is preferred over that of multiple stabbings of the zona in different areas.

Number of Subzonal Sperm Required

The concept that most spermatozoa in the normal ejaculate are unable to fertilize and represent chiasmatic errors occurring during spermatogenesis, is not well founded. The question related to the fertilizing ability of individual human spermatozoa is not only intriguing scientifically, it is also important to know how many spermatozoa from fertile and infertile men can fuse with the oolemma if one wants to use subzonal insertion as a method of alternative choice, rather than regular IVF. Much of our present knowledge of the mechanisms involved in human fertilization is largely derived from observations made during therapeutic IVF. The number of spermatozoa incubated with oocytes varies, depending on the techniques used and the expected fertilizing ability of motile spermatozoa from each individual. With possibly few exceptions, hundreds, or even thousands, of motile spermatozoa will interact with the zona pellucida during several hours. In spite of this, the rate of monospermic fertilization of mature oocytes exceeds 70%, with only 5% incidence of polyspermy. The methodology followed in different laboratories and, hence, the use of varying sperm concentrations for the insemination of oocytes, does not appear to affect the incidence of fertilization and polyspermy. Embryologists in different laboratories inseminate oocytes with sperm concentrations ranging from 0.5×10^5 to 5×10^5/mL. Nevertheless, fertilization rates differ only marginally. The fact that reduced numbers of spermatozoa used for insemination lead to fertilization rates similar to those resulting from insemination with higher numbers of sperm suggests—given the assumption that competition between spermatozoa is not altered by varying concentrations—that a substantial number of human spermatozoa are capable of traversing the zona pellucida and fertilizing the oocyte.

Recently, we performed a subzonal insertion study, in couples with male factor infertility, by inserting between 1 and 20 motile spermatozoa in the perivitelline space of fresh mature oocytes (21). Sixteen percent of individual spermatozoa were able to fuse with the oolemma and form a pronucleus. It is therefore not surprising that fertilization following subzonal insemination increased when more spermatozoa were inserted. However, the incidence of polyspermy also increased, especially when more than two live sperm cells were introduced into the perivitelline space. Insertion of more than eight spermatozoa resulted in 100% polyspermy, indicating that sperm cells derived from infertile men are capable of multiple fusion with the oolemma (Fig. 6.6).

More than half of motile spermatozoa from men with normal semen analyses are able to fuse with the oolemma when inserted directly into the perivitelline space of morphologically normal mature 1-day-old oocytes. This conclusion was reached from the use of subzonal insertion techniques in oocytes that failed to fertilize following insemination in a group of couples with various types of infertility (Table 6.6). Instead of regular reinsemination, subzonal insertion was performed. Sperm–egg fusions were counted by addition of all pronuclei of all zygotes and the final number was diminished by the number of zygotes, to correct for the inclusion of female pronuclei (one per zygote). There were 55 fusions (23%) counted following the insertion of 240 sperm cells. The rate of sperm fusion was higher (39%) when only those patients whose sperm function was considered normal were assessed. The degree of normality was based on the semen analyses and initial fertilization rates following insemination.

To calculate the potential of normally motile spermatozoa to fuse with the oolemma, one has to consider the fertilizing potential of each individual oocyte. It is likely that certain oocytes cannot be fertilized, even if they have an extruded polar body. Some of the subzonally reinseminated oocytes had refractile bodies and others had dark vacuolized cytoplasm. The fusing potential of motile human spermatozoa from men with normal semen analyses should, therefore, be based on potentially fertilizable eggs. Forty-one of 68 subzonally inserted spermatozoa (59%) from such men fused with the oolemma in 13 morphologically normal eggs.

From these results, it can be concluded that the human oolemma has little protective mechanism against multiple sperm fusion, since the vast majority of aged oocytes subjected to subzonal injection became polyspermic. The latter finding is in agreement with previous observations,

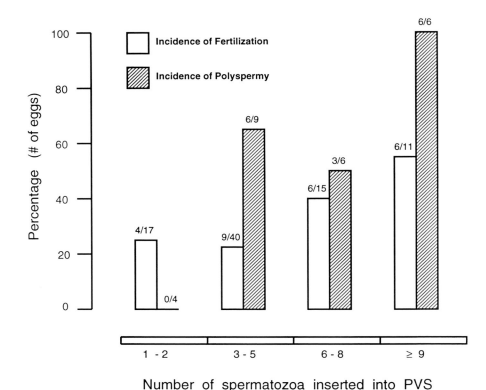

FIG. 6.6. Effect of inserting multiple spermatozoa into the perivitelline space on the frequency of monospermic and polyspermic fertilization.

following zona drilling, assessing the fertilizing capacity of men with abnormal semen (8,21). Others have suggested that the human oolemma, and not the zona pellucida, is the main barrier to polyspermy (22,23). Such conclusions, although drawn from the application of subzonal insemination, were based on sperm populations with a known reduction in fertilizing ability. It is also feasible that swelling sperm heads were present in some of the oocytes studied, but these were possibly unclear due to the nature of zygote assessment. The mechanism of polyspermy can be evaluated by using only normal fertile spermatozoa, and the current observations leave little doubt about the efficiency of the human zona reaction and the relatively poor ability of the oolemma to prevent multiple sperm fusion.

It is recommended that the number of injected spermatozoa from infertile men be limited to a maximum of four, while varying the actual number per oocyte, when large numbers of eggs are available. The maximum is limited to two spermatozoa, when subzonal reinsemination is applied for presumably fertile men.

TABLE 6.6. *Sperm–egg fusion following subzonal insertion (SZI)*

Type of infertility	SZI performed at	No. of fusing sperm/ no. of inserted sperm
Male factor	Insemination	70/438 (16%)
Male factor	Reinsemination	6/108 (6%)
Tubal/idiopathic (all oocytes)	Reinsemination	49/132 (37%)
Tubal/idiopathic (morphologically normal oocytes)	Reinsemination	41/69 (59%)

Identification of Pronuclei and Timing of Fertilization

Pronuclei should be assessed several times through an inverted microscope, while gently rolling the oocyte around with a rounded glass probe. Removal of corona cells from microsurgically treated zygotes should be avoided. Inflation of additional sperm pronuclei several hours following an initial observation is quite common. One of the advantages of reinsemination studies is that the procedures are performed during the morning. This allows early observation of pronuclei at the end of the afternoon or evening. It has been noted that subzonally inserted eggs may reveal pronuclei as early as 6 hours after microsurgery. Rapid cleavage (defined as occurring 20 to 26 hours after the microsurgery) occurs frequently in subzonally inserted zygotes, but it has not been observed following partial zona dissection. This demonstrates that gamete fusion may occur more rapidly if spermatozoa are placed in direct proximity to the oolemma. In our program, several such subzonally reinseminated embryos have implanted.

TREATMENT OF MICROSURGICAL EMBRYOS DURING REPLACEMENT

A disadvantage of any type of zona micromanipulation may be the loss of blastomeres or even the whole embryo during the replacement procedure. Mucus and tissue are frequently collected in the transfer catheter at the time of cervical insertion. Although zona-intact embryos usually squeeze pass such obstacles unharmed, embryos with holes in their zonae are damaged easily and may be lost upon release into the uterine cavity (see Fig. 6.2). Results may improve by patching the artificial hole with a self-digesting biologic gel to improve its strength during embryo replacement. It is recommended that the use of stiff and sharp replacement catheters, some of which may be incompatible with the safe transfer of micromanipulated embryos, be reassessed. It may also be advisable to reassess the vigor and speed of catheter insertion, irrespective of the type of catheter used.

REFERENCES

1. Malter HE, Cohen J. Partial zona dissection of the human oocyte: a nontraumatic method using micromanipulation to assist zona pellucida penetration. *Fertil Steril* 1989;51: 139–148.
2. Brinster RL. A method for in vitro cultivation of mouse ova from two-cell to blastocyst. *Exp Cell Res* 1963;32:205–208.
3. Rafferty KA. *Methods in experimental embryology of the mouse.* Baltimore: The Johns Hopkins Press; 1970.
4. Edwards RG, Fishel SB, Cohen J, et al. Factors influencing the success of in-vitro fertilization for alleviating human infertility. *J In Vitro Fertil Embryo Transfer* 1984;1:3–23.
5. Quinn P, Warnes GM, Kerin JF, Kirby C. Culture factors affecting the success rate of IVF and embryos transfer. *Ann NY Acad Sci* 1985;442:195–204.
6. Purdy JM. Methods for fertilization and embryo culture in vitro. In: Edwards RG, Purdy JM, eds. *Human conception in vitro.* New York: Academic Press; 1982:135.
7. Cohen J, DeVane GW, Elsner CW, et al. Cryopreservation of zygotes and early cleaved human embryos. *Fertil Steril* 1988;49:283–289.
8. Cohen J, Malter HE, Wright G, Kort H, Massey J, Mitchell D. Partial zona dissection of human oocytes when failure of zona pellucida penetration is anticipated. *Hum Reprod* 1989;4:435–442.
9. Pickering SJ, Johnson MH, Braude PR, Houliston E. Cytoskeletal organization in fresh, aged and spontaneously activated human oocytes. *Hum Reprod* 1988;3:978–989.
10. Braude P, Bolton V, Moore S. Human gene expression first occurs between the four- and eight-cell stages of preimplantation development. *Nature* 1988;332:459–461.
11. Kruger TF, Acosta AA, Simmons KF, Swanson RJ, Matta JF, Oehninger S. Predictive value of abnormal sperm morphology in in vitro fertilization. *Fertil Steril* 1988;49:112–117.
12. Cohen J, Edwards R, Fehilly C, et al. In vitro fertilization: a treatment for male infertility. *Fertil Steril* 1985;43:422–432.
13. Cohen J, Aafjes JH. Proteolytic enzymes stimulate human spermatozoa motility and penetration ability into hamster ova. *Life Sci* 1982;30:899–904.
14. Tucker M, Wright G, Bishop F, et al. Chymotrypsin in semen preparation for ARTA. *Mol Androl* 1990;2:179–186.
15. Mahadevan M, Baker G. Assessment and preparation of semen for in vitro fertilization. In: Trounson A, Wood C, eds. *Clinical In vitro fertilization.* Berlin: Springer-Verlag; 1984:83.
16. Ord T, Patrizio P, Marello E, Balmaceda JP, Asch RH. Mini-Percoll: a new method of semen preparation for IVF in severe male factor infertility. *Hum Reprod* 1990;5:987–989.
17. Aitken RJ. Analysis of human sperm function. In: Edwards RG, ed. *Assisted human conception.* Edinburgh: Churchill-Livingstone; 1990:654–674.
18. Cohen J, Weber RFA, van der Vijver JCM, Zeilmaker GH. In vitro fertilizing capacity of human spermatozoa using zona-free hamster ova. Interassay variation of prognostic value. *Fertil Steril* 1982;37:565–572.
19. Cohen J, Fehilly CB, Hewitt J. New developments in in vitro fertilization. In: *Current problems in obstetrics, gynecology and fertility,* Vol 10, no. 5. Chicago: Year Book Medical Publishers; 1986.
20. Malter HE, Talansky BE, Gordon J, Cohen J. Monospermy and polyspermy after partial zona dissection of reinseminated human oocytes. *Gamete Res* 1989;23:377–386.
21. Cohen, J, Talansky BE, Malter HE, et al. Microsurgical fertilization and teratozoospermia. *Hum Reprod* 1991;6(1):118–123.
22. Ng SC, Bongso A, Sathananthan H, Ratnam SS. Micromanipulation: its relevance to human in vitro fertilization. *Fertil Steril* 1990;53:203–219.
23. Fishel S, Jackson P, Antinori S, Johnson J, Grossi S, Versaci C. Subzonal insemination for the alleviation of infertility. *Fertil Steril* 1990;54:828–835.

7

A Review of Clinical Microsurgical Fertilization

Jacques Cohen

Human in vitro fertilization (IVF) is considered a treatment for interrupted conception, since gametes are allowed to interact directly (1). However, sperm and possibly oocyte abnormalities often result in failure of fertilization, despite the cautious use of the standard IVF technique. Various micromanipulation strategies have been suggested for promoting sperm–egg fusion, and their application in animal models has been discussed in Chapter 5. These fall into three basic categories: the direct injection of a single spermatozoon into the ooplasm (microinjection), the placement of spermatozoa into the perivitelline space (subzonal sperm insertion), and the breaching of the zona pellucida to provide an opening through which sperm can more easily gain access to the egg (zona drilling or partial zona pellucida dissection) (2–4). Of these methods, only the latter two have been applied successfully in the human (5–8). Several acronyms have been suggested to describe these techniques. Subzonal sperm insertion for instance has also been called microinsemination sperm transfer (MIST) and subzonal insemination (SUZI) (6,7). To avoid confusion we will refrain from the use of desultory acronyms as much as possible. Where necessary, partial zona dissection is described as PZD and subzonal sperm insertion as SZI.

Potentially, there is a large patient population who may benefit from microsurgical fertilization. Basically, it is aimed at three different patient groups (Fig. 7.1): First, assisted techniques may be applied to couples of whom the male partners have few spermatozoa that are able to fuse with the zona pellucida or penetrate it. A second category includes those patients for whom the oocytes are abnormal. Regular IVF patients constitute the third population for whom microsurgical fertilization could be applied. In general, fertilization does not always occur in all mature oocytes following insemination. Often oocytes are reinseminated, but success rates are usually

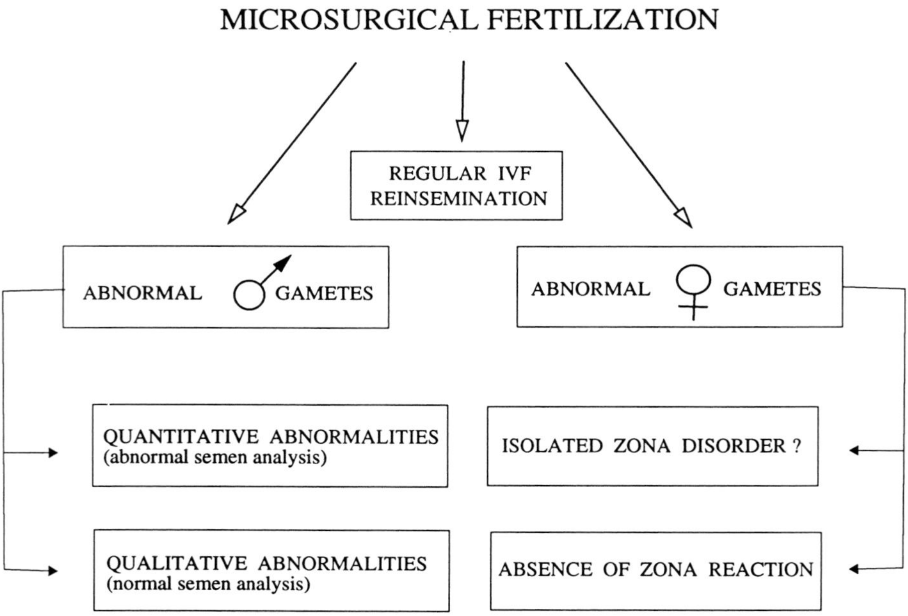

MICROSURGICAL FERTILIZATION

FIG. 7.1. Diagram illustrating three possible patient populations who may benefit from microsurgical procedures.

low. Microsurgical fertilization techniques, especially subzonal sperm insertion, may be beneficial in such cases.

The first group in whom microsurgery can be applied is usually referred to as the male factor population. This relatively large group of men can be divided into two subpopulations. The first includes those who have a *quantitative* spermatogenic or maturational disorder, with consistently abnormal semen analyses and very few normally shaped progressively motile spermatozoa. Second, are men, with apparently normal sperm, who are unable to fertilize (*qualitative* disorder). Quantitative abnormalities are easily revealed, but usually irreversible. A substantial number of such men will not be treated at IVF clinics, although some may be admitted depending on "cutoff" criteria used by individual programs. The failure rate following regular IVF is substantial, since a significant proportion of these couples will not have a single embryo for replacement. The selection criteria and results of microsurgical fertilization techniques in our program are extensively discussed below.

The other subpopulation of infertile men with qualitative disorders is much more difficult to diagnose. These men generally have normal semen analyses, no history of pelvic or urologic disease, and negative antisperm antibody tests. The couples are generally described as having idiopathic infertility, although certain diagnostic tools (hamster egg test or electron-microscopic evaluation, for instance) may now and then indicate a sperm dysfunction. Such patients are frequently identified by cross-fertilization IVF tests using donor semen. Hence, their spermatozoa are considered to be "qualitatively" abnormal or unable to fertilize, in spite of apparently normal semen criteria.

The second population of patients for whom microsurgical fertilization may be applied are those couples in whom the female partners have abnormal gametes. Some women may have morphologically mature oocytes in which the zona pellucida is structurally abnormal; either the sperm receptor may be nonfunctional, or other zona matrix components may be incompatible with sperm passage. Such zona factors must be of a molecular nature and are probably rare, since the absence of zona penetration is usually associated with morphologically abnormal cytoplasm. Therefore, it is unlikely, as will be shown later, that microsurgical fertilization techniques will be successful in this population. Patients with apparently normal gametes and recurrent polyspermy may represent an exception to this hypothesis. In such instances, a single spermatozoon could be injected into the perivitelline space (or vitellus), to eliminate the likelihood of multiple sperm incorporation.

There has been only a handful of publications on the clinical application of microsurgical fertilization, and usually evaluations have been restricted to small mixed populations of the first two groups of patients mentioned (5–7,9–11). It is possible that certain groups of patients may benefit from micromanipulation, whereas others may not. An objective critical assessment of microsurgical fertilization success rates by comparing publications, therefore, is currently unattainable. For this reason we have asked over 30 IVF programs worldwide to provide us with their data on results of micromanipulation. The evaluation of these results is presented in the next section. Nevertheless, it is difficult to compare notes on micromanipulation procedures between laboratories, since patient selection criteria may vary. The results are dependent on the patient's history (e.g., previous standard IVF failure) and on semen abnormalities. The latter criteria cannot be compared objectively among these programs. The only relevant question, therefore, pertains to the proportion of micromanipulated patients with abnormal semen. Evaluation of semen profiles, different microsurgical options, and selection criteria are discussed in a separate section, based on patients who chose microsurgical fertilization in our program. These results are largely unpublished. Moreover, in-depth analysis of procedures relative to oocyte damage and polyspermy rates will be presented. Both published and unpublished results are described.

DAMAGE TO OOCYTE AND EMBRYO DURING AND AFTER MICROSURGICAL FERTILIZATION

Oocytes may be damaged during micromanipulation procedures. The damage may be inflicted during removal of the corona cells, during piercing of the zona pellucida, or by pipetting following micromanipulation. The use of an agent, such as sucrose, which traverses membranes very slowly, has the advantage that the oocyte will compensate for the increased osmolarity by rapidly losing water. Sucrose was chosen, since it has been extensively used as a cryoprotective enhancer during embryo cryopreservation. The use of high amounts (≥ 0.1 M) of sucrose for human oocytes may prolong the recovery period after its removal and, therefore, is not recommended. Both partial zona dissection and subzonal insertion can be performed in a sucrose solution, although experienced micromanipulation technicians may quite easily perform the procedures in regular culture medium. However, we have noticed during recent preliminary experiments, that fertilization may be inhibited when subzonal sperm insertion is performed without sucrose. This is probably due to a local effect on the cytoskeleton following excessive fluid displacement into the perivitelline space of an oocyte (Fig. 7.2).

A number of microsurgical options can be considered for opening the zona pellucida or for inserting spermatozoa into the perivitelline area. Zonae can be locally digested with proteases or acidic Tyrode's solution (9,10). The first technique may enlarge or alter the zona, inhibiting normal integration of precompacted blastomeres. The latter technique does not necessarily affect sperm binding and pronuclear formation; however, it inhibits normal development of the embryo (Fig. 7.3) (5). Inseminated, but unfertilized, oocytes from regular IVF patients were either treated with acidic Tyrode's or their zonae were opened with partial zona dissection. In vitro blastocysts were formed, albeit at a low frequency, only when the oocytes were treated mechanically. That result was the main reason to proceed with partial zona dissection as the clinical form of zona drilling. Results of zona opening with two microhooks were discouraging, and this mode of treatment has not been widely applied in microsurgical fertilization units, probably because it creates large openings, increasing polyspermy and possibly damaging the embryos during or following transfer (12).

Of the first 132 human oocytes treated with partial zona dissection 3 years ago, 5% were damaged (11). Most of the eggs were damaged at the time of corona removal. As is true with most manual techniques, practice improves results. During the first 4 months in 1990, 2% (8/399) of the eggs were damaged in our laboratory when the cells surrounding the oocytes were removed. This decreased to fewer than 0.5% (2/631) during the same period in 1991 (Fig. 7.4). Our most recent results reflect a similar improvement in technique and a decrease in damage rate. In total, fewer than 1% of the

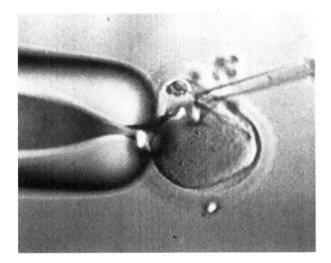

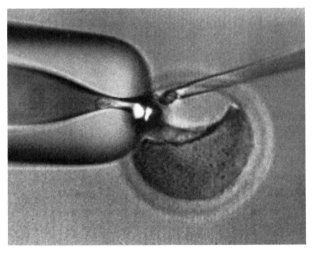

FIG. 7.2. Excessive fluid injection into the perivitelline space when using a large relatively blunt sperm insertion needle. (Courtesy of Mina Alikani, The Center for Reproductive Medicine and Infertility, The New York Hospital–Cornell University Medical Center)

oocytes have been damaged in the last 6 months, a significant reduction from the relatively elevated levels in 1988.

Oocyte damage during micromanipulation is usually visualized immediately, owing to lysis of the vitellus. However, oocytes can also be damaged indirectly without causing immediate lysis. For instance, the cytoskeleton may be affected during subzonal insertion of relatively large amounts of fluid or by inserting seminal debris. In addition, the hatching process may

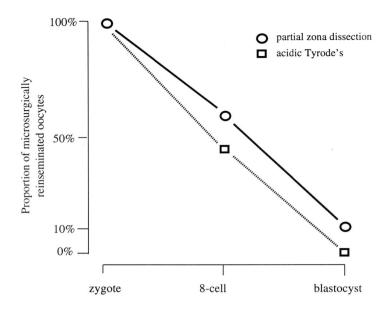

FIG. 7.3. Blastocyst development following zona drilling with acidic Tyrode's or partial zona dissection of unfertilized 1-day-old human oocytes. (From Malter HE, Cohen J. Partial zona dissection of the human oocyte: a nontraumatic method using micromanipulation to assist zona pellucida penetration. *Fertil Steril* 1989;51:139–148, with permission. Reproduced with permission of the publisher, The American Fertility Society.)

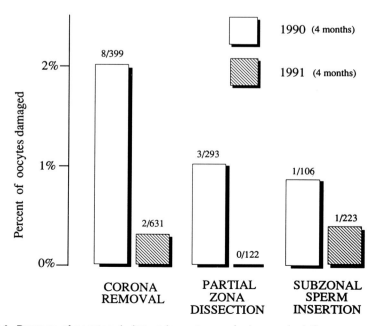

FIG. 7.4. Damage of oocytes during various stages of micromanipulation.

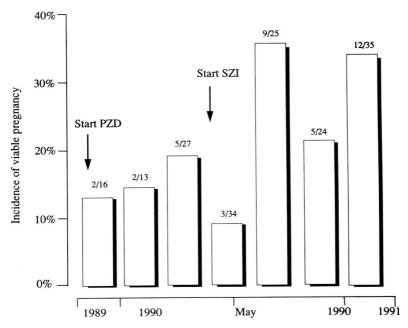

FIG. 7.5. Microsurgical fertilization results (during seven different periods) at The Center for Reproductive Medicine and Infertility, The New York Hospital–Cornell University Medical Center. *Arrows* indicate the start of a new procedure. Proportions refer to number of patients with an ongoing pregnancy and the number of patients treated. PZD, partial zona dissection; SZI, subzonal insertion.

be dramatically altered by using variable-sized needles for aggressive zona entry and withdrawal. This is relatively well described for partial zona dissection of the prefertilization mouse and human zona pellucida (13,14). Conservative application of the same procedure on embryonic zonae may inhibit hatching by causing constriction of the extruding blastocyst (15). This will inhibit not only hatching, but also normal trophoblastic development. Stabbing embryonic mouse zonae with a needle once does not interfere with their hatching. However, although the effect may be similar when subzonal sperm insertion procedures are used, the actual size of openings in the zona depends on the insertion technique and diameter of the needle. It is possible that a relatively large insertion needle will create an opening substantial enough for abnormal premature trophectodermal migration.

Considering all the possible influences of environment and techniques on embryonic viability, it is not surprising that IVF programs will experience learning curves such as the one outlined in Fig. 7.5. Both partial zona dissection and subzonal sperm insertion are now applied in our laboratory. However, we introduced the subzonal procedure 7 months after partial zona dissection was performed. Embryonic viability was reduced during the initial phases of both forms of microsurgical fertilization.

MICROSURGICAL FERTILIZATION WORLDWIDE:
RESULTS OF AN INQUIRY

Twenty-one programs had responded to a questionnaire concerning results of microsurgical fertilization efforts by March 1991. Questions related mostly to overall fertilization and pregnancy results, rather than issues pertaining to, for instance, definitions of semen abnormalities and patient selection criteria. Comparisons of semen cutoff criteria (upper and lower limits) between programs are dependent on parameter settings and judgments. Although sperm concentrations could probably reliably be compared, between programs, scores for motility and especially sperm morphology are laboratory-dependent. Moreover, even if all other factors would be consistent, definitions of abnormal versus acceptable semen for microsurgery would vary considerably. Hence, we did not conduct such an investigation and left it up to the discretion of the program teams to chose patients suitable for micromanipulation. Instead, our survey posed three relatively simple questions: (a) How many patients failed fertilization during regular IVF cycles? (b) How many of the microsurgery patients would not be acceptable for regular IVF in your program? (c) How many had abnormal semen according to the programs criteria? Although the questionnaire could be filled in several times if more than one series had been performed to refine the techniques, only our program had changed its methodology during several large series (see later). An extra series (group K) was included, since these were couples in whom the male partners had presumably normal semen, but fertilization had failed in a previous IVF cycle. A few other programs provided us with data concerning small extra series of fewer than ten patients, varying in one or more techniques. These small series are excluded from the overall results of the 21 larger series presented in Table 7.1.

Results are integrated as four techniques; partial zona dissection ($n=715$), subzonal sperm insertion ($n=703$), zona opening ($n=93$), and single-sperm microinjection into the cytoplasm ($n=22$). Even though fertilization rates were relatively promising in the latter two series, pregnancies were not obtained. Pregnancies from the two other techniques have now been established in at least 17 programs. It is estimated that there are at least five other programs who have pregnancies, but these did not respond to the questionnaire. Cumulative incidences of fertilization, transfer, and clinical pregnancy between the two techniques are very similar. Fertilization rates presented in Table 7.1 are based on monospermy. Fifty patients delivered 64 healthy babies. Most clinical pregnancies are still ongoing, and only one program reported an elevated rate of miscarriage compared with regular IVF patients. The highest rate of fertilization (47%) was reported by one program in a relatively small series of patients. The highest rate of fertilization for programs with series of more than 100 couples was only 30%. Most

TABLE 7.1. Unpublished results from microsurgical fertilization procedures performed in 21 different programs (enquiry March 1991)

Program[a] (main procedure)[b]	Cycles	Previous IVF failure	Unacceptable for regular IVF	Cycles with abnormal semen	Eggs fertilized	Cycles with transfers	Clinically pregnant	Delivered (babies)[a]
A PZD	93	17 (18%)	93 (100%)	93 (100%)	59/370 (15%)	52 (56%)	4 (7%)	4 (4)
B PZD	24	20 (83%)	14 (58%)	24 (100%)	37/142 (26%)	14 (58%)	3 (13%)	3 (4)
C PZD	48	35 (73%)	35 (73%)		78/507 (15%)	35 (73%)	7 (15%)	2 (2)
D PZD	34	18 (53%)	29 (85%)	34 (100%)	46/368 (13%)	14 (41%)	1 (7%)	1 (1)
E PZD	84	62 (74%)	15 (18%)	84 (100%)	147/537 (27%)	52 (62%)	4 (5%)	3 (3)
F PZD	39	26 (67%)	0 (0%)	12 (31%)	63/279 (23%)	23 (59%)	1 (3%)	1 (1)
G PZD	131	63 (48%)	29 (22%)	29 (22%)	141/851 (17%)	67 (51%)	3 (2%)	1 (1)
H PZD	12	6 (50%)	10 (83%)	10 (83%)	14/68 (21%)	7 (58%)	1 (8%)	1 (1)
I PZD	27	7 (26%)	19 (70%)	22 (81%)	62/132 (47%)	22 (81%)	5 (19%)	3 (6)
J PZD	133	29 (22%)	53 (40%)	115 (87%)	250/829 (30%)	98 (74%)	26 (20%)	17 (24)
K PZD	30	30 (100%)	0 (0%)	0 (0%)	55/242 (23%)	26 (87%)	1 (3%)	
L PZD	60	29 (48%)	36 (60%)	60 (100%)	104/282 (37%)	41 (68%)	13 (22%)	5 (6)
Total	*715*	*342 (48%)*	*368 (52%)*	*—*	*855/3841 (22%)*	*404 (57%)*	*69 (10%)*	*41 (53)*
M SZI	118	64 (54%)	54 (46%)	114 (97%)	223/996 (22%)	74 (63%)	3 (3%)	2 (2)
N SZI	27	12 (44%)	7 (26%)	5 (19%)	58/178 (33%)	19 (70%)	1 (4%)	
O SZI	168	168 (100%)	168 (100%)	168 (100%)	261/1376 (19%)	110 (66%)	5 (3%)	1 (1)
P SZI	225	67 (30%)	47 (21%)	47 (21%)	158/1003 (16%)	87 (39%)	12 (5%)	6 (8)
Q SZI	32	8 (25%)	20 (63%)	28 (88%)	50/354 (14%)	20 (63%)	7 (22%)	
R SZI	30	30 (100%)	0 (0%)	26 (87%)	82/308 (27%)	26 (87%)	5 (17%)	
S SZI	103	52 (50%)	72 (70%)	103 (100%)	225/875 (26%)	73 (71%)	26 (25%)	
Total	*703*	*401 (65%)*	*368 (52%)*	*491 (70%)*	*1057/5090 (21%)*	*409 (58%)*	*59 (8%)*	*9 (11)*
T Zona opening	93	71 (76%)	22 (24%)	93 (100%)	133/615 (22%)	53 (57%)	0	
U Microinjection	22	9 (41%)	13 (59%)	21 (96%)	57/158 (36%)	16 (73%)	0	

[a]Key to authors and programs: **A**, Genetics & IVF Institute, Fairfax, Virginia–Thorsell L, Bustillo M, Dorfmann A, Yap S, Fugger E, Schulman JD; **B**, Institute for Reproductive Research, Los Angeles, California–Quinn P, Hirayama T, Marrs RP; **C**, Center for Reproductive medicine, Century City Hospital, Los Angeles,—Hill D; **D**, Mt. Sinai Medical Center, New York,—Garrisi J, Gordon J; **E**, Rambam Medical Center, Haifa, Israel—Itskovitz J, Ievron J; **F**, Dept Obst Gynecol, IVF-unit, Hadassah University Hospital, Jerusalem, Israel—Laufer N, Simon A; **G**, Dept Obst Gynecol, Institut Dexeus, Barcelona, Spain—Veiga A, Calderon G, Barri PN; **H**, Reproductive Genetics Institute, Illinois Masonic Hospital, Chicago—Verlinsky Y; **I**, The Advanced Institute of Fertility, Milwaukee, Wisconsin—Stehlik E, Katayama KP; **J**, Reproductive Biology Associates, Atlanta, Georgia—Elsner C, Kort I, Massey J, Mitchell D, Toledo A, Tucker M, Wiker S, Cohen J, Wright G; **K, L, S**, The Center for Reproductive Medicine and Infertility, Dept Obst Gynecol, The New York Hospital–Cornell University Medical Center, New York—Adler A, Alikani M, Cohen J, Malter H, Reing A; **M**, Sydney IVF, Sydney, Australia—Lippi J, Jansen RPS, Turner M; **N**, Laboratoire de Biologie de la Reproduction Histologie, Embryologie, Cytogenetique, Centre Hospitalier Bicetre, Bicetre, France—Wolf JP, Frydman R, Jouannet P; **O**, National University Hospital, Singapore—Ng Sc, Bongso TA, Ratnam SS; **P**, RAPRU Clinica Nomentana, Rome, Italy—Fishel SB; **Q**, Human Reproduction Unit, St. Leonards, Australia—Krzyminska U, van Gramberg N, Leung P, O'Neill C, Pike I; **R**, Centre for Reproductive Medicine, Academish Ziekenhuis–Vrije Universiteit Brussel, Belgium—van Steirteghem AC, Palermo G; **T**, Reproductive Biology Unit, Royal Women's Hospital, Melbourne, Australia—Bourne H, Odowara Y, Hale L, Vassiliadis A, Liu DY, Lopata A, Johnston WIH, Baker HWG; **U**, Jones Institute for Reproductive Medicine, Norfolk, Virginia—Veeck L.
[b]PZD, partial zonal dissection; SZI, subzonal insertion.

program in a relatively small series of patients. The highest rate of fertilization for programs with series of more than 100 couples was only 30%. Most programs include the use of zona-intact control sibling oocytes for comparison with microsurgical fertilization. Indeed, more than five programs have had pregnancies following replacement of a combination of unmicromanipulated embryos. Consequently, a small proportion of the babies reported here, were derived from such embryos.

The vast majority of patients studied had either failed IVF cycles before or had abnormal semen profiles. One of the larger (>100) partial zona dissection series and two subzonal insertion series, resulted in relatively many embryo replacements; however, few of the embryos implanted.

It can be concluded from evaluating the results of the series presented in Table 7.1 that it is still too early to evaluate the possible impact of microsurgical fertilization on treatment of infertile men. Only six programs reported satisfactory pregnancy rates ($\geq 10\%$ per cycle). To evaluate the value of partial zona dissection and subzonal sperm insertion for various groups of patients, we have now performed relatively large series comparing both techniques simultaneously. Results from these investigations are presented here.

MICROSURGICAL FERTILIZATION: CORNELL

Selection Criteria, Semen Profiles, and Microsurgical Fertilization

Two hundred and five couples with either male factor ($n=163$) infertility (consistent abnormal semen analysis and a duration of infertility longer than 3 years) or normal semen ($n=42$), who failed to fertilize after regular IVF, were selected to have microsurgical fertilization performed in our program. A summary of these studies is presented in Tables 7.2 and 7.3. The patients with abnormal semen were also described in series L and S in Table 7.1. The first 30 of the second group of 42 patients with normal semen was described as series K in Table 7.1. The studies were performed in a period of 18 months between October 1989 and March 1991. The partial zona dissection technique was available during that whole period, whereas subzonal sperm insertion was added only during the last 10 months. Approval for clinical application of both techniques was granted by the Committee of Human Resources of The New York Hospital–Cornell Medical Center.

TABLE 7.2. Summary of microsurgical fertilization results during 18 months at The Center for Reproductive Medicine and Infertility, The New York Hospital–Cornell University Medical Center.

Patients	Abnormal semen	Clinically pregnant	Ongoing pregnant/birth
163	Yes	39 (24%)	35 (22%)
42	No	2 (5%)	2 (5%)

TABLE 7.3. *Summary of microsurgical fertilization results during 18 months in male factor patients (abnormal semen) at The Center for Reproductive Medicine and Infertility, The New York Hospital–Cornell University Medical Center*

Patients	163	(a)	
Monospermic fertilization	334/1371 (24%)		
Replacements	104	64%	(b)
Clinical pregnancy (heart beat)	39	24% (from a)	38% (from b)
From PZD only	7		
From SZI only	14		
From PZD/SZI[a]	1		
From PZD/SZI/IVF[a]	17		
Miscarriage	4/39 (10%)		
Fetal heart/embryo replaced	52/262 (20%)		

[a]PZD, partial zonal dissection; SZI, subzonal insertion; IVF, in vitro fertilization.

Overall results of the male factor couples were satisfactory (22% ongoing pregnancy rate per cycle), although this is considerably lower than that of our regular IVF patients. Results of the patients with normal semen (5% ongoing per cycle) have been disappointing, despite that at least three-quarters of them had embryos for replacement. Only 10% of the pregnant patients of the male factor group miscarried and 20% of the embryos implanted (see Table 7.3).

Three groups of patients were admitted for these studies, according to criteria presented in Table 7.4. The first group (group A, $n=81$) comprised 50% of the total number of patients studied here. These patients had severely abnormal semen analyses ($\leq 10\%$ normal sperm forms according to Kruger's strict criteria, $\leq 20\%$ motile and/or $\leq 10 \times 10^6$ spermatozoa per milliliter) and failed to fertilize all oocytes in a previous IVF cycle (16). Some of these patients failed to fertilize when IVF was repeated several times. Several patients had no normal sperm forms in repeated analyses.

The second group of couples (group B, $n=27$) had not been accepted for regular IVF by any other programs, including our own. These patients' semen analyses were considered highly abnormal; fewer than 2% normal sperm forms (Kruger's strict criteria) in combination with either extreme oligozoospermia ($\leq 5 \times 10^6$/mL) or extreme asthenospermia ($\leq 10\%$ motile). A maximum of only 50,000 motile spermatozoa could be retrieved from their semen, even if the last sperm pellet was resuspended in a small volume of less than 50 μL. The actual sperm count was not available in several of these patients, since the sperm had to be centrifuged first to capture some in the counting chamber.

The third group (group C) of 55 couples had not attempted IVF previously (some were not acceptable for other IVF programs), and all had male factor infertility of intermediate severity. All these men had terato-zoospermia ($\leq 10\%$ normal sperm forms). In addition, their semen was either considered oligozoospermic ($<20 \times 10^6$mL) and/or asthenozoo-

TABLE 7.4. Selection criteria for microsurgical fertilization and regular IVF in instances of male factor infertility

Group	Selection criterium	<50,000 motile sperm recovered	Lowest and highest semen cutoff values			Treatments		
			Count ($\times 10^6$/mL)	Motility	Morphology (normal forms)	PZD	SZI	IVF
A	Previous failure of fertilization	Occasionally	0.1–10	<1–20%	0–10%	+	+	Optional
B	Semen analysis unacceptable for regular IVF	Always	<0.1–5	<1–10%	0–2%	Optional	+	–
C	Semen analysis acceptable for IVF, but reduced prognosis	Not applicable, but reduced progression and survival	0.5–20	1–30%	3–10%	+	+	+
D	Semen analysis acceptable for IVF	Not applicable	2–20	5–30%	4–10%	–	–	+

spermic ($\leq$30% motile with reduced linear progression). Since the chances of fertilization would be somewhat reduced among these patients, micromanipulation was performed on some of their oocytes, while other oocytes were left intact.

Follicular stimulation has been described elsewhere and was performed using either a sequential clomiphene citrate/human menopausal gonadotropin protocol or gonadotropin stimulation following down regulation with leuprolide acetate (17,18).

Study 1: Partial Zona Dissection

During this study, 60 couples were treated, and only partial zona dissection was available as a microsurgical technique (Table 7.5). The majority of patients were considered to have little chance to fertilize spontaneously after standard IVF (groups A and B; see foregoing). Insufficient numbers of motile spermatozoa were retrieved for inseminating oocytes with intact zonae in these cases and, consequently, all the oocytes were micromanipulated. Mature oocytes from the remaining patients were, in each case, divided in two groups. Approximately half the oocytes were subjected to partial zona dissection, whereas the remainder were left zona intact. Each group of oocytes was inseminated separately. In general, zona-dissected oocytes were inseminated with low numbers of motile spermatozoa (0.2–0.5$\times$10^5/mL) to avoid polyspermy. Zona pellucida-intact control oocytes were always inseminated with more spermatozoa (range 1–5$\times$10^5/mL). A maximum of four embryos were replaced, and embryos were cryopreserved if more were available. Five of the 13 pregnancies were derived from replacements with only micromanipulated embryos. Two pregnancies were from embryos whose zonae were intact, and the remainder of pregnancies were from mixed groups of embryos.

Study 2: Subzonal Insertion and Partial Zona Dissection

Study 2 included 103 couples (Table 7.6). Subzonal insertion was performed on all or some of their oocytes. Seventy-six percent of the patients ($n=72$) had severe male infertility (groups A and B). In most of these, partial zona dissection or regular IVF were not contemplated, since fewer than 20,000 motile spermatozoa were recovered for final insemination, and all the oocytes were treated with subzonal sperm insertion. In other patients, more spermatozoa were retrieved (groups A and B) and partial zona dissection was performed on approximately half the patients' oocytes. Subzonal sperm insertion was carried out on the remainder of the oocytes in this group. Oocytes from patients (groups A and C) with approximately 50,000 or more motile spermatozoa/mL per suspension were

TABLE 7.5. Results of the PZD trial performed in 60 cycles using ZP-intact (ZI) control oocytes occasionally as outlined according to criteria presented in Table 7.4 (The Center for Reproductive Medicine and Infertility; The New York Hospital–Cornell Medical Center, New York; October 1989 to December 1990)[a]

Parameter	Group A: IVF failed	Group B: unacceptable for IVF	Group C: reduced IVF prognosis	Total
Fertilization of ZP intact (ZI) eggs	11/77 (14%)	–	64/137 (47%)	n.a.
Fertilization (PZD eggs)	33/136 (24%)	6/28 (21%)	65/118 (55%)	104/282 (37%)
Proportion polyspermic PZD zygotes	8/33 (24%)	2/6	16/65 (25%)	26/104 (25%)
Replacements/cycles	17/29 (59%)	4/7	16/24 (67%)	41/60 (68%)
No. ZI embryos replaced	11		25	36
No. PZD embryos replaced	20	4	43	67
No. fetuses/no. embryos replaced	4/31 (13%)	1/4	12/68 (18%)	17/103 (17%)
Clinical pregnancy	4	1	8	13
Ongoing/delivered	3	1	6	10
Pregnancy from PZD embryos only	2	1	2	5
Pregnancy PZD/ZI mixed	2		6	8
Clinical pregnancy/cycle	4/29 (14%)	1/7	8/24 (33%)	13/60 (22%)
Clinical pregnancy/transfer	4/17 (24%)	1/4	8/16 (50%)	13/41 (32%)

[a]These results were obtained before SZI was routinely available.

TABLE 7.6. Results of the SZI trial performed in 103 cycles using PZD or ZP-intact (ZI) control oocytes occasionally as outlined according to criteria presented in Table 7.4 (The Center for Reproductive Medicine and Infertility: The New York Hospital-Cornell Medical Center, New York; May 1990 to March 1991)

Parameter	Group A: IVF failed	Group B: Unacceptable for IVF	Group C: Reduced IVF prognosis	Total
Fertilization of ZP intact (ZI) eggs	na		33/107 (31%)	na
Proportion polyspermic ZI zygotes	na		1/33 (3%)	na
Fertilization PZD eggs	42/148 (28%)	1/37 (3%)	21/64 (33%)	64/249 (26%)
Proportion polyspermic PZD zygotes	9/42 (21%)	0/1 (0%)	4/21 (19%)	13/64 (20%)
Fertilization SZI eggs	74/261 (28%)	18/138 (13%)	36/120 (30%)	128/519 (25%)
Proportion polyspermic SZI zygotes	11/74 (15%)	3/18 (17%)	16/36 (44%)	30/128 (23%)
Replacements/cycles	43/52 (83%)	9/20 (45%)	21/31 (68%)	73/103 (71%)
No. ZI embryos replaced	9		23	32
No. PZD embryos replaced	17	1	14	32
No. SZI embryos replaced	61	15	19	95
No. fetuses/no. embryos replaced	18/87 (21%)	3/16 (19%)	14/56 (25%)	35/159 (22%)
No. Clinical pregnancy	14	3	9	26
No. Ongoing/delivered	13	3	9	25
Pregnancy from SZI embryos only	11	3	0	14
pregnancy from PZD embryos only	1	0	1	2
Pregnancy from SZI/PZD mixed	1	0	0	1
Pregnancy SZI/PZD/ZI mixed	1	0	8	9
Clinical pregnancy/cycle	14/52 (27%)	3/20 (15%)	9/31 (29%)	26/103 (25%)
Clinical pregnancy/transfer	14/43 (33%)	3/9 (33%)	9/21 (43%)	26/73 (36%)

divided into three subsets. Some of the oocytes were not micromanipulated, some were subjected to partial zona dissection, and others were manipulated by subzonal sperm insertion.

Twenty-two percent of replaced embryos implanted, and only one of the 26 clinical pregnancies thus far miscarried. Results of groups A and C were almost identical, except that subzonally inserted oocytes from group C patients had higher polyspermy rates. The lowest success rate (15% clinical pregnancy per cycle) was found in group B patients. Seventeen of the 26 pregnancies resulted from replacements of microsurgically treated embryos only, most of them ($n=14$) from subzonally inserted embryos (see Table 7.6).

A Comparison of Partial Zona Dissection and Subzonal Sperm Insertion

The only consequential comparison between the two techniques would either be a trial of randomization of patients or by performing both techniques simultaneously in sibling oocytes. The first option, although certainly attractive, is somewhat impractical, since an interesting subgroup of patients yield insufficient sperm numbers for insemination. In addition, some of the patients requesting subzonal sperm insertion previously failed partial zona dissection. The second option can be practiced only when sufficient numbers of sperm and eggs are available. Hence, a direct comparative study has not been implemented in our program. However, valuable indirect comparisons can be made, since the subzonal insertion technique was implemented only 8 months after partial zona dissection was already routinely available. The impact of subzonal sperm insertion on a microsurgical program can, therefore, be evaluated by comparing similar groups of patients during both periods (Tables 7.7–7.9) or by analyzing results of patients who had sufficient numbers of gametes available to perform both techniques simultaneously (Table 7.10).

TABLE 7.7. *Summary of microsurgical fertilization results in male factor patients who failed to fertilize following regular IVF (group A)*

	Available techniques	
	PZD only	PZD and SZI
Monospermic fertilization	36/213 (17%)	96/409 (25%)
Polyspermic frequency	8/44 (18%)	20/116 (17%)
Replacements/cycles	17/29 (59%)	43/52 (83%)
Fetal heart beat/embryos replaced	4/31 (13%)	18/87 (21%)
Clinical pregnancy/cycle	4/29 (14%)	14/52 (27%)
Ongoing pregnancy/cycle	3/29 (10%)	13/52 (25%)
Exclusive microsurgical pregnancy[a]	2/4	13/14

[a]No zona-intact embryos transferred

TABLE 7.8. *Summary of microsurgical fertilization results in male factor patients who were not acceptable for regular IVF (group B)*

	Available techniques	
	PZD only	PZD and SZI
Monospermic fertilization	4/28 (14%)	16/175 (9%)
Polyspermic frequency	2/6	3/19
Replacements/cycles	4/7	9/20
Fetal heart beat/embryos replaced	1/4	3/16
Clinical pregnancy/cycle	1/7 (14%)	3/20 (15%)
Ongoing pregnancy/cycle	1/7 (14%)	3/20 (15%)
Exclusive microsurgical pregnancy[a]	1/1	3/3

[a]No zona-intact embryos transferred.

Spermatozoa from patients who failed to fertilize zona-intact oocytes (group A), more frequently fused with the oolemma when subzonal insertion was available than following the exclusive application of partial zona dissection (25% versus 17%, respectively). This resulted in a significant increase in the proportion of patients who had monospermic embryos replaced (see Table 7.7). The incidence of embryonic implantation also increased from 13% to 21% when subzonal sperm insertion was added to the microsurgical program. Consequently, the incidence of ongoing pregnancy per cycle improved from 10% to 25%. It is obvious from these results that the introduction of subzonal insertion has been an advantage for group A patients. Such a trend has not been found in patients who were not acceptable for regular IVF (group B) and those who were, but whose prognosis was considered reduced (group C). Monospermic fertilization in both groups declined when subzonal sperm insertion was added to the microsurgery program (see Tables 7.8 and 7.9). However, the proportions of patients with embryo replacement and clinical pregnancies was not affected by this conversion.

TABLE 7.9. *Summary of microsurgical fertilization results in male factor patients with reduced IVF prognosis (group C)*

	Available techniques	
	IVF/PZD only	IVF/PZD and SZI
Monospermic fertilization	113/255 (50%)	72/291 (25%)
Polyspermic frequency	16/129 (12%)	21/93 (23%)
Replacements/cycles	16/24 (67%)	21/31 (68%)
Fetal heart beat/embryos replaced	12/68 (18%)	14/56 (25%)
Clinical pregnancy/cycle	8/24 (33%)	9/31 (29%)
Ongoing pregnancy/cycle	6/24 (25%)	9/31 (29%)
Exclusive microsurgical pregnancy[a]	2/8	1/9

[a]No zona-intact embryos transferred

TABLE 7.10. *A comparison of partial zona dissection and subzonal sperm insertion in patients in whom both techniques were performed on sibling oocytes*

Group	Parameter	Partial zona dissection	Subzonal insertion
A	Oocytes fertilized	29/121 (24%)	54/176 (31%)
	Fertilization per cycle	12/34 (35%)	22/34 (65%)
B	Oocytes fertilized	1/37 (3%)	3/62 (5%)
	Fertilization per cycle	1/8	1/8
C	Oocytes fertilized	19/64 (30%)	19/72 (26%)
	Fertilization per cycle	11/19 (58%)	6/19 (32%)
Combined	Oocytes fertilized	49/222 (22%)	76/310 (25%)
	Fertilization per cycle	24/61 (39%)	29/61 (48%)
Fertilization only by one method		11/61	16/61

Of the 103 couples treated during the second period, 61 had both techniques performed on sibling oocytes (see Table 7.10). Once more, oocytes from group A patients were more frequently fertilized when subzonal sperm insertion was added to the program, resulting in a significant increase in replacements from 35% to 65%. However, in group C patients, the opposite results were found. Consequently, overall rates of fertilization for all groups combined remained rather similar. In 27 of the 61 patients (44%), fertilization occurred only following one of the two techniques. Therefore, it can be concluded that both techniques should be applied when sufficient gamete numbers are available, whereas subzonal sperm insertion should be primarily considered for group A patients.

Microsurgical Fertilization and Teratozoospermia

In addition to the foregoing comparisons, the embryonic morphology and implantation potential of partial zona-dissected and subzonally inserted embryos from couples with teratozoospermia were compared using retrospective analyses of videotapes of micromanipulated embryos shortly before replacement (8). The morphology of these micromanipulated embryos was compared with those of zona-intact embryos cultured under identical conditions and replaced concurrently. Previously, it was demonstrated that the percentage of spermatozoa with normal forms, as assessed by strict criteria, was the only semen parameter correlated with the implanting capacity of partially zona-dissected embryos (18,20).

Recently, we correlated the implanting ability of 74 embryos derived from microsurgical fertilization with teratozoospermia (8). Subzonally inserted embryos ($n=15$) from men with extreme teratozoospermia ($\leq 5\%$ normal forms) were able to implant at a significantly higher rate than PZD embryos ($n=18$) from a comparable group of men (Table 7.11). Because of the possi-

TABLE 7.11. *Correlation between sperm morphology and ability of SZI and PZD embryos to implant*

Mode of Micromanipulation	Percentage normal sperm in semen			
	0–5%		6–10%	
	Incidence of embryonic implantation		Incidence of embryonic implantation	
	Minimum	Maximum	Minimum	Maximum
Partial zona dissection	0/18 (0%)[a]	3/18 (20%)[b]	5/25 (20%)	7/25 (28%)
Subzonal sperm insertion	6/15 (40%)[a,c]	7/15 (47%)[b,d]	1/16 (7%)[c]	1/16 (7%)[d]

[a,b]$p < .05$
[c]$p < .05$
[d]$p < .02$

bility of mixed embryo transfers, the range of minimum and maximum implantation rates was compared for each group; both analyses were significant. If it is assumed that a minimum number of embryos from microsurgical fertilization implanted, then none of the 18 zona-dissected embryos from couples with extreme teratozoospermia implanted. Under these conditions, subzonal sperm insertion appeared significantly more successful; at least 6/15 (40%) of the embryos implanted. The same significance was found when the assumption was made that the maximum number of embryos implanted was derived from microsurgery. Again subzonal sperm insertion appeared more effective than partial zona dissection in this particular group of patients. With the same mode of comparison, partial zona dissection appeared more successful than subzonal sperm insertion in men with moderate teratozoospermia (6% to 10% normal forms); however, the trend was not significant due to the small sample size.

The total number of abnormal embryo characteristics (score between 0 and 11) in partial zona-dissected embryos was no different from that of subzonally treated embryos (an average of 2.4 and 2.9, respectively). However, the distribution of abnormal embryos in both groups was different when it was correlated with teratozoospermia (Fig. 7.6). For example, partial zona-dissected embryos from extreme teratozoospermic patients were more frequently abnormal (defined as having at least two abnormalities) than embryos from moderate teratozoospermic patients (94% versus 56%, respectively). On the other hand, most abnormal subzonally manipulated embryos (87%) were associated with cases of moderate teratozoospermia. Plausible explanations for these observations have been given elsewhere and are summarized here (8,20).

The fact that embryos derived from routine IVF as well as partial zona dissection rarely implant when the spermatozoa are obtained from extreme

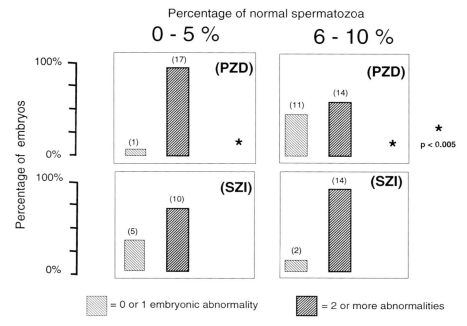

FIG. 7.6. Effect of sperm morphology on embryonic morphology following partial zona dissection or subzonal sperm insertion. Sperm morphology was assessed with strict criteria, whereas embryonic morphology was based on retrospective analyses of videotapes, scoring 11 parameters for each embryo. (Adapted from Cohen J, et al. Partial zonal dissection or subzonal sperm insertion: microsurgical fertilization alternatives based on evaluation of sperm and embryo morphology. *Fertil Steril* 1991;56 [in press]).

teratozoospermic men, whereas subzonally manipulated embryos appear unaffected, may be the result of the insemination procedure. The first two groups of embryos are inseminated with large numbers of spermatozoa, many of which are immotile owing to the complexity of the semen profiles. These ostensibly normal spermatozoa may interfere with subsequent development of zona-intact or zona-dissected embryos by releasing toxic elements, such as free radical oxygen species (21). The intact zona may normally function as a partial filter, protecting the oocyte and zygote from environmental damage. This protection may become ineffective by partial or complete removal of the zona pellucida. Embryos from subzonal sperm insertion are less likely to be affected by the environment, as they are not exposed to heterogeneous sperm populations and other seminally derived components, but are presented with only a few spermatozoa during micromanipulation.

It is more difficult, however, to provide an explanation for the frequent abnormality and lack of viability of subzonally treated embryos from couples in whom the men had moderate teratozoospermia. Polyspermy possibly occurs more frequently when more normal specimens are used (see Table 7.9). Similarly, some of the apparently monospermic and subzonally treated embryos may have been polyspermic, and this was possibly overlooked by the observers, especially since pronuclei may have formed very rapidly in some of these embryos. In addition, embryos from spermatozoa of infertile men with "relatively normal" semen parameters (such as percentage motility and concentration) may, in general, be less viable than those derived from spermatozoa of patients with extremely low semen

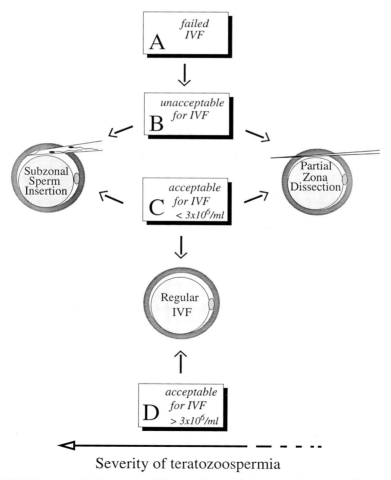

FIG. 7.7. Diagram outlining current IVF and microsurgical approaches in the different populations of patients.

values. The first population of spermatozoa may represent men with quantitative as well as qualitative disorders, whereas the second population of spermatozoa represents men with mostly quantitative disorders. Selection of rare viable spermatozoa by subzonal sperm insertion would, therefore, circumvent the major problem in these men, that of severely decreased sperm numbers.

In conclusion, subzonal sperm insertion should be applied to extreme forms of teratozoospermia, whereas partial zona dissection may be more beneficial in cases of moderately abnormal teratozoospermia. A diagram outlining these findings and indicating pathways of treatment when IVF as well as both microsurgical approaches are available, is provided in Fig. 7.7.

Frequency of Polyspermy

Zona-drilling techniques provide the experimental embryologist with information on the efficiency of the block to polyspermy on the level of the plasmalemma and zona reaction. Breaching the zona of mouse eggs, for instance, leads to high levels of monospermic fertilization, whereas similar procedures in hamster oocytes will induce polyspermy uniformly. It

TABLE 7.12. *Incidence of polyspermy following microsurgical fertilization*

Source	Type of procedure	Incidence of fertilization			Relative incidence of polyspermy
		Monospermy	Polyspermy	Total	
Gordon et al (9)	Drilling	5/31 (16%)	5/31 (16%)	10/31 (32%)	5/10 (50%)
Malter and Cohen (5)	Zona dissection	23/34 (68%)	4/34 (12%)	27/34 (79%)	4/27 (15%)
Cohen et al (11)	Zona dissection	28/50 (56%)	6/50 (12%)	34/50 (68%)	6/34 (18%)
Cohen et al (22)	Zona dissection	55/138 (40%)	20/138 (15%)	75/138 (54%)	20/75 (27%)
Cohen et al (19)	Zona dissection/	25/160 (16%)	22/160 (14%)	47/160 (29%)	22/47 (47%)
	Subzonal insertion				
Tucker et al (23)	Zona dissection	73/281 (26%)	31/281 (11%)	104/281 (37%)	31/104 (30%)
Cohen et al (8)	Zona dissection	23/148 (16%)	8/148 (5%)	31/148 (21%)	8/31 (26%)
	Subzonal insertion	52/254 (21%)	13/254 (5%)	65/254 (26%)	13/65 (20%)
Fishel et al (7)	Subzonal insertion	53/369 (14%)	2/369 (1%)	55/369 (15%)	2/55 (4%)
Garrissi et al (10)	Drilled	4/40 (10%)	3/40 (8%)	7/40 (18%)	3/7 (43%)
	Chymotrypsin	12/84 (14%)	9/84 (11%)	21/84 (25%)	9/21 (43%)
	Zona dissection	26/143 (18%)	5/143 (4%)	31/143 (22%)	5/31 (16%)
Combined		379/1732 (22%)	128/1732 (15%)	507/1732 (29%)	128/507 (25%)

appears, although this is disputed by some, that the block to polyspermy in the human, is similar to that of the hamster model (7,9,11). Rates of polyspermy following microsurgical procedures are elevated to approximately 25% of fertilized eggs (Table 7.12). This level is especially high, if one considers that the populations of spermatozoa used represent those with decreased-fertilizing ability. Only one group of researchers reported relatively low rates of polyspermy following subzonal sperm insertion (7). Rates of polyspermy following partial zona dissection in instances of normal sperm function may be as high as 50% (24). However, a weak block to polyspermy is likely to be in place on the level of the plasmalemma. One would expect equal levels of 3, 4, and 5, pronucleate embryos and so on after zona drilling, if the membrane block was completely inactive. However, most multinucleate zygotes are dispermic, and the degree of multinucleation diminishes with each additional sperm being incorporated (Fig. 7.8). The actual number of fertilizing spermatozoa is not necessarily reduced following the decondensation of two spermatozoa, but it is dependent on how many functional spermatozoa are present in the perivitelline space.

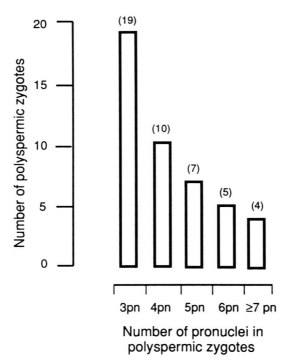

FIG. 7.8. Frequency of spermy (number of spermatozoa integrated into the oocyte) in polyspermic zygotes following partial zona dissection.

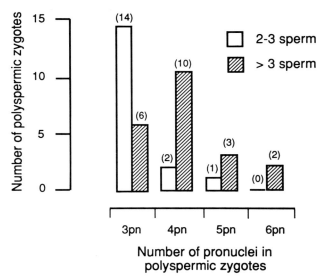

FIG. 7.9. Frequency of spermy (number of spermatozoa integrated into the oocyte) in polyspermic zygotes following subzonal sperm insertion with either two and three spermatozoa or with more than three spermatozoa injected.

The level of dispermy is actually lower than trispermy when three or more spermatozoa are deposited into the perivitelline area (Fig. 7.9).

Sperm Selection and Microsurgical Fertilization

The selection process that precedes fertilization is equally, if not more, important than capacitation and acrosome reaction. Although millions of sperm are present at the distal region of the female reproductive tract, only a few of these eventually contact the vitelline membrane. The outer vestments of the egg, such as the follicular cells, cumulus complex, and zona pellucida, all contribute to the selection process by various biologic mechanisms, some of which are poorly understood. By interrupting the contiguity of the zona, we are bypassing the oocyte's natural ability to exert selection on the overwhelming numbers of approaching sperm and are, therefore, allowing a heterogeneous population of spermatozoa direct access to the oocyte.

The ability to penetrate an oocyte and form a male pronucleus does not prove that a given spermatozoon is genetically fit. The role of the sperm cell is certainly not complete at the moment of fertilization. In fact, it has been shown, in the human embryo, that transcription is not initiated until a point between the four- and eight-cell stage of development (see Chap. 4) (25). Therefore, since the contribution of the paternal genome is not immediately evident, a successful fertilization may not necessarily be predictive of a genetically normal embryo. Some form of selection for genetically healthy sperm is probably functional at the level of the various oocyte barriers. Since it creates a direct channel to the oolemma, zona micromanipulation by partial zona dissection somewhat reduces the oocyte's natural control over sperm selection. However, in our laboratory, it has been observed that most spermatozoa in the perivitelline space of partial zona-dissected oocytes had normal morphology. This possibly indicates that the hole can be traversed only by relatively normal spermatozoa. The hole created is relatively narrow and rarely allows free movement of the sperm cell. Spermatozoa usually block the open area, inhibiting each others passage (Fig. 7.10).

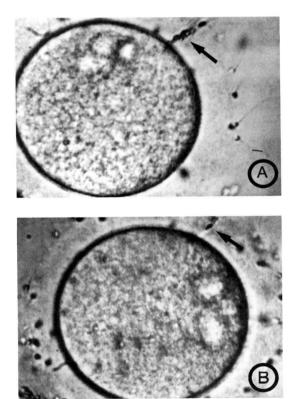

FIG. 7.10. Selection of viable spermatozoa following partial zona dissection. Spermatozoa block each others passage through the gap. The first spermatozoon usually has some free access to the perivitelline space and, presumably, binds to the zona inside the gap, where it may undergo its normal conversions, leading to zona traversion. The *arrow* indicates the row of trapped spermatozoa in the artificial gap **(A)**. Only a single sperm may be trapped in some instances **(B)**. (Courtesy of Mina Alikani, The Center for Reproductive Medicine and Infertility, The New York Hospital–Cornell University Medical Center.)

Following subzonal insertion, the role of the zona pellucida in the selection process is completely bypassed. There is a greater chance for an abnormal sperm to fuse with the egg after subzonal insertion, since it would be selected from a relatively heterogeneous population. Therefore, not only does natural selection play a more influential role in partial zona dissection, but the increased numbers of sperm favor fertilization by a normal sperm. However, miscarriage rates from subzonal procedures are not elevated, and the 11 babies born worldwide so far, and the many prenatal genetic analyses performed on our relatively large population of patients with an ongoing pregnancy, do not reveal an increased trend of abnormal karyotypes. Hence, it is likely that if abnormal embryos are created from these procedures, they generally do not implant.

CONCLUDING REMARKS

Over 60 babies have now been born worldwide from microsurgical fertilization. Reported fertilization rates are generally lower than 30% and, hence, the proportions of patients with embryo replacements are reduced when compared with regular IVF. Nevertheless, miscarriage and implantation rates appear unaffected in a number of the larger programs, and the babies born are healthy and karyotypically normal. The only two successful techniques are partial zona dissection and subzonal sperm insertion. Both methods seem relatively equal in terms of fertilization and implantation when comparing data from several programs. Direct comparisons between these two microsurgical techniques have been made only in our program.

Since only partial zona dissection was available in our program when the first group of 60 male factor patients were treated, and subzonal sperm insertion was added only during the last 103 male factor couples, the impact of the latter technique on the treatment of such patients could be evaluated. Moreover, 61 of these couples had sufficient gamete numbers to allow the simultaneous use of both techniques on sibling oocytes. Patients who failed regular IVF before (50% of this population) clearly benefited from the addition of subzonal manipulation to the microsurgical program. The incidence of fertilization was increased, resulting in more embryo replacements. Embryonic viability was enhanced, resulting in a higher clinical pregnancy rate. The other two populations of selected patients, those who were unacceptable for regular IVF, and others, who had sufficient sperm numbers for IVF, but a poor prognosis, did not benefit from the addition of subzonal sperm insertion.

In 44% of those cases in which both methods were applied simultaneously, only one of the two techniques was successful. Although results suggest that subzonal insertion should be preferentially applied to patients who failed regular IVF, partial zona dissection will be the only useful method in many patients whose gametes do not respond to subzonal insertion. How these patients can be identified is as yet unknown. Hence, it is suggested that both techniques be applied when a sufficient number of mature oocytes are available.

The number of normal sperm forms assessed by using strict criteria is the only semen parameter currently correlated with the outcome of microsurgical fertilization. Analyses of embryonic morphology and implantation rates of embryos derived from the various methods revealed that oocytes from patients with extreme teratozoospermia should be preferentially allocated to subzonal sperm insertion, whereas oocytes from moderate teratozoospermic patients should be treated with partial zona dissection.

REFERENCES

1. Cohen J, Edwards RG, Fehilly CB, et al. In vitro fertilization: a treatment for male infertility. *Fertil Steril* 1985;43:422–433.
2. Hosoi Y, Miyake M, Utsumi K, Iritani A. Development of rabbit oocytes after microinjection of spermatozoa. In: *Proceedings 11th International Congress on Animal Reproduction and Artificial Inseminations* 1988:3.
3. Mann J. Full-term development of mouse eggs fertilized by a spermatozoon microinjected under the zona pellucida. *Biol Reprod* 1988;38:1077–1083.
4. Gordon J, Talansky BE. Assisted fertilization by zona drilling: a mouse model for correction of oligozoospermia. *J Exp Zool* 1986;239:347–354.
5. Malter HE, Cohen J. Partial zona dissection of the human oocyte: a nontraumatic method using micromanipulation to assist zona pellucida penetration. *Fertil Steril* 1989;51:139–148.
6. Ng SC, Bongso A, Sathananthan H, Ratnam SS. Micromanipulation: its relevance to human in vitro fertilization. *Fertil Steril* 1990;53:203–219.
7. Fishel S, Jackson P, Antinori S, Johnson J, Grossi S, Versaci C. Subzonal insemination for the alleviation of infertility. *Fertil Steril* 1990;54:828–835.
8. Cohen J, Alikani M, Malter HE, Adler A, Talansky BE, Rosenwaks Z. Partial zona dissection or subzonal sperm insertion: microsurgical fertilization alternatives based on evaluation of sperm and embryo morphology. *Fertil Steril* 1991;56 (in press).
9. Gordon JW, Grunfeld L, Garrisi GJ, Talansky BE, Richards C, Laufer N. Fertilization of human oocytes by sperm from infertile males after zona drilling. *Fertil Steril* 1988;50:68–73.
10. Garrisi GJ, Talansky BE, Grunfeld L, Sapira V, Gordon JW. Clinical evaluation of three approaches to micromanipulation-assisted fertilization. *Fertil Steril* 1990;54:671–677.
11. Cohen J, Malter H, Wright G, Kort H, Massey J, Mitchell D. Partial zona dissection of human oocytes when failure of zona pellucida penetration is anticipated. *Hum Reprod* 1989;4:435–442.
12. Odawara Y, Lopata A. A zona opening procedure for improving in vitro fertilization at low sperm concentrations: a mouse model. *Fertil Steril* 1989;51:699–704.
13. Cohen J, Malter H, Elsner C, Kort H, Massey J, Mayer MP. Immunosuppression supports implantation of zona pellucida dissected human embryos. *Fertil Steril* 1990;53:662–665.
14. Malter H, Cohen J. Blastocyst formation and hatching in vitro following zona drilling of mouse and human embryos. *Gamete Res* 1989;24:67–80.
15. Cohen J, Feldberg D. Effects of the size and number of zona pellucida openings on hatching and trophoblast outgrowth in the mouse embryo Moles Reprod Dev (in press).
16. Kruger TF, Acosta AA, Simmons KF, Swanson RJ, Matta JF, Oehninger S. Predictive value of abnormal sperm morphology in in vitro fertilization. *Fertil Steril* 1988;49:112–121.

17. Cohen J, DeVane GW, Elsner CW, Kort HI, Massey JB, Norbury SE. Cryopreserved zygotes and embryos and endocrinologic factors in the replacement cycle. *Fertil Steril* 1988;50:61–67.
18. Droesch K, Muasher SJ, Brzyski RG, et al. Value of suppression with a gonadotropin-releasing hormone agonist prior to gonadotropin stimulation for in vitro fertilization. *Fertil Steril* 1989;51:292.
19. Cohen J, Talansky BE, Malter HM, et al. Microsurgical fertilization and teratozoospermia. *Hum Reprod* 1991;6(1):118–123.
20. Cohen J, Malter HE, Talansky BE. Microsurgical fertilization. In: Brinsden P, Rainsbury P, Yovich J, eds. *Assisted reproduction.* (in press.)
21. Aitken, RJ. Evaluation of human sperm function. In: Edwards RG, ed. *Assisted human conception.* Edinburgh: Churchill-Livingstone; 1990:654–674.
22. Cohen J, Malter H, Talansky B, Tucker M, Wright G. Gamete and embryo micromanipulation for infertility treatment. In: Mars RP, Speroff L, eds. *In Vitro Fertilization: Seminars in Reproductive Endocrinology.* New York: Thieme, Inc., 1990; 8(4):290– 295.
23. Tucker MJ, Bishop FM, Cohen J, Wiker SR, Wright G. Routine application of partial zona dissection for male factor infertility. *Hum Reprod* 1991; (in press).
24. Malter H, Talansky BE, Gordon JW, Cohen J. Monospermy and polyspermy after partial zona dissection of reinseminated human oocytes. *Gamete Res* 1989;23:377–386.
25. Tesarik J. Developmental control of human preimplantation embryos: a comparative approach. *J In Vitro Fert Embryo Transfer* 1988;5:347–362.

8

Zona Pellucida Micromanipulation and Consequences for Embryonic Development and Implantation

Jacques Cohen

Micromanipulation imposes artificial conditions upon gametes and embryos. Gaps are created in the zona pellucida may affect fertilization as well as further embryonic development. Sperm cells are compressed and possibly damaged in the lumen of sperm injection needles. Enucleation needles enter and disrupt the ooplasmic cytoskeleton. Biopsy procedures may interfere with intracellular communication, cellular polarity, and other factors needed for normal differentiation. Furthermore, it is often necessary to modify media compositions for particular procedures (for instance Ca^{2+}/Mg^{2+}-free medium during blastomere biopsy). A range of enzymes, such as hyaluronidase and chymotrypsin, and substances, such as cytochalasin B and sucrose, that are not necessary for regular in vitro fertilization (IVF), are used during micromanipulation procedures. These and other potentially negative factors must be considered in the development and management of clinical micromanipulation.

Breaching of the zona pellucida is associated with both benefits and disadvantages. Although some procedures, such as subzonal sperm insertion (SZI) do not entail substantial zona disruption, other more invasive methods, such as blastomere biopsy, may permanently alter the stability of the zona. Artificially induced modifications in the thickness and integrity of the zona pellucida may affect not only normal fertilization, but also cleavage, compaction, blastocyst formation, and hatching. Zona changes may become obvious only after prolonged in vitro culture, during embryo transfer, or as a result of an altered ability to implant (Table 8.1). This

TABLE 8.1. *Possible disadvantages of zona micromanipulation*

Disadvantage	Before cleavage	After cleavage	During transfer	After transfer
Polyspermy	+			
Nonselective fertilization	+	+		+
Seminal toxins	+	+		
Environmental toxins	+	+	+	+
Manipulation damage	+	+	+	+
Abnormalities of hatching			?	+

Based on Refs. 3, 23, 26, 28, 49.

chapter will discuss some current micromanipulation methods and attempt to address the potential benefits and problems that may have consequences for the application of clinical microsurgery.

POLYSPERMY REPAIR AND IDENTIFICATION OF PRONUCLEAR GENDER

Polyspermic fertilization—a natural error of the fertilization process—occurs when more than one sperm cell enters the oocyte. Polyspermy is inhibited by changes in the zona pellucida and oolemma following fusion with the first sperm cell (see Chap. 4). The occurrence of polyspermy in human IVF is low and reportedly varies between 2% and 12% (1–3). Approximately 75% of all polyspermic zygotes are tripronucleate. Some of these become diploid owing to either the absence of functional nucleoli or errors of syngamy. Fortunately, this represents a minor disadvantage for IVF patients; rates of monospermic fertilization are generally high. In rare cases, IVF cycles have been observed with a high degree of polyspermy in the absence of zona micromanipulation.

Any procedure that involves the physical disruption or circumvention of the oocyte's natural protective barrier will leave the egg's plasma membrane susceptible to multiple sperm. In the human oocyte, it is the zona pellucida, not the plasma membrane, that is believed to be largely responsible for limiting supernumerary sperm penetration (4–6). Opening the zona pellucida, as in zona-drilling methods, may jeopardize the egg's principal selective barrier, and the oocyte may become fertilized by multiple spermatozoa. This polyspermic state may result in an excessive genetic complement and a nonviable embryo.

It is difficult to prevent polyspermy when performing partial zona dissection (PZD), since it is necessary to inseminate the oocyte with as high a sperm concentration as possible. Although this will vary according to the requirements of individual cases, a general risk of partial zona dissection is that multiple sperm will enter the gap. On the other hand, if subzonal sperm insertion is used as a means by which to achieve fertilization, the risks of polyspermy could probably be more easily managed, since exact sperm numbers are determined by the individual performing micromanipulation. However, this is a complex issue. Within a given population of sperm from a patient with compromised fertility, apparently "normal" cells may be incapable of completing capacitation and the acrosome reaction. Consequently, such spermatozoa will be unable to fuse with an oocyte. Therefore, it is necessary to artificially induce capacitation and the acrosome reaction in entire populations of sperm to be used for subzonal sperm insertion, to ensure selection of a fertilizable cell. However, even if very few sperm are inserted into the perivitelline space, there is still no guarantee that polyspermy will be avoided.

Preventing or correcting polyspermy will be an important factor in using micromanipulation to assist human IVF. Biochemical or biophysical methods might eventually be used to limit polyspermy by controlling oocyte activation. Agents acting on the oocyte membrane could be used to prevent multiple-sperm binding (7). Although attractive, such precise control over the events of the fertilization process is presently beyond the grasp of embryological technology.

The rescue of polyspermic zygotes by removing, destroying, or inactivating supernumerary male pronuclei, thereby recovering physiologic potential and restoring diploidy, is a plausible means of correcting polyspermy. A large body of animal research exists based on techniques for the vital, intact removal of mammalian pronuclei (see Chap. 2). Normal development and offspring were obtained when the extra female pronucleus was removed from potentially triploid digynic mouse zygotes (8). We have investigated whether similar methods could be used for the safe removal of extra male pronuclei in the human in over 250 polyspermic zygotes (Malter H, Cohen J, unpublished).

The enucleation procedure uses a holding pipette for stabilizing the zona pellucida while the vitellus is penetrated with an enucleation needle (Fig. 8.1.). The tip of the needle is positioned adjacent to the target pronucleus, which is then aspirated into the needle lumen. In human zygotes, the zona presents a thick and resilient barrier to the passage of the needle. It is advantageous to first create a dent in the zona to permit needle entry. Most zygotes survive this procedure, but not all exhibit further cleavage. There may be an optimum period during pronuclear and cytoskeletal development when enucleation will be least traumatic. The use of cytoskeletal relaxants, such as cytochalasin B, may be required to reduce trauma. However, these compounds are highly toxic and may be undesirable for use with human embryos (9).

The survival rate in our enucleation work is 87% (60 of the last 70 micromanipulations), and most of the surviving embryos exhibit further development (Malter H, unpublished observations). An assessment of embryonic

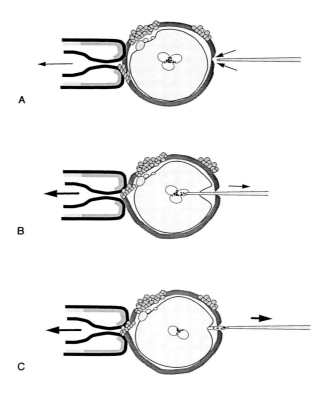

FIG. 8.1. Polyspermy correction. Diagram representing the steps during enucleation. **A:** A small hole is made in the zona with acidic Tyrode's. The flow of medium is stopped and some suction is steadily maintained. **B:** The needle is inserted in one straight move into the target pronucleus. **C:** Suction is resumed and maintained until the pronucleus is removed.

development was compromised by the desire to perform ultrastructural and genetic analysis. The embryos of those patients who consented to provide blood for genetic analysis were cryopreserved at the two- to four-cell stage for subsequent polymerase chain reaction (PCR) screening of genetic makeup. Most of the embryos of those patients who did not consent were fixed for ultrastructural analysis; either 3 hours postenucleation or at syngamy. The remaining embryos were left in vitro and observed for development. Cleavage was positively observed in 62% of the enucleated embryos. However, accounting for those that appeared healthy, but were fixed prematurely, this rate could increase to 79%. Both the ultrastructural and genetic analyses are in progress, and no data are yet available.

An important issue in using clinical enucleation to correct polyspermy is the correct identification of the supernumerary male pronuclei, to avoid the potential of hydatidiform moles. Moles are usually diploid and are genetically entirely paternal. In classic moles, the female pronucleus has been inactivated or has not participated in syngamy. Such moles are usually derived from a single diploid sperm, although dispermic moles have been reported (10,11). The cause of molar development can be studied, in part, by assessing triploid forms. Cytogenetic studies to determine the origin of triploid hydatidiform moles have shown that the extra chromosome set is essentially always of paternal origin and is usually the result of dispermy (12,13). The second most frequent source of error appears to be a paternal first meiotic one, whereas maternally derived triploid moles are rare. Certain types of trisomy may also result in swollen villi, characteristic of molar activity, indicating that hydatidiform moles adhere to genomic imprinting principles (14).

There are several possibilities for a paternal origin of triploidy. Triploidy most likely arises by dispermic fertilization of a haploid oocyte, or by a diploid sperm resulting from first and second meiotic failure. Triploid androgenesis may be explained by fertilization of an "anucleate" egg either by three haploid or one haploid and one diploid sperm. Diploid sperm are apparently not very common. Surti et al. (11) proposed that partial molar development is primarily associated with an excess of paternal over maternal chromosomal sets in the conceptus. A complete molar change contains only paternal chromosomes and is irrespective of ploidy. However, one complete mole has been described with one set of maternal and three sets of paternal chromosomes (11).

Pronucleus gender identification is simple in rodent zygotes, in which nuclear size and the presence of sperm tail remnants, as well as position in relation to the second polar body, are all valid criteria (Fig. 8.2). In human zygotes, size appears to be a random variable and sperm tail remnants can almost never be identified by vital microscopic observation (Table 8.2) (3,15). In a current study, pronuclei that are farthest from the second polar body are being selected for removal, and we hope that genetic analysis will vindicate this as being a valid criteria for identification. Ultrastructural analysis will hopefully show that the procedure does not result in damage to the cytoskeleton or other components of the ooplasm. Until it is certain that this procedure produces normal, diploid embryos, with both a maternal and paternal component, clinical application would be highly ill-advised, despite the apparent physical success of the enucleation procedure.

Polyspermic zygotes could also theoretically be rescued through the in situ destruction of the extra male pronucleus or through interference with syngamy-related pronuclear movement. Effective destruction could be accomplished by the injection of agents that affect nuclear physiology or DNA and its related proteins. Likely candidates would be DNA- or protein-degrading enzymes, lectins, or antibodies. The injection needle is likely to cause less trauma than the enucleation device. However, potential general

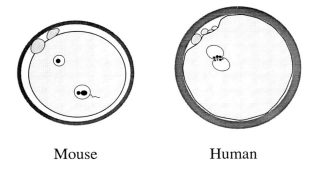

Mouse   Human

FIG. 8.2. Pronuclear size and position. Recognition of male pronucleus in mouse and human. The paternal pronucleus in the mouse zygote is large, opposite the second polar body, and may have tail remnants. The human male pronucleus is possibly the farthest from the second polar body.

toxic effects of the injectant would have to be determined and minimized. Such toxic effects would depend upon the intrinsic nature of the injectant, the precision of the injection procedure, and the amount of diffusion through the nuclear pores or membrane into the cytoplasm or other pronuclei. In preliminary experiments (Malter H, Cohen J, unpublished) involving the injection of a variety of substances, such as endonucleases, proteolytic enzymes, and polyethylene glycol, into the male pronucleus of diploid mouse zygotes, survival and cleavage were excellent. These treatments appeared to have little affect on nuclear status, as all embryos in which ploidy level could be determined remained diploid. Success with this method will obviously require careful selection of the nature and dosage of the injectant.

Electromagnetic laser-generated energy could possibly be used to destroy the unwanted pronucleus, either alone or as a mediator for a photochemical reaction involving a pronucleus-injected agent. Preliminary experiments using a laser directed through the optics of a microscope and focused on the pronucleus have resulted in some success (Tadiry, unpublished results). If the cytoplasmic movement of the extra male pronucleus was hampered, exclusion from syngamy could result. This could effectively negate the genetic contribution of this pronucleus. Movement could be affected by simply dragging the pronucleus across the cytoplasm with a needle. This procedure might be less traumatic than complete enucleation.

As this section demonstrates, the zona pellucida plays an important role in preventing polyspermy in humans. However, the protective function of the zona becomes particularly apparent during preimplantation development.

TABLE 8.2. *Relative sizes and positions of pronuclei in zygotes containing two or three inflated pronuclei*

Number of pronuclei in zygote	Position of pronucleus	Size of pronucleus compared with others			Presence of sperm tail remnants
		Smallest	Largest	Similar	
2	Close to PB2	64/133 (48%)	55/133 (41%)	14/133 (10%)	0/133 (0%)
2	Away from PB2	60/133 (45%)	59/133 (44%)	14/133 (11%)	2/133 (2%)
3	Close to PB2	8/39 (21%)	13/39 (33%)	18/39 (46%)	0/39 (0%)
3	Farthest away from PB2	18/37 (49%)	8/37 (22%)	11/37 (30%)	1/37 (3%)

Adapted from Wiker S, et al. Recognition of paternal pronuclei in human zygotes. *J In Vitro Fertil Embryo Transfer* 1990;7:33–37.

THE ROLE OF THE ZONA PELLUCIDA FOLLOWING FERTILIZATION

The zona pellucida plays an important role in maintaining the three-dimensional integrity of the precompacted embryo. Edwards (16) was one of the first to suggest that blastomeres may be weakly connected, when he reported that rabbit embryos would occasionally disaggregate when cultured in vitro without their zonae from the one- and two-cell stage. Several years later, Schlafke and Enders (17) described intracellular connections that first appeared in rat blastocysts. Modlinski (18) performed transfers to the oviduct of zona-free mouse embryos between the zygote and blastocyst stages. It was demonstrated that these zona-free embryos would adhere to the oviductal walls, become wedged between the numerous folds, or would adhere to one another (Fig. 8.3). Cleavage divisions were inhibited in those embryonic blastomeres that adhered to the oviduct. Implantation occurred only after transfer of compacted embryos. Whereas zona-free morulae and blastocysts were able to implant, almost all precompacted embryos were found adhered to one another and immobilized. It was assumed that embryos found freely dispersed in the oviductal lumen eventually became conjoined, since none implanted. From these studies, it was concluded that the zona may be needed to facilitate free passage of the embryo through the oviduct. Recently, it was shown that the size of the breach in the zona pellucida determines the fate of transferred micromanipulated precompacted mouse embryos (19). Empty zonae, derived from micromanipulated mouse embryos in which relatively large holes had been produced in their zonae, were flushed from the reproductive tract. It was suggested that contractions of the reproductive tract may cause the precompacted embryos to escape through the holes. Bronson and McLaren

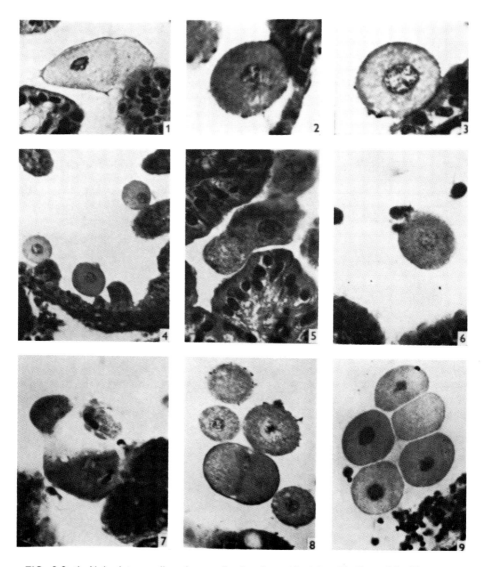

FIG. 8.3. 1: Naked two-cell embryo adhering to oviductal epithelium. **2,3:** Blastomeres adhering to epithelium. **4:** Blastomeres adhering to a fold in the oviduct. **5:** Two-cell embryo between folds. **6:** Blastomere in lumen of oviduct, with leukocytes on its surface. **7:** Degenerate blastomere. **8:** Group of naked blastomeres and one two-cell embryo in zona pellucida. **9:** Group of blastomeres from two-cell embryos adhering together in large groups. (From Modinski JA. The role of the zona pellucida in the development of mouse eggs in vitro. *J Embryol Exp Morphol* 1970;23:539–547, with permission of Company of Biologists Ltd.)

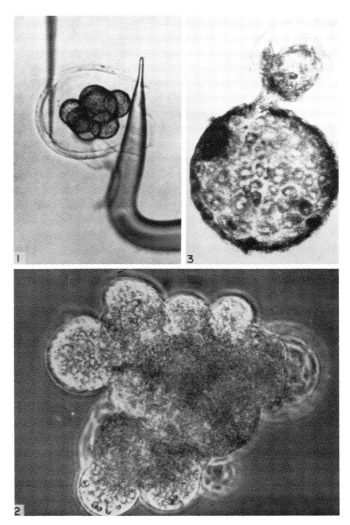

FIG. 8.4. Glass crook and needle in the process of removing a portion of the zona of a 3-day-old sheep embryo. Note extensive tearing of the zona. (From Trounson AO, Moore NW. The survival and development of sheep eggs following complete or partial removal of the zona pellucida. *J Reprod Fertil* 1974;44:97–105, with permission.)

(20) compared the embryonic zona pellucida to a shock absorber, preventing the separation of blastomeres within the cleaving embryo.

Trounson and Moore (21) postulated that a secondary mechanism could also be responsible for the demise of precompacted micromanipulated sheep embryos transferred to recipient ewes. Mechanical removal of a portion of the zona was achieved using sterile glass needles and crooks (Fig. 8.4). Removal or thinning with a protease had no effect on embryonic development in vitro. However, survival rates of the manipulated embryos after transfer to recipients were low. The authors suggest that this was due to either a loss of the integrity of the precompacted embryo or to the inability of the damaged zona to protect the embryos from hostile uterine factors. The authors suggested that an immune response may have been partially responsible for embryonic degeneration. This was later confirmed by the work of Willadsen (22,23).

Microbial Organisms and Intrauterine Hostility

Invasion of toxins through the artificial gap in the zona may occur at any point after early embryonic cleavage. For instance, even after replacement, the manipulated embryo is still susceptible to invasion by any foreign cells present in the uterine environment. Application of micromanipulation to precompacted embryos of rabbit, bovine, and sheep may cause cell death, possibly as a result of immune cell penetration through the artificial gap (23,24). An elegant way of avoiding contact with immune cells in the female reproductive tract was introduced by Willadsen (22), who applied an insoluble agar layer around the micromanipulated embryo. The agar embedding sealed any holes in the zona pellucida, thereby allowing normal development in the reproductive tract. As a result of this work, invasive procedures involving dissection of zonae in embryos of larger domestic species are either applied following compaction, or after agar embedding. Several problems need to be addressed before application of such methods in micromanipulated human embryos. The use of a temporary recipient or host uterus is impractical, for many reasons. The ingredients of the agar or coating may need to be adjusted to ensure timely disintegration of the embedding material before blastocyst expansion. Precompacted human embryos with small incisions in their zonae are currently replaced without physical protection and apparently implant normally.

The hypothetical possibility of immune cell invasion into micromanipulated human embryos or the release of cytotoxins from neighboring noninvasive immune cells cannot be excluded, even when the incisions are smaller than 5 μm, as in partial zona dissection. Uterine polymorphonuclear leukocytes or segmented neutrophils may change in size and shape, a flexibility that could allow them to gain access to the precompacted embryo through the narrow incision (25). Therefore, the effect of immunosuppression with methylprednisolone on potential immune cell invasion was investigated in alternative IVF patients who had PZD-embryos replaced (26).

Methylprednisolone (Medrol) and tetracycline were administered to alternate patients who had monospermic fertilization following PZD. Methylprednisolone (16 mg daily) treatment was commenced on the evening following oocyte collection and continued until 4 days later. The patients also received a 4-day course of tetracycline (250 mg, four times daily). The control patients were not aware of the methylprednisolone trial and received only 2 days of tetracycline as a routine prophylactic following egg retrieval. Four patients had micromanipulated embryos replaced and were not allocated to receive medication. They did not become pregnant and returned for a second attempt of partial zona dissection. These patients received medication during this second cycle. The treatment group ($n=18$) was therefore larger than the control group ($n=14$).

Thirty-two patients had between one and three micromanipulated embryos replaced. Eight clinical pregnancies (defined by fetal heart activity) were obtained in the 24 patients who had more than one embryo for replacement. Twin pregnancies occurred only after replacement of three embryos. Five of the eight clinical pregnancies had ultrasound evidence of twins with cardiac activity in both gestational sacs. In a patient with Cushing's syndrome, both sacs were reabsorbed in the first trimester after cardiac activity had been documented. One patient had evidence of the vanishing twin syndrome, but, subsequently, delivered a healthy girl. Another patient miscarried a single fetus. Six patients delivered healthy babies.

Only one twin pregnancy was obtained in the control group (Table 8.3). Two micromanipulated and one zona-intact embryo were replaced in this patient. She delivered nonidentical twins. The incidence of embryonic

TABLE 8.3. *Methylprednisolone (M) and tetracycline (T) administration to patients receiving partial zonal dissected embryos and effects on implantation*

Number of embryos replaced	Incidence of implantation in patients		Incidence of implantation per embryo	
	M/T treatment	Control	M/T treatment	Control
1	0/5	0/3	0/5	0/3
2	2/5	0/5	2/10	0/10
3	5/8	1/6	9/24	2/18
Total	7/18 (39%)[a]	1/14 (7%)[a]	11/39 (28%)[b]	2/31 (7%)[b]

From Cohen J, Malter H, Elsner C, Kort H, Massey J, Mayer MP. Immunosuppression supports implantation of zona pellucida dissected human embryos. *Fertil Steril* 1990;53:664. Reproduced with permission of the publisher, The American Fertility Society.
[a]Fisher's exact test, $p<.05$.
[b]Fisher's exact test, $p<.05$.

implantation of embryos in patients receiving medication was 28%. The incidence of implantation of embryos from non-male factor IVF patients in this program during the same period was 12%. There were no side effects reported in any of the patients receiving corticosteroids, other than vaginal yeast infections.

Implantation of PZD embryos in immunosuppressed patients was four times higher than in those patients who did not receive exogenous corticosteroids. Broad-spectrum antibiotics (4 days) and corticosteroids (4 days) have been administered to more than 400 patients prophylactically when micromanipulation methods were performed. Administration of antibiotics to the recipients of micromanipulated embryos is recommended, considering that vaginal microbial organisms may occasionally be carried into the uterine cavity by means of the replacement catheter.

Further insight into the actual mechanisms of immunosuppression in IVF patients is needed to understand the interaction between immune cells and the micromanipulated embryo. In general, administration of exogenous corticosteroids for long periods will initially induce a paradoxical rise in blood lymphocytes, lasting several weeks (27). This phenomenon represents a compartmental shift from tissues to blood, which subsides as the body pool of lymphocytes diminishes after prolonged treatment. It may be postulated that the current therapy diminishes the presence of uterine lymphocytes, thereby allowing the embryo to develop normally.

The incisions following subzonal sperm insertion and partial zona dissection are narrow and it is unlikely that monocytes or macrophages will invade through these gaps, as happened in microsurgically treated precompacted rabbit and sheep embryos in which the blastomere number was reduced or altered (23). This technique requires the presence of very large gaps in the zona pellucida, often exceeding 30 μm. However, segmented neutrophils are able to change shape markedly, possibly invading the perivitelline space by ameboid-type movements through the incision in the zona pellucida. Despite their diameter of 13 μm, they are designed to insinuate and push their way through narrow gaps between endothelial lining cells of capillaries. They are attracted to their target by chemical signals. Embryo replacement might be causing minor trauma to the endometrium, resulting in an increase in the number of segmented neutrophils. Moreover, it is possible that microbial organisms or foreign cells are incorporated with the embryos, attracting even larger numbers of immune cells.

Direct invasion of immune cells through the artificial incisions may possibly occur in embryos in which the incision diameter increased in size following replacement. This could be caused by contractions of the reproductive tract or excessive swelling of the blastomeres (19). Blastomeres of PZD embryos cultured on bovine endometrial fibroblasts may swell considerably, causing the incision to open (28). This same phenomenon may occur in the fallopian tube when noncocultured PZD embryos are replaced.

Immunosuppression probably has an advantage, as it decreases the number of peripheral immune cells, especially segmented neutrophils.

Blastocyst Expansion, Trophoblast Extrusion, and Hatching

Expansion and thinning of the blastocyst zona pellucida occurs before hatching, in most mammalian species, including the human. Whitten (29) was the first to describe lobes extruding from the trophoblast, which penetrate the zona of mouse blastocysts in vitro. Cinemicrographic studies performed by Cole showed that mouse blastocysts contract and reexpand in cycles (Fig. 8.5)(30). Contraction is achieved in 4 to 5 minutes, whereas expansion requires several hours. The zona thickness also diminishes elastically during the contraction cycle. In species, in which marked expansion occurs before lysis and implantation, as in the rabbit, bovine, mouse, and human, the zona pellucida becomes extremely attenuated and almost invis-

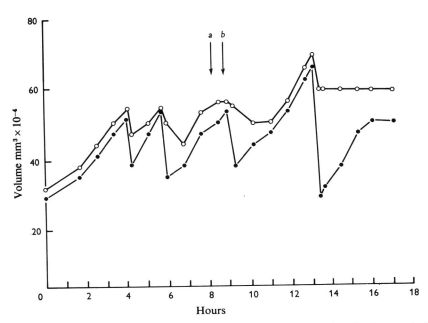

FIG. 8.5. Time course of volume changes in an individual blastocyst related to the penetration of the zona. The record began 98 hours after the estimated time of ovulation. The *upper line* connecting the *open circles* represents volume changes of the zona pellucida. The *lower line (closed circles)* reflects volume changes of blastocyst. *(a)* The beginning of partial rotations of the blastocyst, and *(b)* the initial penetration. (From Cole RJ. Cinemicrographic observations on the trophoblast and zona pellucida of the mouse blastocyst. *J Embryol Exp Morphol* 1967;17:481–490, with permission of Biologists Ltd.)

ible (Fig. 8.6). However, mouse and human embryos with artificial holes do not enlarge, and their zonae do not thin (Fig. 8.7)(31). In the rat, guinea pig, and hamster, the zona diameter is not greatly enlarged during cavitation and hatching (32).

Rupture of the zona is regulated by lysins (either embryonic or uterine in origin), by an Na^+K^+ ATPase that pumps sodium into the blastocoele, by cell proliferation, and by pulsatile movements of the blastocyst (30,33,34). In the mouse and human, complete expansion of the blastocyst must occur before the escape of the embryo from the zona. The timing of cleavage and hatching in vivo in the Siberian hamster is similar to that of the mouse (32). However, full expansion of the blastocoele does not take place. Both hatched and unhatched uterine blastocysts have small cavities and visible perivitelline spaces. The authors suggest that the Na^+/K^+ ratio may be low in the uterus of the Siberian hamster, reducing sodium pump activity.

Several studies have been conducted to elucidate the metabolic requirements of the hatching process. Mouse embryos decrease their endogenous protein content by 26% between the two-cell and the blastocyst stages (35); later, they rely upon exogenous reserves (36). Hatching, attachment, and outgrowth of mouse blastocysts in vitro are dependent upon the presence of specific free amino acids in the medium (37). Essential amino acids are required for normal development during and after hatching, whereas nonessential amino acids do not stimulate these processes (Table 8.4). During the postblastocyst period, the mouse embryo becomes dependent upon a specific exogenous fixed nitrogen source, which includes essential amino acids and a nondialyzable component from serum. Recently, it was shown in our laboratory that lysis without hatching can occur when mouse blastocysts are maintained in sera-free media (Alikani M, Cohen J, unpublished).

Early studies of mouse blastocyst development suggested that loss of the zona in utero is a combined result of embryonic and uterine functions (33,38). When implantation is interrupted by lactation or ovariectomy, escape from the zona is delayed for 24 hours. Furthermore, shed zonae remain within the uterus without lysing, but once implantation has been induced, lysis of zonae occurs (39). These observations suggested that two mechanisms of zona removal occur in vivo, including a hormone-dependent uterine lytic event and a process in which the mature blastocyst escapes from the zona, independent of hormonal stimuli. The uterine and embryonic components can be sequentially separated following ovariectomy. In such mice, evacuated zonae and hatched blastocysts coexist in utero. Within a few hours, the zonae will disappear, presumably by lysis, after the implantation stimulus is given. The fact that blastocysts in lactating females retain their zonae for up to 24 hours longer than in normal pregnancy suggests that zona loss by hatching alone is a more extended process than when uterine lytic factors facilitate the process. Unfertilized eggs in pseudopregnant females provide the converse situation. Hatching is

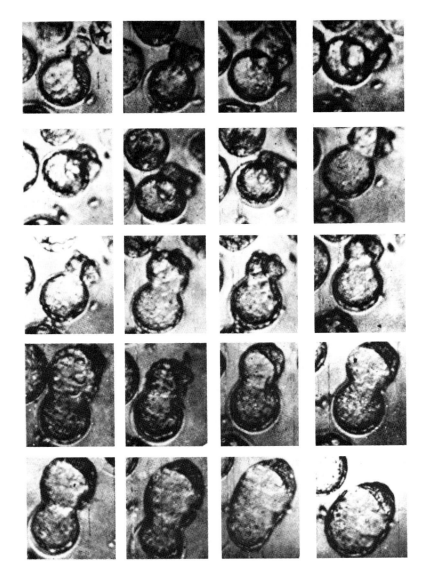

FIG. 8.6. Successive stages in the escape of a mouse blastocyst from the zona pellucida beginning 98 hours after the estimated time of ovulation and ending 17 hours later. (From Cole RJ. Cinemicrographic observation on the trophoblast and zona pellucida of the mouse blastocyst. *J Embryol Exp Morphol* 1967;17:481–490, with permission of Biologists Ltd.)

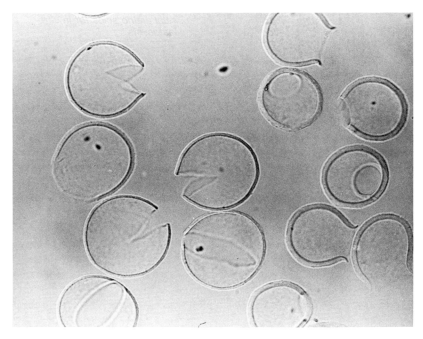

FIG. 8.7. Zonae shed by normally hatched mouse blastocysts are shown on the *left* and zonae from embryos that were zona drilled with acidic Tyrode's at the eight-cell stage on the *right.* The holes in spontaneously shed zonae are large and wedge shaped, whereas the holes in micromanipulated embryos were round and small. The zonae of shed micromanipulated embryos are thicker and smaller than those of spontaneously shed zonae.

not possible, because the egg is "inactive." The egg degenerates, and the zona is eliminated by lysis. The zona persists longer than in normal pregnancy, probably because embryonic lysins are not produced. Another possibility is that the egg zona does not stretch. As the diameter of the expanding mouse embryo increases from 70 to 100 μm, the thickness of the zona must be halved, without the intervention of a lytic process. A postulated model of the factors involved in hatching in the mouse is presented in Table 8.5.

During pregnancy in the mouse, coordination of blastocyst activity and lytic factors regulates zona loss on the fourth or fifth day of pregnancy. In the absence of either factor, zona loss is delayed. McLaren (39) was unable to demonstrate activity of an embryonic zona lysin and thus concluded that lysis of the mouse blastocyst zona occurs with the assistance of a uterine factor and the expansive activity of the blastocyst. Subsequently, it was postulated that a lytic agent is produced by the mouse blastocyst cultured in vitro (40). Hatching in vitro rarely occurred when embryos were singly cultured. When they were cultured in groups, hatching occurred frequently. Individually cultured mouse embryos hatched more frequently when they

TABLE 8.4. *Optimal concentrations of essential amino acids for in vitro development of mouse blastocysts*

L-amino acid	Concentration relative to Eagle's BME	Molar concentration
Arginine	1×	1×10^{-4}
Cystine	10×	5×10^{-4}
Histidine	20×	1×10^{-3}
Isoleucine	1×	2×10^{-4}
Leucine	5×	1×10^{-3}
Lysine	10×	2×10^{-3}
Methionine	5×	2.5×10^{-4}
Phenylalanine	5×	5×10^{-4}
Threonine	10×	2×10^{-3}
Tryptophan	5×	1×10^{-4}
Tyrosine	1×	1×10^{-4}
Valine	5×	1×10^{-3}

From Spindle AI, Pedersen RA. Hatching, attachment, and outgrowth of mouse blastocysts in vitro: fixed nitrogen requirements. *J Exp Zool* 1973; 186:305–318. Copyright © 1973, reprinted by permission of Wiley-Liss, a division of John Wiley and Sons, Inc.
[a]Concentrations are relative to Eagle's basal essential medium (BME) for HeLa cells.

were kept in conditioned medium derived from highly concentrated groups of blastocysts. This conditioned hatching medium had no effect on the zonae of cleaved embryos.

It has been postulated that human cleaved embryos produce an active component that reduces the thickness of the zona in preparation for hatching (41,42). Nieder et al. (43) showed that mouse embryos secrete a set of glycoproteins, beginning at the early blastocyst stage on the morning of day 4. The number of proteins secreted increases with time. In vitro the secretion is influenced by the macromolecular component of the culture medium. It is suggested that these glycoproteins, specifically produced by the trophectoderm, are involved in hatching and uterine attachment. More specific information on the nature of the hatching enzyme is available from studies in several nonmammalian species. The sea urchin blastula, for instance, produces a chymotrypsinlike enzyme, which is a 51- to 57-kd glycoprotein (44,45). Teleost hatching, on the other hand, is executed by an

TABLE 8.5. *Factors affecting loss of the zona pellucida in the mouse*

Situation	Activity of embryo	Zona lysin	Time of zona loss
Ovariectomized or lactating animals	Present	Absent	Late on fifth day
Pseudopregnant females (unfertilized eggs)	Absent	Present	Late on fifth day
Normal pregnancy	Present	Present	Beginning of fifth day

From McLaren A. The fate of the zona pellucida in mice *J Embryol Exp Morph* 1970; 23:1–19. With permission of Biologists Ltd.

enzyme system composed of two distinct zinc proteases, which solubilize the hard egg envelope (chorion). One choriolytic enzyme swells the inner layer of the chorion; another solubilizes the swollen outer portion (46). Similar roles for hatching have been described in unicellular algae, gastropods, ascidians, fish, and amphibians (44).

Number and Size of Artificial Gaps in the Zona and Hatching

The absence of zona thinning and expansion during expulsion of the blastocyst through an artificial zona opening may cause constriction of the trophoblast and the inner cell mass (28,31,47). Trophoblast tissue may be lost when the blastocyst squeezes through the narrow gap. Two sets of twins resulting from clinical micromanipulation were monozygotic and both miscarried; one in the first and the other in the second trimester of gestation. Another hazard is that apparently healthy embryos with several small gaps in their zonae may attempt to hatch prematurely through several openings, before expansion and growth of the blastocyst. Several clinical techniques are now being employed that involve repeated piercing of the zona. For instance, the reliability of polar body biopsy for preconception genetic diagnosis involves confirmation with blastomere biopsy and, hence, reintroduction of a microneedle. Another example is subzonal insertion, during which the sperm injection needle may be passed through the zona several times in the event of technical difficulties. An animal model for assessing abnormalities of hatching after application of techniques like subzonal insertion and partial zona dissection has recently been developed in our laboratory (48).

Two types of distinctively different holes were made in 1,190 eight-cell mouse embryos. Limited partial zona dissection (conservatively applied) produced small narrow incisions and zona drilling with acidic Tyrode's across a larger area in the zona was performed to create larger round holes. Some embryos were micromanipulated only once, others several times, to simulate repetitive zona-breaching techniques occasionally applied in human IVF. Blastocysts tended to hatch through the artificial gaps, but completion of hatching was entirely dependent on the size of the hole. Whereas 16% of the embryos entirely emerged from the narrow PZD incisions, the remainder of them became trapped in a typical figure-8 configuration (see Chap. 5). Seventy-two percent (43/60) of those migrating through larger PZD holes hatched completely. However, trophoblast outgrowth was not observed in any of the hatched PZD-embryos. Significantly ($p<.001$) more acidic Tyrode's-exposed-blastocysts hatched (248/270;92%), and 70% (176/248) showed trophoblast outgrowth. Hatching through several openings simultaneously was rarely observed among acidic Tyrode's-exposed embryos (14/167; 8%), but it did occur in 36% (73/201) of the partially zona

TABLE 8.6. *Abnormal hatching and trophoblast outgrowth following the introduction of narrow holes in the zonae of eight-cell mouse embryos and attempts to rescue such embryos by drilling larger holes elsewhere in the zonae*

Experimental group	Trapped hatching embryos	Eight-cell embryos that hatched	Trophoblast outgrowth
A Zona-intact control	0/78 (0%)	78/91 (86%)	74/78 (95%)
B Conservative PZD (≤5-μm hole)	104/136 (77%)	33/149 (22%)	0/33 (0%)
C Agressive AT (11- to 25-μm hole)	4/75 (5%)	62/76 (83%)	42/62 (68%)
D Simultaneous PZD and AT (PZD-rescue)	4/158 (3%)	135/158 (85%)	123/135 (91%)
χ^2 between group B versus A, C, and D	$p < .0001$	$p < .0001$	$p < .0001$

Data from Cohen J, Feldberg D. Effects of the size and number of zona pellucida openings on hatching and trophoblast outgrowth in the mouse embryo. *Mol Reprod Dev* (in press).
[a]PZD, partial zonal dissection; AT, acidic Tyrode's solution.

dissected embryos. The occurrence of trapped embryos could be almost entirely avoided by performing zona drilling with acidic Tyrode's elsewhere on the zona, following the partial zona dissection procedure(s) (Table 8.6). Only 3% (4/158) of zona-dissected embryos, also drilled with acidic Tyrode's, became trapped during hatching. This is significant improvement over the frequency of embryo trapping that occurred after partial zona dissection (77%; 104/136; $p<.0001$).

Embryos with multiple holes in their zonae preferentially hatched through the largest opening. It is suggested that practitioners of human IVF carefully (re)assess the ability of micromanipulated embryos to fully hatch in vitro, prior to application of clinical micromanipulation systems. Micromanipulated embryos with small holes in their zonae may be rescued by performing a subsequent, more aggressive opening procedure elsewhere on the zona, before transfer.

Zona Hardening and Facilitation of Hatching

The zona reaction results in an increased resistance to dissolution by various chemical agents, a phenomenon termed *zona hardening*. Various substances, including proteases, disulfide-bound reducing agents, sodium periodate, as well as low pH and high temperature, have been used to study the zona reaction. It has been shown that the zona is more readily removed from unfertilized oocytes than from embryos. The human zona seems to change in its receptivity to decreased pH. That is, using an acidic solution, it is easier to create a hole in the zona of a zygote than in that of an unfertilized oocyte (28,49). The human zona becomes more brittle and loses its elasticity after fertilization. In addition to fertilization-induced hardening, spontaneous hardening also occurs after in vitro culture (50,51) and in vivo aging (52).

Zona hardening may be important for three postfertilization events, including the block to polyspermy (53), protection of the developing embryo (54), and oviductal transport (55). Although the process is believed to be a physical change, assays usually involve solubilization techniques. Drobnis et al. (56) studied the extent of zona distortion after aspiration into a narrow micropipette as an assay for zona hardening (Fig. 8.8). Their studies revealed that mechanical deformability occurred in both the hamster and the mouse. Hamster oocytes do not show zona hardening following regular solubilization methods.

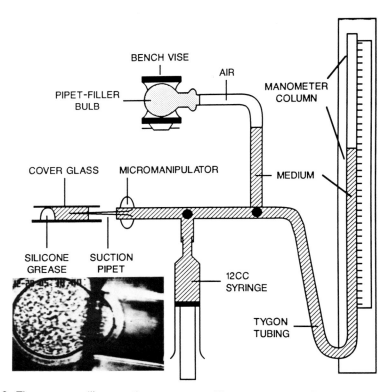

FIG. 8.8. The zona capillary-suction apparatus. The manometer indicates the pressure exerted upon the zona of the oocyte or embryo, which is held on the micropipette. Gross changes in pressure are controlled with the syringe, whereas small changes in pressure are controlled with a pipette-filling bulb. The photograph *(insert)* was taken from the video monitor of a hamster oocyte deformed into the suction pipette. The measure deformation for this frame was 32 μm. (From Drobnis EZ, et al. Biophysical properties of the zona pellucida measured by capillary suction: is zona hardening a mechanical phenomenon? *J Exp Zool* 1988;245:206–219, with permission. Copyright © 1988, reprinted with permission of Wiley-Liss, a division of John Wiley and Sons, Inc.)

Prolonged exposure of human oocytes and embryos to artificial conditions appears to impair their ability to implant. The incidence of birth following culture of embryos for several days in vitro is generally believed to be lower among fertile couples who conceive naturally or infertile couples whose zygotes are returned to the fallopian tube (57). One can only speculate about the causes of embryonic failure. In general, four areas are considered to play a key role: These are, first, the follicular environment and endometrial receptivity, which are both under endocrinologic control (58); second, embryonic implantation can be influenced by the replacement procedure; and, third, as many as 38% of early conceptuses are genetically imbalanced (59,60). The fourth cause of embryonic demise lies entirely in the domain of the embryology laboratory. The artificial conditions to which gametes and embryos are exposed may cause either a delay of the cell cycle or an overall breakdown of cellular processes, which can be measured by the general presence of cellular fragmentation (61).

Recently, we suggested a fifth factor that may cause embryonic death after IVF (28). Failure of zona rupture and shedding following complete blastocyst expansion may be a consequence of either in vitro-induced zona hardening or a phenomenon inherent to a substantial number of human embryos, irrespective of their conception in vivo or in vitro. What is the rationale for suggesting such a hypothesis? One of the most important reasons is derived from the study of implantation following microsurgical fertilization. Both the timing and morphology of the in vitro-hatching process of mouse and human zona-dissected embryos are altered (31). The zona does not thin as it does normally during blastocyst expansion, and hatching occurs earlier (Fig. 8.9). Evidence is accumulating from relatively large series of observations that human embryos that were partially zona-dissected before fertilization implant to a higher extent than zona-intact embryos (26,49,62). The incidence of implantation of such embryos in patients who received corticosteroids and antibiotics ranged from 20% to 28%.

Another important observation leading to the study of "assisted hatching" was the finding that some cleaved human embryos had uniform zonae, whereas others had thin patches. Cleaved embryos with thinned areas in their zonae appear to implant more frequently then embryos with uniform zonae. This morphologic characteristic is reliable and consistent and provides a significant factor by which to predict embryonic implantation. The zonae of 25% of human embryos actively thin between the zygote and four-cell stages (42). However, many embryos have not thinned their zonae at the time of replacement, 2 days following oocyte collection. Consequently, it may be postulated that the ability of some human embryos to undergo hatching could be enhanced by artificial thinning or opening of the zona.

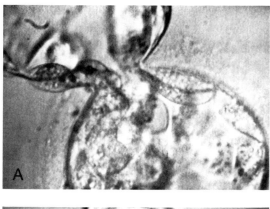

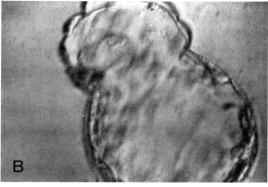

FIG. 8.9. Five-day-old human embryo (day 1 is day of egg collection) zona drilled with acidic Tyrode's at the eight-cell stage **(A)**. Note that the hole is sufficiently large to allow free migration of blastocyst cells. In comparison a nonmicromanipulated spare blastocyst **(B)**, in which hatching commences late on day 6. The hatching area is considerably larger than in the micromanipulated embryo. Normal hatching in the human occurs following complete expansion and zona thinning.

A number of other findings in recent years support the hypothesis that some human IVF embryos lack the ability to produce zona lysins or that their zonae pellucidae withstand normal dissolution. Only one in four fully expanded blastocysts derived from in vitro-fertilized ovarian oocytes will hatch (63,64). This provides evidence that human blastocysts are capable of hatching in the absence of uterine lysins, but it also demonstrates that zonae are often resilient to dissolution. The incidence of blastocyst formation and hatching can be increased by culturing human embryos on monolayers of reproductive tract cells (61,64). This finding supports the argument that many in vitro-fertilized embryos are deficient in the amount of zona lysins needed to initiate and complete hatching.

Assisted Hatching: Which Methods Can Be Used?

There are several issues to consider prior to routine opening of human zonae for therapeutic purposes. Thawed human cleaved embryos with large gaps in their zonae do not develop into viable fetuses. This may be due to embryonic cell loss through the zona as a result of uterine contractions. Similar results were obtained when precompacted mouse embryos with large openings in their zonae were transferred into the oviduct (19). However, other investigators reported high rates of implantation following biopsy of eight-cell human embryos using acidic Tyrode's solution (65). Test results of the preimplantation diagnosis were obtained only after 6 or more hours. Biopsied embryos were therefore replaced at the time of early compaction. It may be advantageous to transfer embryos with substantial holes in their zonae after increased adherence of the blastomeres.

Although development of mouse embryos is not affected following the use of acidic Tyrode's to open the zona before fertilization, application in human oocytes appears limited, owing to the increased size and resilience of the zona pellucida and the limited buffering capacity of the small amount of perivitelline fluid. Microvilli on the plasma membrane were reduced by the acidic solution, and blastocyst formation was inhibited (3). These disadvantages should not necessarily be extrapolated to the fertilized human egg. Zona hardening improves the efficiency of acidic dissolution markedly, and the total volume of the perivitelline space in zygotes and embryos is increased. These differences may be sufficient to reconsider the application of acidic dissolution of the embryonic zona pellucida. Moreover, the use of acidic dissolution for blastomere biopsy in Ca^{2+}/Mg^{2+}-free medium has the advantage that the blastomere directly exposed to the micropipette will be removed.

The creation of a narrow slit following partial zona dissection of four-cell human embryos shortly before transfer may be advantageous, but could lead to trophoblast constriction or cell loss before the formation of junctional mechanisms between the blastomeres. Indeed, human embryos with narrow artificial slits in the zona hatch frequently in vitro, but most of these blastocysts will extrude and escape from the zona in several small trophectoderm vesicles. Blastocysts with larger acidic Tyrode's openings made at the early eight-cell stage usually hatch completely (see Fig. 8.9). The absence of zona thinning and expansion during expulsion of the blastocyst through the artificial opening may cause constriction of the trophoblast and the inner cell mass. The majority of micromanipulated blastocysts in the mouse with small partial zona dissection openings will become trapped in the zona, forming a figure-8 configuration (see Table 8.6). The human blastocyst appears much more fragile than that of the mouse, and the integrity of the trophoblast and the inner cell mass may be jeopardized during expulsion through a narrow opening. Consequently, the blastocyst may be dissected into several parts, or the inner cell mass may split and adhere to different areas of the trophoblast. Thus, it is not surprising that two twin pregnancies following assisted hatching were identical (28). Two fetuses with fetal heart activity were seen in a single sac in each case; however, both pairs miscarried.

Assisted hatching of cleaved embryos was applied to 99 patients, using partial zona dissection as the technique by which to open the zona (49). Embryos allocated for replacement were micromanipulated in alternate patients. This resulted in an experimental group (patients whose embryos were micromanipulated) and a control group (patients whose embryos had intact zonae). The zonae of a total of 144 fresh two- to eight-cell embryos were thus micromanipulated 2 days after egg collection. All embryos appeared intact following micromanipulation and none of the blastomeres were damaged. A maximum of three embryos were replaced per patient. Positive human β-chorionic gonadotropin (βhCG) was confirmed in 17/51 (34%) of the control patients who received zona-intact embryos, and 24/48 (50%) of the assisted-hatching patients (Table 8.7). The incidence of clinical pregnancy increased from 26% in the control group to 46% per embryo replacement in the experimental group, a significant improvement ($p < .05$). Moreover, embryonic implantation increased from 13% to 22% ($p < .05$). Half of the pregnancies in the experimental group were either twin or triplet pregnancies. From these experiments, it has been postulated that approximately one-quarter of all IVF embryos have the ability to implant, that a substantial number of IVF embryos are unable to breach the zona at the time of hatching, and that many can be rescued by opening their zonae several days earlier. It is as yet unclear whether assisted hatching by partial

TABLE 8.7. *Assisted-hatching with partial zona dissection of fresh (prospective randomized) and freeze-thawed (not randomized) 2-day-old human embryos (trial 1)*[a]

Status of the embryo	Definition of pregnancy	Zona pellucida	
		Intact	With incision
Fresh	Biochemical (per patient)	17/51 (34%)	24/48 (50%)
Fresh	Fetal heart beat (per patient)	13/51 (26%)	22/48 (46%)
Fresh	Per embryo	16/129 (13%)	32/144 (22%)
Thawed	Biochemical (per patient)	6/23 (26%)	7/19 (37%)
Thawed	Fetal heart beat (per patient)	6/23 (26%)	7/19 (37%)
Thawed	Per embryo	6/43 (14%)	8/35 (23%)

Data reprinted from Cohen J, et al. Gamete and embryo micromanipulation for infertility treatment. In: Mars RP, Speroff L, eds. *In Vitro Fertilization—Seminars in Reproductive Endocrinology.* New York: Thieme, Inc., 1990; 8(4):290–295.
[a]Performed at Reproductive Biology Associates

zona dissection should be applied as part of the standard IVF procedure. Only 7% of human embryos treated with assisted hatching implanted when we applied PZD in 20 couples at the IVF program at Cornell in 1989 (66). This series of investigations was not performed as part of a prospective randomized trial. However, the implantation rate of zona-intact embryos in this program normally exceeds 10%, indicating that narrow holes in the zonae may also have an adverse effect on implantation. This may have been due to many differences between culture methods and replacement procedures between the two IVF programs at the time. Others have also been unable to improve implantation with this method in small series. It may not always be advantageous to perform assisted hatching on an embryo, using the partial zona dissection technique, 2 days after egg collection. Zona hardening alters the resilience of the zona pellucida to the partial zona dissection technique; the incisions are easier to make and may be smaller than those made before fertilization.

Alternatively, embryos may be micromanipulated with acidic medium to increase the size of the opening after the formation of constructional junctions between the blastomeres. This may avoid the hazards imposed on the precompacted embryos during replacement and would facilitate trophoblast expulsion during hatching. Sixty regular IVF couples consented to have assisted hatching on the basis of a prospective randomized trial (30 experimental and 30 control couples). We present here the results of the first 2 months of this second assisted-hatching trial. The average age of the female partners was 38 (range 31–43). Patients with highly elevated day 3 follicle-stimulating hormone levels and those selected for microsurgical fertilization were excluded from the study. Limited sections of the zonae of all embryos from experimental patients were exposed to small amounts of acidic Tyrode's (Table 8.8). The diameter of the sizable holes ranged from 15 to 30 μm. The incidence of clinical pregnancy of the experimental and control groups of patients was 57% (17/30) and 40% (12/30), respectively (see Table 8.8). The incidence of implantation of zona-drilled embryos was 32% (33/103). Although this compared favorably with the implanting ability of zona-intact embryos (19%; 19/98), the difference was only slightly signifi-

TABLE 8.8 *Preliminary results of a randomized trial of assisted hatching performed with acidic Tyrode's applied to 3-day-old embryos in 60 patients at The Center for Reproductive Medicine and Infertility, The New York Hospital–Cornell Medical Center*

Parameter	Zona drilled	Zona intact
Mean age of female partner (range)	37 (31–43)	38 (31–43)
Positive human β-chorionic gonadotropin	18/30 (60%)	13/30 (43%)
Fetal heart beat (per patient)	17/30 (57%)	12/30 (40%)
Implantation per embryo	34/103 (33%)[a]	19/98 (19%)[a]

Cohen J, Alikani M, Rosenwaks Z, unpublished results.
[a]$p < .05$

cant ($p<.05$). We conclude from these and other preliminary findings that (a) large artificially made holes in the zona pellucida following the third cleavage division probably promote implantation, (b) there is a difference between the oocyte and the embryo in the sensitivity to acidic Tyrode's, and (c) it is the embryos with evenly shaped zonae (conclusions derived from retrospective measurements of zonae from videotapes) that especially benefit from assisted-hatching procedures.

Assisted Hatching: Step by Step

Presently, two methods, partial zona dissection and zona drilling with acidic Tyrode's, have been used for promoting hatching. Both methods have advantages and disadvantages, but it is likely that two important principles will prevail for the safe application of these techniques in the future. First, large holes are more efficient for supporting hatching than small holes and, second, embryos with large gaps in their zonae should be replaced after the onset of compaction. Whether the use of acidic solution will be a reliable mode for routine application is somewhat doubtful. It is possible that its use is detrimental to blastomere(s) adjacent to the exposure area in the zona and that other blastomeres may be affected as well. The latter is especially likely when acidic solution is used after intracellular communication systems are already in place.

The procedure used for performing assisted hatching during our first trial closely follows that of the partial zona dissection technique described previously, except that hyaluronidase and sucrose were not used to pretreat the embryos. Excessive amounts of corona cells were removed with hypodermic needles or by suction from the holding pipette. Embryos were micromanipulated in droplets of sucrose-free culture medium under oil in glass-well slides. The oil, culture medium, and slide were kept at 37°C before micromanipulation. Oil and medium were preequilibrated with 5% CO_2, 5% O_2, and 90% N_2. The micromanipulation was performed between 5 and 200 minutes before replacement. Only one embryo at a time was pipetted into the well slide. Each micromanipulation procedure required 1 to 5 minutes. All embryos allocated for replacement were micromanipulated.

Micromanipulations were performed on a heated stage, attached to an inverted microscope equipped with Nomarski optics. Embryos were secured onto the holding pipette in such a way that the indentation between two adjacent blastomeres was between the 2- and 3-o'clock positions (Fig. 8.10). The zona pellucida was then pierced with the microneedle on that side until the needle tip was visible in the perivitelline space. The zona pellucida was moved upward, and the microneedle was pushed tangentially through the space between the zona and blastomere until it pierced the zona again. The zona pellucida often hardens following fertilization, and it may

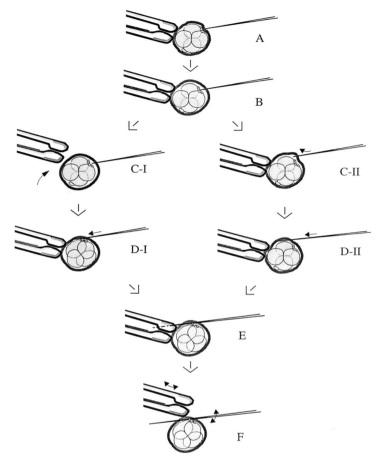

FIG. 8.10. Assisted-hatching step by step using partial zona dissection. See text for explanation.

not be possible to move the needle through both sides in one smooth movement. Moreover, if the blastomeres are swollen the embryo may have to be moved before it can be pierced again. The suction on the holding pipette can be released after the zona is pierced once and the embryo can be rolled around slightly before the second piercing (see Fig. 8.10).

Extracellular fragments were occasionally pierced during this procedure, if this facilitated micromanipulation. The suction was discontinued, and the holding pipette was rubbed over the small part of the zona trapped against the microneedle. The procedure was completed when the area between the two sides pierced by the microneedle was opened, leaving a narrow incision in the zona. The actual openings could rarely be seen following micromanipulation, as opposed sides along the incision remained rigid (unlike that of the unfertilized egg). The procedure was never repeated at a different side of the zona pellucida.

Zona drilling with acidic Tyrode's (Table 8.9) was performed approximately 72 hours following egg collection. Transfers were performed 5 to 7 hours later. The scope of this procedure was to drill before the formation of intracellular mechanisms and to replace the embryos after these connections had been established. The procedures were either performed in PBI supplemented with 10% Plasmanate or in equilibrated human tubal fluid extended with 15% homologous serum. Micromanipulations were performed with straight microtools, and the embryo was contained in a small microdroplet under mineral oil in a depression slide. Embryos were micromanipulated individually and immediately washed four times to remove acidic medium.

Embryos were clamped onto the holding pipette (syringe suction system) in such a way that the acidic Tyrode's-filled microneedle at the 3-o'clock area was exposed to empty perivitelline space or to cellular fragments (Fig. 8.11). The microneedle was front loaded before each micromanipulation, using mouth-controlled suction. Acidic medium was expelled gently over a small area (30 μm) by holding the needle tip very close to the zona. Small circular motions were sometimes made to avoid excess acid in a single area. The inside of the zona is more difficult to pierce and the expulsion pressure must frequently be increased. It is recommended that the optical system be optimized for this part of the procedure, since the stream of acidic medium may be relatively invisible, and the piercing of the inside of the zona may go by unnoticed. Expulsion of acidic medium should be ceased immediately when the inside of the zona is pierced or softened. Suction is recommended at this point. A small "inside" hole may be widened mechanically by moving the microneedle through the opening in a tearing motion while continuing gentle suction. Small fragments may be removed, since this does not seem to interfere with further development.

TABLE 8.9. *Preparation of acidic Tyrode's (pH is varied between 2.3 and 2.5)*

Compound	For 1L
NaCl	8.00 g
KCl	0.20 g
$CaCl_2 \cdot 2H_2O$	0.20 g
$MgCl_2 \cdot 6H_2O$	0.10 g
$NaH_2PO_4 \cdot H_2O$[a]	0.05 g
Glucose	1.00 g
PVP (polyvinylpyrrolidone)	4.00 g
H_2O	1.00L
Titrate to pH 2.3–2.5 with HCl	

[a] If anhydrous NaH_2PO_4 is used, 0.04 g

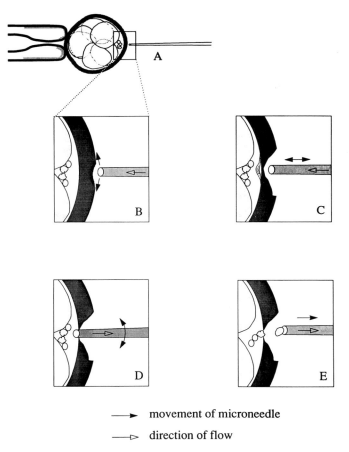

——▶ movement of microneedle

——▷ direction of flow

FIG. 8.11. Assisted-hatching step by step using acidic Tyrode's. *Closed arrows* represent movements of tools. *Open arrows* indicate suction. See text for further explanation.

REFERENCES

1. Wentz AC, Repp JE, Maxson WS, Pittaway DE, Torbit CA. The problem of polyspermy in in vitro fertilization. *Fertil Steril* 1983;40:748–754.
2. Kola I, Trounson A, Dawson G, Rogers P. Tripronuclear human oocytes: altered cleavage patterns and subsequent karyotypic analysis of embryos. *Biol Reprod* 1987;37:395–401.
3. Malter HE, Cohen J. Embryonic development after microsurgical repair of polyspermic human zygotes. *Fertil Steril* 1989;52:373-380.
4. Gordon JW, Grunfeld L, Garrisi BJ, Talansky BE, Richards C, Laufer N. Fertilization of human oocytes by sperm from infertile males after zona pellucida drilling. *Fertil Steril* 1988;50:68–73.
5. Cohen J, Malter H, Wright G, Kort H, Massey J, Mitchell D. Partial zona dissection of human oocytes when failure of zona pellucida penetration is anticipated. *Hum Reprod* 1989;4:435–442.

6. Cohen J, Alikani M, Malter HE, Adler A, Talansky BE, Rosenwaks Z. Partial zona dissection or subzonal sperm insertion: microsurgical fertilization alternatives based on evaluation of sperm and embryo morphology. *Fertil Steril* 1991;56 (in press).
7. Malter H, Talansky B, Gordon J, Cohen J. Monospermy and polyspermy after partial zona dissection of reinseminated human oocytes. *Gamete Res* 1989;24:377–386.
8. Surani MAH, Barton SC. Development of gynogenetic eggs in the mouse: implications for parthenogenetic embryos. *Science* 1983;222:1034–1036.
9. Gordon JW, Grunfeld L, Garrisi GJ, Navot D, Laufer N. Successful microsurgical removal of a pronucleus from tripronuclear human zygotes. *Fertil Steril* 1989;52:367–372.
10. Kajii T, Ohama K. Androgenetic origin of hydatidiform mole. *Nature* 1977;268:633–634.
11. Surti U, Szulman AE, O'Brien S. Complete (classic) hydatidiform mole with 46 XY karyotype of paternal origin. *Hum Genet* 1979;51:153–155.
12. Jacobs PA, Szulman AE, Funkhouser J, Matsuura JS, Wilson CC. Human triploidy: relationship between parental origin of the additional haploid complement and development of partial hydatidiform mole. *Ann Hum Genet* 1982;46:223–231.
13. Lawler SD, Fisher RA, Pickthall VJ, Povey S, Wyn Evans M. Genetic studies on hydatidiform moles. I. The origin of partial moles. *Cancer Genet Cytogenet* 1982;5: 309–320.
14. Vejerslev LO, Dissing J, Hansen HE, Poulsen H. Hydatidiform mole: genetic origin in polyploid conceptuses. *Hum Genet* 1987;76(1):11–19.
15. Wiker S, Malter H, Wright G, Cohen J. Recognition of paternal pronuclei in human zygotes. *J In Vitro Fert Embryo Transfer* 1990;7:33–37.
16. Edwards RG. Cleavage of one-and two-celled rabbit eggs in vitro after removal of the zona pellucida. *J Reprod Fertil* 1964;7:413–415.
17. Schlafke S, Enders AC. Cytological changes during cleavage and blastocyst formation in the rat. *J Anat* 1967;102:13–32.
18. Modlinski JA. The role of the zona pellucida in the development of mouse eggs in vitro. *J Embryol Exp Morphol* 1970;23:539–547.
19. Nichols J, Gardner RL. Effect of damage to the zona pellucida on development of preimplantation embryos in the mouse. *Hum Reprod* 1989;4:180–187.
20. Bronson RA, McLaren A. Transfer to the mouse oviduct of eggs with and without the zona pellucida. *J Reprod Fertil* 1970;22:129–137.
21. Trounson AO, Moore NW. The survival and development of sheep eggs following complete or partial removal of the zona pellucida. *J Reprod Fertil* 1974;41:97–105.
22. Willadsen SM. A method for culture of micromanipulated sheep embryos and its use to produce monozygotic twins. *Nature* 1979;277:298–301.
23. Willadsen SM. *Micromanipulation of embryos of the large domestic species* [Dissertation]. Copenhagen, 1982.
24. Moore NW, Adams CE, Rowson LEA. Developmental potential of single blastomeres of the rabbit egg. *J Reprod Fertil* 1968;17:527–531.
25. Oliver JM, Berlin RD: Surface cytoskeletal events regulating membrane topography. *Semin Hematol* 1983;20:282–304.
26. Cohen J, Malter H, Elsner C, Kort H, Massey J, Mayer MP. Immunosuppression supports implantation of zona pellucida dissected human embryos. *Fertil Steril* 1990;53: 662–665.
27. Jandl JH. Chronic lymphatic leukemia. In: *Blood.* Boston: Little Brown & Co; 1987:769.
28. Cohen J, Wright G, Malter H, et al. Impairment of the hatching process following in vitro fertilization in the human and improvement of implantation by assisting hatching using micromanipulation. *Hum Reprod* 1990;5:7–13.
29. Whitten WK. Culture of tubal ova. *Nature* 1957;179:1081.
30. Cole RJ. Cinemicrographic observation on the trophoblast and zona pellucida of the mouse blastocyst. *J Embryol Exp Morphol* 1967;17:481–490.
31. Malter H, Cohen J. Blastocyst formation and hatching in vitro following zona drilling of mouse and human embryos. *Gamete Res* 1989;24:67–80.
32. Nieder GL, Caprio TL. Early development in the Siberian hamster (*Phodopus sungorus*). *Mol Reprod Dev* 1990;27:224–229.
33. McLaren A. The fate of the zona pellucida in mice. *J Embryol Exp Morphol* 1970;23:1–19.
34. Wiley LM. Cavitation in the mouse preimplantation embryo: Na/K-ATPase and the origin of nascent blastocoele fluid. *Dev Biol* 1984;105:330–342.

35. Brinster RL. Protein content of the mouse embryo during the first five days of development. *J Reprod Fertil* 1967;13:413–420.
36. Cholewa JA, Whitten WK. Development of two-cell mouse embryos in the absence of a fixed-nitrogen source. *J Reprod Fertil* 1970;22:553–555.
37. Spindle AI, Pedersen RA. Hatching, attachment, and outgrowth of mouse blastocysts in vitro: fixed nitrogen requirements. *J Exp Zool* 1973;186:305–318.
38. Mintz B. Control of embryo implantation and survival. *Adv Biosci* 1971;6:317–342.
39. McLaren A. A study of blastocysts during delay and subsequent implantation in lactating mice. *J Endocrinol* 1968;42:453–463.
40. Wright RW, Watson JG, Chaykin S. Factors influencing the in vitro hatching of mouse blastocysts. *Anim Reprod Sci* 1978;1:181–188.
41. Cohen J, Inge KL, Suzman K, Wiker SR, Wright R. Videocinematography of fresh and cryopreserved embryos: a retrospective analysis of embryonic morphology and implantation. *Fertil Steril* 1989;51:820–827.
42. Wright G, Wiker S, Elsner C, et al. Observations on the morphology of pronucleoli in human zygotes and implications for cryopreservation. *Hum Reprod* 1990;5:109–115.
43. Nieder GL, Weitlauf HM, Suda-Hartman M. Synthesis and secretion of stage specific proteins by peri-implantation mouse embryos. *Biol Reprod* 1987;36:687–692.
44. Post LL, Schuel R, Schuel H. Evidence that hatching enzyme of the sea urchin *Stronylocentrotus pupuratus* is a chymotrypsin-like protease. *Biochem Cell Biol* 1988;66:1200–1209.
45. Lepage T, Gache C. Purification and characterization of the sea urchin embryo hatching enzyme. *J Biol Chem* 1989;264:4787–4793.
46. Yasumasu S, Katow S, Umino Y, Iuchi I, Yamagami K. A unique proteolytic action of HCE, a constituent protease of a fish hatching enzyme: tight binding to its natural substrate, egg envelope. *Biochem Biophys Res Commun* 1989;161:58–63.
47. Talansky BE, Gordon JW. Cleavage characteristics of mouse embryos inseminated and cultured after zona pellucida drilling. *Gamete Res* 1988;21:277–287.
48. Cohen J, Feldberg D. Effects of the size and number of zona pellucida openings on hatching and trophoblast outgrowth in the mouse embryo. *Mol Reprod Dev* 1991; (in press).
49. Cohen J, Malter H, Talansky B, Tucker M, Wright G. Gamete and embryo micromanipulation for infertility treatment. In: Marrs RP, Speroff L, eds. *In Vitro Fertilization—Seminars in Reproductive Endocrinology.* New York: Thieme Inc; 1990:8(4):290–295.
50. DeFelici M, Siracusa G. "Spontaneous" hardening of the zona pellucida of mouse oocytes during in vitro culture. *Gamete Res* 1982;6:107–113.
51. Downs SM, Schroeder AC, Eppig JJ. Serum maintains the fertilizability of mouse oocytes matured in vitro by preventing hardening of the zona pellucida. *Gamete Res* 1986;15:115–122.
52. Longo FJ. Changes in the zonae pellucidae and plasmalemmae of aging mouse eggs. *Biol Reprod* 1981;25:399–411.
53. Austin CR. *The mammalian egg.* Oxford: Blackwell Scientific Publications; 1961:89–97.
54. Gwatkin RBL. *Fertilization mechanisms in man and mammals.* New York: Plenum Press; 1977:91–108.
55. Betteridge KJ, Flood PF, Mitchell P. Possible role of the embryo in the control of oviductal transport in mares. In: Harper MJK, Pauerstein CJ, Adams CE, Coutinho EM, Croxatto HB, Paton DM, eds. *Ovum transport and fertility regulation.* Copenhagen: Scriptor; 1976:381–389.
56. Drobnis EZ, Andrew JB, Katz DF. Biophysical properties of the zona pellucida measured by capillary suction: is zona hardening a mechanical phenomenon? *J Exp Zool* 1988;245:206–219.
57. Yovich JL, Yovich JM, Edirisinghe WR. The relative chance of pregnancy following tubal or uterine transfer procedures. *Fertil Steril* 1988;49:858–864.
58. Keenan D, Cohen J, Suzman M, Wright G, Kort H, Massey J. Stimulation cycles suppressed with gonadotropin-releasing hormone analog yield accelerated embryos. *Fertil Steril* 1991; (in press).
59. Plachot M, De Grouchy, Junca AM, Mandelbaum J, Salat-Baroux J, Cohen J. Chromosomal analysis of human oocytes and embryos in an in vitro fertilization program. *Ann NY Acad Sci* 1988;451:384–397.

60. Martin RH, Rademaker A. The frequency of aneuploidy among individual chromosomes in 6821 human sperm chromosome complements. *Cytogenet Cell Genet* 1990;53:103–107.
61. Wiemer KE, Cohen J, Wiker SR, Malter HE, Wright G, Godke RA. Coculture of human zygotes on fetal bovine uterine fibroblasts: embryonic morphology and implantation. *Fertil Steril* 1989;52:503–508.
62. Tucker MJ, Bishop FM, Cohen J, Wiker SR, Wright G. Routine application of partial zona dissection for male infertility. *Hum Reprod* 1991;56: (in press).
63. Fehilly CB, Cohen J, Simons RF, Fishel SB, Edwards RG. Cryopreservation of cleaving embryos and expanded blastocysts in the human: a comparative study. *Fertil Steril* 1985;44:638–644.
64. Lindenberg S, Hyttel P, Sjogren A, Greve T. A comparative study of attachment of human, bovine and mouse blastocysts to uterine epithelial monolayer. *Hum Reprod* 1989;4:446–456.
65. Handyside AH, Kontogianni EH, Hardy K, Winston RML. Pregnancies from biopsied human preimplantation embryos sex by Y-specific DNA amplification. *Nature* 1990;344:378–770.
66. Cohen J, Grifo J, Malter HE, Talansky BE. Gamete and embryo micromanipulation. In: Marrs RP, ed. *The assisted reproductive technologies.* Oxford: Blackwell Scientific Publications; (in press).

9

Preconception and Preimplantation Genetic Diagnosis: Polar Body, Blastomere, and Trophectoderm Biopsy

Jamie Grifo

Thirty-five years have passed since the classic article was published by Watson and Crick in which a model was described for the structure of DNA (1). Gene cloning and DNA sequencing are now routine techniques. The application of gene therapy becomes more realistic as our knowledge of gene regulation increases. Concurrent with this increased understanding of molecular biology has been significant progress in the area of assisted reproductive technology. Increased implantation rates in excess of 20% per embryo have been reported (see Chap. 8). In vitro fertilization has created an opportunity to study the genetics and developmental potential of the preimplantation embryo.

Access to the preimplantation human embryo has enabled the embryologist to perform genetic analysis by removing polar bodies, blastomeres, or trophectodermal cells. Increased sensitivity of DNA analyses permits certain genetic diagnoses to be made utilizing a single cell. Currently, it is possible to determine the sex of an embryo by removing a blastomere and analyzing it by the polymerase chain reaction (PCR) or by in situ hybridization. As molecular geneticists map the human genome, it will be possible to perform genetic diagnosis during the preimplantation period for a variety of diseases. The purpose of this chapter is to review current methods of preimplantation diagnosis. A variety of techniques for evaluating the early embryo, such as polar body biopsy, blastomere removal, and trophectoderm sampling, have been investigated. In addition, methods for genetic analysis of single cells or small numbers of cells have been utilized. The polymerase chain reaction amplifies a single fragment of known DNA to as many as 1 million copies (2,3). In situ hybridization allows one to visualize a sequence of DNA present in a cell and may be of important diagnostic value in the future (4).

PREEMBRYO BIOPSY TECHNIQUES

The first successful preimplantation genetic diagnosis was performed by Gardner and Edwards in 1968 (5). Rabbit blastocysts were sexed by the removal of trophectodermal tissue, followed by the examination of sex chromatin. They confirmed these gender diagnoses in newborn rabbits following transfer of the blastocysts to host mothers. These techniques have been further refined to routinely determine the gender of cattle blastocysts for use in commercial embryo transfer (6). Because of the increased cell number, trophectodermal biopsy would be an advantageous alternative for preimplantation diagnosis. However, this method appears to have limited use in humans. Currently, in vitro fertilization (IVF) technology and culture methods do not permit the routine recovery of human blastocysts. Only 30% to 40% of human embryos cultured in vitro will proceed to the blastocyst stage. Although some blastocysts can be recovered from the uterus by transcervical flushing, this is an inefficient procedure (7,8).

Despite these advantages, embryo biopsy technology is currently focused on the precompaction embryo. This is due to the widespread availability of four- to eight-cell embryos from in vitro fertilization. One group of investigators is testing polar body biopsy as a possible method for preconception genetic diagnosis (9). Since it involves study of the oocyte, this method may be used only in those instances in which the disease is maternally derived.

There are a number of animal models available for studying preimplantation genetic diagnosis. Monk and coworkers (10) described the preimplantation diagnosis of hypoxanthine phosphoribosyltransferase (HPRT) deficiency in the mouse as a model for Lesch–Nyhan syndrome. In this study they mated females, heterozygous for HPRT deficiency, with normal males. Offspring from this mating either include 50% normal and 50% affected males, or 50% normal and 50% carrier females. Embryos were obtained and sampled at the eight-cell stage. A microenzyme assay was used by the investigators to analyze the activity of HPRT and adenosine phosphoribosyltransferase (APRT) in single blastomeres and categorized the embryos as affected or normal. The *APRT* gene is autosomally located. In the male, the presence of only one X chromosome directs synthesis of

HPRT, whereas in the female two X chromosomes are involved. The differential expression of the ratio of HPRT to APRT in the male and female embryos permitted both gender determination and the detection of an HPRT-deficient male. However, since there was great variability in the assay, a single measurement of only HPRT would not be sufficient for determination of HPRT deficiency. Only when the HPRT/APRT ratio was assessed could the distribution be evaluated. This requirement for a second enzyme limits the potential of the microenzyme assay. Results of the analyses were rapidly available so that the embryos could be transferred in the same cycle. Subsequent analyses of the resulting offspring showed that the selective procedure had been successful. This work was further characterized by trophectoderm biopsy performed in mouse embryos at the blastocyst stage (11). Embryos were flushed from the uterus, diagnosed, and returned within 2 days without the need for cryopreservation. As before, affected male embryos as well as carrier females were identified among the offspring. These two studies utilized microenzyme assays for diagnosing the presence or absence of gene products; here an enzyme activity.

Trophectodermal biopsy was also performed in marmoset monkeys (12). With micromanipulation techniques, a tear was made in the zona pellucida opposite the inner cell mass of eight-day blastocysts. This tear facilitated the controlled herniation of trophectodermal cells as the blastocysts expanded in vitro. The herniated trophectoderm was cut off and the biopsied blastocysts were transferred to recipients. Normal offspring were born. Biopsies from 30 to 50 cells from day-10 blastocysts were cultured in vitro, and trophoblast vesicles with an excess of a thousand cells were obtained. However, biopsies from day-9 blastocysts contained fewer than 20 cells and formed a monolayer of binucleated cells, with limited cell replication. Viable pregnancies were obtained by this method. A pregnancy was also derived from a biopsied blastocyst that had been frozen. This technique is of potential use in the human.

A mouse model was utilized to develop four- to eight-cell embryo biopsy techniques. Wilton and Trounson (13) reported a successful single-cell biopsy and cryopreservation of preimplantation mouse embryos. They described a method of removing a single blastomere from a four-cell mouse embryo, which did not compromise further development in vitro or in vivo. When transferred to pseudopregnant mice, 60.3% and 64.3% of biopsied and control embryos, respectively, implanted. In addition, 52.6% and 52.4% of biopsied and control embryos, respectively, developed into fetuses. Embryos biopsied in this fashion could be successfully cryopreserved by ultrarapid freezing, even though there was a puncture site in the zona pellucida. Implantation rates and fetal formation rates of biopsied, thawed embryos were identical with those of controls. Wilton, Shaw, and Trounson (14) biopsied the successful culture of a single blastomere removed from an early embryo.

More than 90% of biopsied and control embryos reached the blastocyst stage after 48 hours of culture. Implantation rates of biopsied embryos were in excess of 53%. Individual blastomeres were cultured in vitro on extracellular matrix components, such as fibronectin, laminin, and a complex of laminin and nidogen, to enhance proliferation. After 6 days in culture, between 10 and 20 cells were obtained. These techniques would allow the introduction of embryo biopsy, coupled with cryopreservation, to enhance preimplantation diagnosis of a single blastomere. Many copies of the genetic material could be obtained for the application of various techniques, including karyotyping, in situ hybridization, and DNA amplification.

Currently, there is limited experience with human embryo biopsy. The landmark article by Handyside et al. (15) demonstrates the ability to sample a human embryo at the four-cell stage and determine the sex of the embryo before implantation. Embryos undergoing these micromanipulation techniques had similar viability and proceeded to the blastocyst stage at similar rates, when compared with control embryos. This work was used as the basis for a clinical trial of preimplantation sexing of embryos from couples at risk for transmitting sex-linked disorders. Gender determination of biopsied embryos was performed by amplifying Y chromosome-specific repeat sequences from a single blastomere, utilizing the polymerase chain reaction. The presence of a 149-base pair fragment denoted a male karyotype. Since 50% of the male embryos are affected, they were not transferred. Since female embryos were either carriers or homozygous for the normal allele (thus unaffected in both cases), female embryos were transferred exclusively. Pregnancies were established and viable normal female offspring have resulted (16). Additional pregnancies utilizing this method are also still in progress. This method serves as a model for preimplantation diagnosis for any disorder that can be assessed at the single-cell level.

This technology is, at present, rather limited. Although it is unlikely that the eight-cell embryo contains mosaicism, it is possible. In addition, genetic modification may occur after the eight-cell stage. For example, loss or inactivation of DNA following the analysis is possible, thus negating the analysis. Single-gene PCR and in situ hybridization are encumbered by hazards, such as maternal loss or contamination. Understanding all of these problems and solving them will, no doubt, expedite the expansion of this technology.

BIOPSY METHODS

Polar Body Removal

The polar body of an oocyte is removed for DNA analysis to determine if the oocyte contains the abnormal gene for a particular disease. This method is limited because it is an indirect method for analyzing the secondary oocyte. The first polar body from the oocyte of a woman who is a carrier for a particular genetic disorder will contain either the normal gene or the abnormal gene and, therefore, genetic analysis of the polar body will indirectly predict which gene is present in the egg. Assuming that no crossing-over has occurred, and that the genetic principles that occur in plants and lower animals apply to humans, analysis of the polar body can serve as method of preimplantation diagnosis. This also assumes that the mother is a carrier of a particular disorder that can be detected with a single copy as a template for DNA analysis. The first polar body is extruded from the developing oocyte during the first meiotic division and is not required for successful fertilization or normal embryonic development. Normal newborn offspring have resulted following the loss or destruction of the first polar body during partial zona dissection as treatment for male factor infertility. Ethically, the oocyte is preferred for micromanipulation since its loss or destruction is not equivalent to the loss or destruction of an embryo.

To perform polar body removal, a holding pipette and a beveled micropipette, approximately 12 to 15 µm in diameter are used. A description of microtool construction is presented in Chapter 10. The best pipette for polar body removal is the same as that used for subzonal insertion of sperm, although with a slightly larger inside diameter. The beveled pipette is filled with silicone oil before attaching it to the micromanipulator holder. The micropipettes are lowered into the depression slide, which contains a droplet of medium covered with mineral oil that has been equilibrated with the biopsy medium. A number of different media have been described and are detailed in Table 9.1. Excess oil is removed from the outer surface of the instruments and a small amount of medium is aspirated into the beveled pipette. Once the oocyte has been gently aspirated into place with the holding pipette, the oocyte is rotated, using the beveled pipette, until the polar body is at the 12-o'clock position. Careful attention is paid to avoid aspirating any corona cells that may still be attached to the zona pellucida. The beveled micropipette is passed through the zona, and the polar body is aspirated into the pipette. If the polar body is still attached to the ooplasm, further incubation is required before complete detachment. The beveled pipette is lifted out of the dish and handed to an assistant who is wearing gloves to avoid contamination with DNA from exfoliated cells. Procedures should be performed in a laminar flow hood when mineral oil is not used. The tip of the beveled pipette is lowered into a microcentrifuge tube containing high-performance liquid chromatography (HPLC)-grade, autoclaved, filtered water and the polar body is expelled. The pipette tip is then crushed on the bottom of the microcentrifuge tube. The oocyte is released from the holding pipette and transferred back to its original dish. This procedure is illustrated in Fig. 9.1.

TABLE 9.1. *Embryo biopsy media*

Medium 1: micromanipulation medium (mm)

Component	Concentration
NaCl	136.90 mM
KCl	2.68 mM
Na_2HPO_4	8.17 mM
KH_2PO_4	1.47 mM
$MgCl_2 \cdot 6H_2O$	0.50 mM
$CaCl_2 \cdot 2H_2O$	0.9 mM
Glucose	5.56 mM
100 U/mL penicillin-G	
0.001% phenol red	
Na pyruvate 0.0185 g/500 mL	
Osmolarity: 280–285 mOsm; pH: 7.35–7.4 (adjust with 1 N NaOH)	
For MM: 6% volume/volume plasmanate: phosphate-buffered saline (Dulbeccos; PBI) + Plasmanate	

Medium 2: PESB

Calcium, magnesium-free phosphate buffered saline (10 × stock from Sigma)
   Make a 1× solution with sterile double-distilled water
   Add the following reagents to a final concentration as indicated

Component	Concentration
Sucrose	0.1M
EDTA	0.01% (w/v)
Bovine serum albumin (BSA; fraction 5)	4 mg/mL

Medium 3[a]

Component	Concentration
NaCl	106 mM
KCL	2.7 mM
KH_2PO_4	1.5 mM
Na_2PO_4	8.1 mM
Glucose	5.6 mM
Sodium lactate	25 mM
Sodium Pyruvate	0.33 mM
EDTA	2.0 mM
Sucrose	100 mM
BSA (Fraction)	3 mg/mL

[a]Developed by J. Gordon and I. Gang.

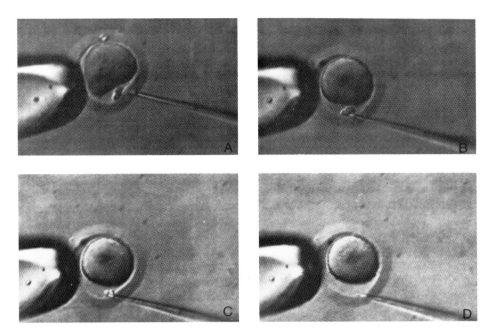

FIG. 9.1. Polar body removal. **A:** The sampling pipette is placed through the zona pellucida. **B,C:** The sampling pipette reaches the first polar body, and it is aspirated into the pipette. **D:** The pipette is removed, and its tip is broken into a microfuge tube for genetic analysis. (From Verlinsky Y, et al. Analysis of the first polar body: preconceptual genetic diagnosis. *Hum Reprod* 1990;5:826–829. By permission of Oxford University Press.)

Embryo Biopsy

Embryo biopsy may be performed on the same day as embryo transfer, if the DNA analysis is done rapidly and efficiently. The procedure can be carried out as soon as the embryo reaches the three-cell stage, but it is preferable to biopsy an embryo at a later cleavage stage, when the loss of one blastomere will pose a smaller threat to the viability of the embryo. There is evidence derived from studies with mouse embryos that the eight-cell stage is optimal. In fact, there have been human pregnancies with normal offspring from embryos biopsied at the eight-cell stage.

Since the embryo has been incubated in the insemination medium containing between 50,000 and 200,000 sperm, it is imperative that the embryo be thoroughly rinsed in fresh medium to remove contaminating sperm. It is essential that at least five transfers into microdrops of fresh medium (under oil) be performed, since analysis of the initial wash droplets has tested positive for DNA contamination.

The microtools used for embryo biopsy can be the same as for polar body removal; although it is preferable to use a beveled pipette with a larger-diameter (approximately 18 to 25 μm). We use a two-step procedure in which a hole is made in the zona pellucida by a method similar to that used for assisted hatching (see Chap. 8). However, a larger hole is required for blastomere removal. We perform this at the eight-cell stage and make a hole that is about half the diameter of the blastomere. A second pipette is then placed in the hole. It has an inside diameter of approximately one-third to one-half the diameter of the blastomere to be removed. During the aspiration of a blastomere, its membrane may break. Therefore, special care is taken that the nucleus is drawn into the pipette. For this reason, it is best to choose a blastomere with a clearly visible nucleus. Once aspirated, the blastomere and its nucleus are expelled into the microcentrifuge tube. It is preferable that the blastomere remain intact so that it can be rinsed in a series of microdrops to remove residual sperm or corona cells. We usually rinse the blastomere in at least five microdrops. A fresh sterile pipette is used to transfer the blastomere to the microdrops and to the PCR vessel. Figure 9.2 demonstrates this procedure.

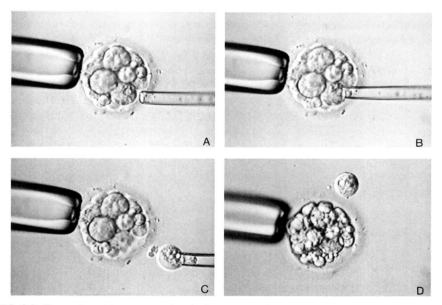

FIG. 9.2. The embryo biopsy procedure is demonstrated on an abnormal polyspermic human embryo. The embryo is picked up with a holding pipette and a hole is made in the zona pellucida. This is done with a fine micropipette filled with acidic Tyrode's solution. **A,B:** A second pipette about one-third the diameter of the blastomere is aspirated. **C,D:** It is removed from the embryo, released into the medium, and rinsed. Finally, it is placed into the microfuge tube for genetic analysis.

Blastocyst Biopsy

Trophectodermal biopsy is best accomplished when the hatching blastocyst extrudes through the zona pellucida. Since only a percentage of embryos in culture hatch spontaneously, it is advantageous to make a hole or slit in the zona using the methods of partial zona dissection or assisted

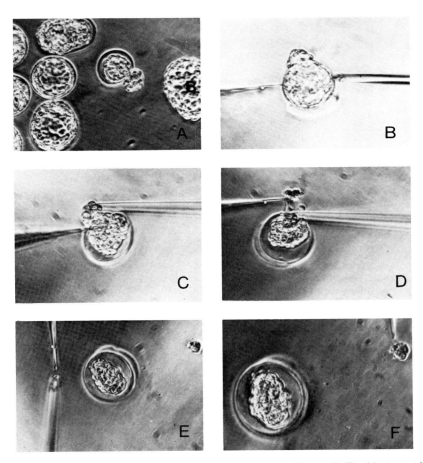

FIG. 9.3. A hatching blastocyst is selected for trophectoderm biopsy. **B:** The blastocyst has been manipulated by the microinstruments to extrude a number of cells through the zona pellucida. **C,D:** The micropipette sucks a number of cells away from the trophectoderm cell layer while the microneedle cuts the cell contacts. **E:** A clump of five to ten cells is placed on one side. **F:** The collapsed blastocyst within the zona pellucida is removed from the medium and cultured before transfer. (From Monk M, et al. Preimplantation diagnosis of HPRT-deficient male and carrier female mouse embryos by trophectoderm biopsy. *Hum Reprod* 1988;3:377–381, with permission.)

hatching (i.e., mechanically or with acidic Tyrode's solution) to increase the number of embryos available for this type of analysis.

The procedure is performed in two steps. First, using the same setup used for partial zona dissection, the zona is breached above the trophectoderm, opposite the inner cell mass. Alternatively, the hole in the zona pellucida can be made with a 2- to 3-μm inside-diameter microneedle loaded with acidic Tyrode's solution. The Tyrode's solution is delivered by gentle pressure until a small opening is made in the zona pellucida. Subsequently, the blastocyst is placed in culture until it begins to hatch through the opening made in the zona. Second, with a microneedle, herniated trophectodermal cells are pressed to the bottom of the petri dish. While moving the needle back and forth, assurance is made that the "neck" of the herniated blastocyst is sealed. The herniated piece is cut away by a razor blade attached to a metal arm held by the micromanipulator. This procedure can also be performed under a dissecting microscope by hand using a scalpel blade (N15). The biopsied cells are transferred into a microcentrifuge tube for genetic analysis, using a Pasteur pipette. Media supplemented with either bovine serum albumin (BSA) or another protein are preferred, since cells obtained by this method are "sticky." However, it is imperative that these substances are tested for contaminating DNA (see Fig. 9.3 for a representation of this procedure).

GENETIC ANALYSIS OF SINGLE CELLS

Microenzyme Assay

A microenzyme method has been utilized for preimplantation diagnosis of hypoxanthine phosphoribosyltransferase (HPRT) deficiency in the mouse. This methodology requires a sensitive assay that can measure specific enzyme activity to a level of femtomoles (10^{-15} mol) produced per hour. It also requires that the enzyme activity measured is adequately reflected by RNA synthesis and translation of that particular mRNA into active enzyme. In general, the microenzyme assay will have limited value. Recently, it has been used to obtain a preimplantation diagnosis of sex and detection of HPRT-deficient males (see earlier discussion).

Polymerase Chain Reaction

The polymerase chain reaction has opened a new frontier in genetic analysis. This method permits the amplification of a specific sequence of DNA by as much as 1 million times, and it now makes analysis of DNA from a single cell possible. The method capitalizes on the thermostability of *Thermus aquaticus,* polymerase (*Taq* polymerase), a thermophilic bacterium that can survive extended incubation above 90°C. The reaction is divided into three separate components: the melting reaction, the primer-annealing reaction, and the primer-extension reaction. A thermal-cycler permits the orderly progression from each step to the next. In the first reaction, the double-stranded target DNA is denatured at 94°C to single-stranded DNA. In the primer-annealing step, the temperature is lowered to a level, usually between 37° and 60°C, at which the specific primers can anneal to single-stranded DNA. Since the primers are in molar excess, they preferentially anneal to the DNA, rather than allowing the DNA to reform double strands. The primers are chosen such that they recognize a specific sequence of DNA of a length 50 to 2,000 base pairs (bp). Any known sequence of DNA can have primers constructed that will flank the region of interest. Most primers are from 15 to 25 bases in length and are easily produced on a DNA synthesizer. Each primer recognizes one of the two complementary strands of DNA. After annealing has been accomplished, the primer extension is started, whereby the primer serves as the start point of the *Taq* polymerase to synthesize a complementary copy of the DNA template. This reaction is usually carried out at 72°C, but each specific template may have an optimal temperature, which is determined empirically. In the first cycle, the length of the newly synthesized DNA extends beyond the boundary set by the primer pair (Fig. 9.4). At this point, the denaturation step is repeated, making all of the DNA single stranded. Now four single-stranded copies of DNA are present, including the original DNA template and two newly synthesized long fragments. All of these can now serve as templates for another round of annealing and primer extension. Thus, at the end of the second cycle of PCR, eight single-stranded fragments of DNA are present; the original template (two strands), a fragment of length defined by the region at which the primers flank (two stands, called the short fragments), and a fragment that polymerase was able to copy beyond the site at which the opposite primer flanks when the original DNA served as template (four strands, called long fragments) (Fig. 9.5).

As the reaction goes through several cycles there is a logarithmic increase in the number of short fragments, as the newly made short fragments become templates for the synthesis of others. There is an arithmetic increase in the number of long fragments, and there is no change in the number of copies of the original template. Thus, at the end of many cycles, the predominant DNA contained in the reaction vessel is a fragment of DNA of length defined by the number of base pairs separating the primer pair (Fig. 9.6).

For specific gene defects, PCR enables one to amplify a sequence of DNA that contains the site of the defect (deletion, mutation). Further strategies are being developed that allow a single gene from a single cell to be analyzed. Currently, the most useful application of PCR for preimplantation genetics is embryo sexing, using a single cell removed by biopsy. The strategy is based on chromosome-specific repeat sequences present on either the X or Y chromosome.

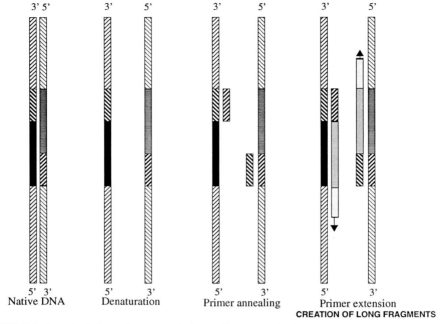

3' 5'   3'   5'   3'   5'   3'   5'

5' 3'   5'   3'   5'   3'   5'   3'
Native DNA   Denaturation   Primer annealing   Primer extension
CREATION OF LONG FRAGMENTS

FIG. 9.4. In cycle 1, the polymerase chain reaction occurs in three parts: denaturation, primer annealing, and primer extension. These steps constitute a cycle and are repeated many times. In the first cycle, the native template DNA is denatured allowing the primers access to bind in the annealing step. Polymerization follows as *Taq* polymerase extends the sequence. Extension continues beyond the end of the sequence flanked by the primers and, thus, long fragments are synthesized. This step occurs in each subsequent cycle.

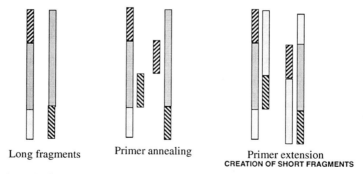

Long fragments   Primer annealing   Primer extension
CREATION OF SHORT FRAGMENTS

FIG. 9.5. In cycle 2, the long fragments also serve as template; however, when the end is reached, extension stops, thereby short fragments are created. These are the length that the primers flank.

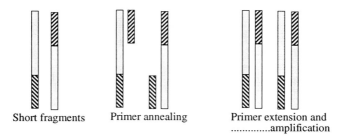

Short fragments   Primer annealing   Primer extension and
..............amplification

FIG. 9.6. In cycle 3, the short fragments serve as template, and primer extension results in the creation of a complimentary short fragment. In every subsequent cycle the steps in cycle 1, using native DNA as template, and in cycle 2, using long fragments as template, are duplicated. However, short fragments are duplicated geometrically, long fragments arithmetically, and native DNA not at all. The result after many cycles is a population of DNA fragments, mainly of a short fragment length.

In particular, two Y chromosome-specific primer sets have been utilized on blastomeres obtained from human embryo biopsy. Both primer pairs flank Y chromosome-specific repeat sequences, thus amplification of DNA is enhanced by the fact that 800 to 1,500 copies of the sequence of interest are contained in a single cell. In one instance, the additional strategy of utilizing nested primers also increases the level of sensitivity of the assay (16). This strategy involves a second amplification with a second primer set that anneals to a sequence contained within the first amplification product. Thus, the second amplification increases the product by another order of magnitude, making visualization using ethidium bromide and ultraviolet light more feasible. The other Y chromosome-specific primer pair described does not require nested primers to amplify DNA from a single cell (17).

Single-gene defect disorders could also potentially be identified with PCR analysis of single cells (Table 9.2). The DNA from single human oocytes has been genetically analyzed. Gene markers have been identified closely linked to the genes affected in cystic fibrosis and Duchenne muscular dystrophy. Thus, it is feasible to amplify DNA from a haploid cell. The β-hemoglobin sequences have been amplified in single oocytes and polar bodies. A 680-base pair sequence was obtained by first amplifying a 725-base pair fragment. The utilization of nested primers in this fashion offers a more sensitive method of analysis. Moreover, since the sickle cell mutation destroys the *Dde1* site, a method of distinguishing normal from sickle cell genotype is provided. Restriction analysis of the 680-base pair fragment amplified by this method and then digested by *Dde1* results in one 210- and one 180-base pair fragment when the normal gene is analyzed, and a diagnostic 381-base pair fragment when the sickle cell mutation is present (18).

TABLE 9.2. *Heritable disorders that could be diagnosed by embryo biopsy and the polymerase chain reaction*

X-Linked diseases
Lesch–Nyhan syndrome
Duschenne muscular dystrophy
X-Linked mental retardation
Adrenoleukodystrophy
Single-gene defects
Sickle cell anemia
Thalassemia
Cystic fibrosis
Tay–Sachs disease

Additionally, allele-specific oligonucleotide probes offer a very sensitive and specific method for detecting the hemoglobin *HbS, HbC,* and *HbA* genotypes and could be coupled with PCR analysis of single cells to provide a preimplantation diagnosis (19). Drawbacks of these methods are that the duration of analysis is prolonged and radioactively labeled probes are required. Cystic fibrosis has been diagnosed in embryos by analyzing the first polar body, as well as a blastomere (20). An embryo homozygous for the delta 508 deletion (affected) was thus identified and not replaced. Improvement of techniques for detection of single-gene disorders will be necessary before wide-scale application of preimplantation genetics.

In Situ Hybridization

In situ hybridization permits direct visualization of DNA sequences of interest in metaphase or interphase nuclei. Previously, this method utilized radiolabeled probes, coupled with autoradiography, to visualize specific binding of DNA probes to the cell. More recently, nonisotopic methods for in situ hybridization have provided a more rapid and direct method for visualization (21). In situ hybridization is ideal for numerical chromosomal analysis using chromosome-specific probes. In addition, it is not fraught with the hazards of contamination that plagues PCR technology.

Several factors have contributed to the improved techniques for nonisotopic in situ hybridization. First, probes can be modified by directly incorporating reporter molecules (i.e., biotin, digoxigenin, dinitrophenol) into the probe by utilizing nick translation (Fig. 9.7). Nonisotopic methods are considerably faster than autoradiographic methods. In addition, since signals are visualized directly under the microscope and not by capture into emulsion overlay, as in autoradiography, localization of signal is more precise. This factor also accounts for an increased sensitivity. Nonisotopic

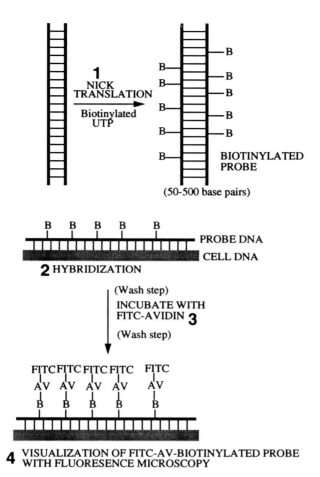

FIG. 9.7. A schematic representation of in situ hybridization. **1:** The DNA probe is nick-translated in the presence of biotinylated UTP, thereby incorporating biotin in the probe. **2:** The probe is then hybridized to the cell DNA. **3:** The biotin is bound by avidin, which is conjugated to a fluorescent molecule, here, fluorescein isothiocyanate (FITC). Unbound FITC-avidin is rinsed away by a washing step. **4:** Fluorescence microscopy is performed. This allows direct visualization of the DNA sequences present in the cell.

probes can be stored for years in the freezer. A major advantage of in situ hybridization is the ability to localize multiple signals using different reporter–detection systems. We have performed sexing of single cells using X and Y chromosome-specific probes with different reporter molecules [fluorescein isothiocyanate (FITC) and rhodamine], which give different color signals (Grifo JA, Boyle A, Ward DC, unpublished). Images were created using computer-enhanced signal detection coupled to a photomultiplier detector, with laser excitation of chromophobes on a confocal microscope.

We have used this system to perform in situ hybridization on blastomeres obtained from mouse preembryos by micromanipulation techniques. We are able to image the sodium/potassium ATPase gene on chromosome 3, as well as the X chromosome, and to determine if one or two copies (i.e., male versus female) are present in a single cell. In addition, we have been able to perform in situ hybridization on human embryos and image the X and Y chromosome (4). Other investigators have utilized in situ hybridization for rapid sexing of human embryos using nonisotopic methods of detection (22). Although this technology needs further development and better efficiency, it offers the potential for rapid, direct determination of gender and trisomy.

New and exciting developments in molecular genetics are allowing earlier prenatal diagnoses to be made. As reproductive technologies improve and as novel genetic techniques become more widespread, preimplantation diagnosis will become a feasible option for patients at genetic risk.

Polymerase Chain Reaction: Specific Methods

The polymerase chain reaction is relatively simple to perform. However, there are a number of details that must be addressed to ensure efficiency and reproducibility. Clearly, each set of primer pairs has an optimum concentration, magnesium ion concentration, and annealing temperature, which must be determined empirically. Primers must be synthesized consistently and prepared in the same solutions, such that they do not interfere with the PCR reaction. Differences obtained in amplification with the same primer sequences synthesized by different laboratories may reflect the fact that small and incomplete primer sequences contaminate the primers. These can be removed by an HPLC ion-exchange purification step after the primers are synthesized. In addition, differences have been noted when comparing native *Taq* polymerase with Amplitaq (recombinant *Taq* polymerase), as well as enzyme preparations from different manufacturers. Finally, there are a number of different thermal-cyclers available, and one must evaluate them and choose the one that is most suitable. The reaction is performed in 500-μL polypropylene microcentrifuge tubes that have been washed and autoclaved. Tubes that are not properly handled can be a source of DNA contamination, which will negate the analysis. Reactions are carried out in a final volume of 25 to 100 μL. Obviously the smaller volume requires using less of the expensive reagents, but is more susceptible to pipetting error. It is preferable to prepare a master mixture that contains all of the reagents in common for a particular assay and then to aliquot the necessary amount into each reaction vessel. Usually, this contains the nucleotide triphosphates, reaction buffer, magnesium chloride, and primers. The reaction buffer is usually prepared as a 10× stock, consisting of 100 mM Tris-HCl (HCl-neutralized tris[hydroxymethyl]aminomethane), pH 8.3,

500 mM potassium chloride, 15 mM magnesium chloride, and 0.01% (w/v) gelatin (Sigma Chemical Co.). A 1:10 dilution of this mixture gives the proper final concentration in the reaction vessel. The nucleotide triphosphates are usually added to a final concentration of 200 μM. (However, an optimum level can be determined empirically.) Since the optimal magnesium concentration can vary with triphosphate concentration, it is important to consider these variables together. The *Taq* polymerase is generally used at a level of 2.5 units/100 μL reaction. However, the optimal level may vary with the specific primer pair. If high levels of enzyme are used, artifacts may result. The order of additions is critical when performing single-cell PCR. It is preferable to make the master mixture first, in an area separate from where the samples are kept. The *Taq* polymerase should be added to the master mixture last and vortexed gently, with care taken not to raise bubbles, which can denature the enzyme. Unknown test samples should be

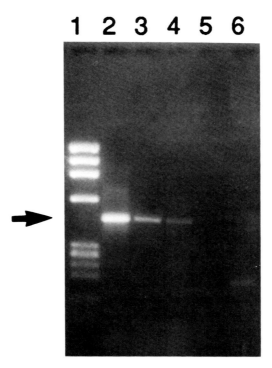

FIG. 9.8. Amplification of Y chromosome-specific sequences by the polymerase chain reaction/DNA titration curve. Varying amounts of genomic DNA were subjected to the polymerase chain reaction under standard conditions. *Lanes 2–4* contain amplification products, using male genomic DNA as template (*lane 2:* 1 ng; *lane 3:* 50 pg; *lane 4:* 10 pg). *Lanes 5* and *6* show amplification products using 100 ng of female genomic DNA as template. A single cell contains approximately 5 pg of DNA. The specific 500-base pair fragment amplified by this primer set is depicted by the *arrow*.

kept separate from the control samples, and a fresh pipette tip should be used to add the master mixture to each reaction tube. In addition, the master mixture should be added to tubes with the least amount of DNA first, then to the negative control, and, finally, to the positive control. It may be useful to have dedicated mechanical positive-displacement micropipettors. It is useful to have specific micropipettors for known samples of high DNA content and specific micropipettors for the unknown samples of single cells. Performing all manipulations under a laminar flow hood guards against the possibility of exfoliated cells contaminating the reaction vessel. Figure 9.8 demonstrates gel electrophoresis of DNA amplification products using a primer pair specific to a repeat sequence on the long arm of the Y chromosome. The remainder of this chapter presents detailed instructions for agarose gel electrophoresis and in situ hybridization.

DNA Electrophoresis Using a Minigel Apparatus

Precooling the Unit and Casting the Gel

1. To fill the interior, use pliers to unscrew the small plug located beneath the unit. Using a 50-mL syringe or pump, fill the cavity with approximately 60 mL of 50% ethylene glycol, leaving as little air as possible. Adding a drop or two of India ink makes the sample wells more visible for loading. Replace the plug. Once the unit has been filled, the coolant does not need to be removed. Whether or not you intend to run the minigel chilled, you should fill the interior with ethylene glycol (50%) or other suitable liquid. The liquid acts as a heat sink and protects the unit from the adverse effects of heating.
2. Place the filled unit in an ice bucket, refrigerator, or freezer to chill. Cooling takes 15 minutes in an ice bucket or about an hour in the refrigerator or freezer.
3. Set the casting tray on a level surface and insert the running plate. The running plate will extend over the rim of the casting tray.
4. Select a comb with the desired number of teeth and attach it to the comb backing by aligning the three slots in the comb with the smaller holes in the comb back. Place the small screws supplied with the comb back through the aligned holes and tighten loosely.
5. Position the comb across the width of the casting tray. If desired, two combs can be placed across the tray, one at the end and the other between the running plate handles. Adjust the depth of the comb to provide about 1 mm of space between the ends of the teeth and the surface of the running plate. This can be done by loosening the screws and moving the comb up or down on the comb back. Once the comb is at the proper depth, tighten the screws.

TABLE 9.3 *Agarose DNA buffers*

TCH buffer	Components	pH
Tris-borate (TBE)	89 mM boric acid 89 mM Tris base 2 mM EDTA	8.2
Tris-phosphate (TPE)	80 mM phosphoric acid 80 mM Tris base 8 mM EDTA	8.1
Tris-acetate (TAE)	20 mM acetic acid 40 mM Tris base 2 mM EDTA	8.4

6. Prepare a solution of agarose in running buffer. See Table 9.3 for the composition of the buffer solutions and Table 9.4 for the choice of agarose concentrations. Melt the agarose and allow it to cool to 50°C before pouring. For a 3-mm gel, you will need to prepare approximately 25 mL of agarose. **Warning:** Do not pour agarose hotter than 50°C or you may warp the casting unit.
7. Pour the agarose into the casting unit. (Some may seep under the casting plate.) Allow the agarose to harden for at least 30 minutes. (This time depends on the gel thickness.) Further hardening can be accomplished by pouring the running buffer over the gel.
8. The comb must be removed carefully so as not to disturb the gel. A vacuum has been created, and pulling the comb out gently at an angle avoids lifting the gel off the casting plate.

Running the Gel

1. After the gel tray is placed in the center of the unit, it is covered by at least 1 mm of running buffer. Adding 0.5 mg/mL of ethidium bromide to the bottom chamber will allow staining of the gel while the electrophoresis is

TABLE 9.4 *Agarose concentration for specific DNA fragment lengths*

% Agarose	DNA fragment length (kb)
0.3	60–50
0.6	20–10
0.7	10–0.8
0.9	7–0.5
1.2	6–0.4
1.5	4–0.2
2.0	3–0.0

in progress. This allows one to stop the gel at any point and monitor the progress of separation.

2. The sample is mixed with loading buffer that has a higher density than the running buffer and allows easy placement into the sample wells (composition: 0.35% bromophenol blue, 0.25% xylene cyanol, and 15% Ficoll 406). The sample may be diluted by as much as one-fifth with sample buffer.

3. The volumes of the sample wells are dependent upon the gel thickness, the comb size, and the number of wells that the comb makes. This must be checked for each individual apparatus.

4. The gel apparatus is attached to the power supply, making sure that the correct polarity is obtained. DNA is negatively charged and migrates toward the positive pole. The power setting and the running time depend upon the desired resolution. The *Hin*dIII digestion standard, which has fragments ranging from 100 to 23,000 base pairs, separates nicely on a 1% agarose gel run at a constant voltage of 150 volts for 30 minutes. The cooling system of the gel apparatus allows one to run the gel at high voltage for shorter times, with adequate resolution.

DNA Detection

1. The DNA may be visualized during the electrophoresis run using a hand-held UV lamp to monitor the separation.*

2. At the end of the run, the gel may be transferred to a transilluminator that delivers UV light from below the gel and allows efficient detection as well as a means to photograph the gel. Destaining the gel with 0.01 M $MgCl_2$ for 10 minutes aids in removing background ethidium bromide[†] and allows detection of nanogram quantities of DNA.

In Situ Hybridization: Specific Methods

Preparation of Samples for In Situ Hybridization

Sperm Preparation

Liquefy sperm
Pellet sperm in an IEC clinical centrifuge setting 5 for 10 min
Resuspend in 3 mL of phosphate-buffered saline (PBS)
Spin down
Resuspend in 3 mL of PBS

---

*When using UV light it is imperative that one wear goggles to protect the eyes from UV-mediated damage.
†Ethidium bromide is a potent carcinogen and must be handled appropriately. Consult your chemical safety department for its proper handling.

Remove 100 µL into microfuge tube
Add 100 µL acetic acid/methanol (1:3) for 10 min
Spin in a microfuge at 13,500 rpm for 5 min
Remove supernatant
Add 100 µL acetic acid/methanol (1:3) and incubate for 5 min
Resuspend by vortexing
Spread by dropping 10 µL on clean acid-washed glass slides
Dry in 55°C warm oven for 10 min

Permeabilize
(0.5% Triton X-100 and 0.5% saponin) in PBS
Incubate the slide for 10 min
Dip in liquid nitrogen for 30 sec
Remove and repeat two times
Rinse with PBS
Air-dry
   The slide is ready for in situ hybridization.

Blastomere Preparation

Remove blastomeres, taking care that they remain intact throughout the
   procedure.
   *Blastomere loss is the biggest problem associated with this method. Each
   step should be performed under a dissecting microscope and care should
   be taken to keep the blastomeres in sight at all times.*
   *The fixation method is a modification of the Tarkowski air-drying
   method (24), which has been improved upon by Dyban (25).*
Incubate blastomere in a hypotonic solution such as 0.5% sodium citrate for
   5 min.
Pick up blastomere using a clean, sterile pulled pipette and transfer in a
   small droplet to a clean acid-washed glass slide.
   *The slide may be treated with poly-d-lysine (10mg/mL) and oven-dried
   (55°C), before use to aid in cell adherence.*
Allow excess solution to evaporate or aspirate with a fine-pulled pipette.
When the blastomere is almost dry, add a fine drop of acetic acid/methanol
   (3:1).
Allow to dry.
Repeat addition of acetic acid/methanol (3:1), until a total of 5 drops have
   been added.
   *This crucial step allows adequate fixation and permeabilization. It is
   easy to lose a blastomere during this step if too much fixative is added.*
Repeat procedure until a number of blastomeres have been applied to the
   slide.
On the opposite side of the slide, mark the approximate location of each
   blastomere with a diamond-tipped pencil.

Dehydrate the slide by equilibrating in:
   70% ethanol for 5 min
   90% ethanol for 5 min
   100% ethanol for 5 min
   Methanol may also be used for this step.
Allow slide to air-dry.
Store in a clean slide holder at 4°C.
   If permeabilization is a problem, the slides may be incubated in 0.5%
   Triton X-100 and 0.5% saponin, dipped into liquid nitrogen treated, as
   described in the section on sperm preparation.
Dehydrate the slide through the methanol series described above.
   The blastomeres are now prepared for in situ hybridization.

In Situ Hybridization Methods

In Situ Hybridization Protocol Using Biotinylated Probes.
Slides. These should be acid-washed and precleaned in ethanol. Slides
should be air-dried and stored in a dust-free container. There is no need for
routine RNase treatment, although it might be useful for certain probes. For
best results use fresh slides within a month. Slides may also be frozen in a
sealed box to prolong their freshness. After thawing, do not refreeze slides.
   Probes. For detection of single-copy sites, probes should be greater than
10 kb, since smaller ones produce a signal less consistently. Competition
with genomic human DNA is necessary to suppress background hybridization of repetitive sequences present in long probes (26). Chromosome-
specific libraries are used to detect specific chromosomes or chromosomal
domains.

Labeling Probes

Nick-translation stock solutions

[A]10× Nick-translation buffer:
   0.5 M Tris-HCl; pH 7.8–8.0
   50.0 mM $MgCl_2$
   0.5 mg/mL bovine serum albumin (BSA)
[B]Nucleotide stock:
   0.5 mM dATP
   0.5 mM dGTP
   0.5 mM dCTP
   0.5 mM biotin-11-dUTP
[C]0.1M β-mercaptoethanol
[D]1µg/mL DNase 1
   1 mg/mL in 50% glycerol at stored −20°C. Dilute fresh each time 1 µL in
   1 mL of ice-cold sterile distilled water immediately before use and
   discard afterwards

Reaction Mix for 100 μL

Add reagents in following order, all on ice:

Probe DNA *(clean, RNase treated)*	2 μg
Sol [A]	10 μL
Sol [B]	10 μL
Sol [C]	10 μL
Sol [D]	1–12 μL
E. coli DNA polymerase (10 U/μL) need 5 U/μg DNA	1 μL

Add double-distilled sterile water to final volume→100 μL
Immediately place tube into 15°C waterbath for 2 hr
Terminate reaction by adding EDTA to final conc. of 10–15 mM
   e.g., add 2.5 μL of 0.5 M EDTA
Add sodium dodecyl sulfate (SDS) to final conc. of 0.1%
   e.g., add 1 μL of 10% SDS
Incubate at 65–68°C for 15 min

Spin-Column to Separate Unincorporated Nucleotides (see Maniatis Manual [23])

Equilibrate Sephadex G-50 and wash column with:
   50 mM Tris
   1 mM EDTA
   0.1% SDS
Run aliquot of labeled probe, after heat denaturation (5 min boiling water bath, then 2 min on ice) in 2% agarose test gel with 1-kb ladder marker.
   Probe size should be smaller than 500 base pairs, best size is around 200 bp.

Hybridization Solutions

Stocks

Formamide (Aldrich or Boeringer):
Deionize by ion-exchange column *(BioRad AG 501-× 8(D)*
Check conductivity to monitor level of deionization
Freeze in aliquots after deionization
   For washes use formamide as supplied
Dextran sulfate (Pharmacia): 50% stock in water
   Autoclave (15–30 min) to reduce background
20× SSC (autoclaved)
   Before use make 20% dextran sulfate solution in 2× standard saline citrate (SSC)
   Mix well
   Warm to 42°C

Volume of hybridization solution needed

For small coverslip (18×18 mm): 10 μL/slide
For large coverslip (24×50 mm): 30 μL/slide

DNA:Total DNA concentration: 10 µg/10 µL hybridization solution

Labeled cosmid DNA: 50 ng/µL *(30–40 ng if more than one probe used)*

Human competitor DNA: 1–3 µg/10 µL
> *Start with 1.5 µg and increase if background is too high; incomplete suppression of Alu sequences produces R-banding patterns useful for chromosome identification.*

Salmon sperm DNA
> *Use this as nonspecific carrier DNA to bring the final concentration of DNA to 10 µg/10 µL.*

(*Note:* Competitor, human, and salmon-sperm DNA must be digested with DNase I to 200-bp fragment size. Use 1 mg DNA for 5-mL reaction, in 1× nick-translation buffer, DNase I, at 15°C for 1–2 hr. Check aliquots on 2% agarose minigel gel for size. If too large, digest for more time to get the right size.)

Mix DNAs

Ethanol precipitate

Leave at −70°C for 30 min or at −20°C overnight

Spin

Wash in 70% EtOH

Spin

Dry tube in Speed-Vac 5–15 min
> *For DNA volumes of less than 10 µL, Speed-Vac only*

Resuspend in one-half final vol. 100% deionized formamide, vortex extensively

Add one-half final vol of prewarmed 20% dextran sulfate in 2× SSC
> *Mark pipette tip after test with water to assure pipetting exact amount.*

Mix by lightly vortexing

Denature Probe/Competitor DNA

5 min at 75°C *(heatblock)*

Incubate 37°C for 5–15 min *(to reanneal with competitor)*
> or place on ice *(without competitor)*

Denature Slides

Prewarm slides in oven at 60°C

Incubate in 70% formamide, 2× SSC for 2 min at 70°C
> *For 50 mL Coplin jar, mix 35 mL formamide, 5 mL 20× SSC, 10 mL H$_2$O*

Dehydrate in 70%–90%–100% EtOH, Coplin jars on ice, 3 min each

Air-dry

(*Note:* For single-copy probes or chromosome-specific repetitive probes without competitor DNA, probes and slides can be denatured together: Place probe in hybridization solution on slide, coverslip, seal with rubber cement, place in 75°C oven for 8 min to denature (optimal time can vary), then incubate at 37°C for hybridization overnight.

Hybridization

During the entire in situ hybridization procedure, slides should never be allowed to dry.

Prewarm slides in stainless-steel pan floating on a 42°C waterbath
Pipette hybridization solution onto center of slide *(or premarked area)*
Carefully lower coverslip to avoid air bubbles *(bubbles can be squeezed out)*
Seal with rubber cement from 10 mL plastic syringe
Incubate in moist chamber at 37°C overnight *(16–20 hr)*

Washes

50% formamide in 2× SSC, three times for 5 min each, Coplin jars in shaking waterbath, prewarmed to 42°C
0.1× SSC, three times for 5 min each, at 60°C in shaking waterbath (slides can sit in last wash, do not let them dry out)

Blocking Nonspecific-Binding Sites

Need: 200 µL/slide, extralarge coverslip, moist chamber
Blocking agents differ depending on detection system.
For bio-dUTP/avidin-FITC: 3% BSA, 4× SSC, 30 min at 37°C
For detection with fluorochrome-conjugated antibodies: As above *or* if antibody reacts with BSA, use 4% nonfat dry milk, 4× SSC, 30 min at 37°C.
Milk does not dissolve completely, therefore, it is essential to centrifuge the blocking solution before use.
After incubation, drain blocking solution. There is no need to wash it off.

Detection

These steps are done in the dark as the chromophobes are easily photobleached.
200 µL/slide, moist chamber covered with aluminum foil
Avidin-FITC (fluorescein isothiocyanate-conjugated avidin: Vector Labs) supplied as 2 mg/mL, freeze small aliquots, cover with foil once thawed; keep at 4°C for several weeks in the *dark*)
For final conc. of 5 µg/mL dilute stock 1:400, in 4× SSC, 1% BSA, 0.1% Tween 20
Incubate at 37°C for 15–30 min
Wash in 4× SSC, 0.1% Tween 20, three times for 5 min at 42°C *(shaking waterbath).*
(*Note:* Fluorochrome-conjugated antibodies: freeze aliquots at −20°C
At room temperature fluorochromes can come off the antibody, and free fluorochromes cause background. This can be avoided by removing free

fluorochromes from antibody-bound fluorochromes using a spin-column if necessary.)

Amplification

The avidin–FITC signal can be amplified by incubating slide in 1–5 μg/mL biotin-conjugated goat anti-avidin D antibodies (Vector Labs) at 37°C for 30 min. Wash. Incubate again with avidin–FITC as above. Wash. This process can make a weak signal more pronounced, but background fluorescence may also increase.

Conterstain: Immediately after last wash

Propidium iodide, 200 ng/mL in 2× SSC for 10 min at room temperature
DAPI (4,6-diamidino-2-phenylindole dihydrochloride), 200 ng/mL, 2×
    SSC, for 5 min at room temperature
Wash in 2× SSC, 0.05% Tween 20 once for 2 min at room temperature

Mount in antifade

For 10 mL stock:
    0.233 g DAPCO (1,4-diazobicyclo (2.2.2.)octane) [Sigma]
    800 μL double-distilled H_2O
    200 μL 1 M Tris-HCl, pH=8.0
    9 mL glycerol
    Store at 4°C in aluminum foil
    Add 30 μL slide and use large coverslip
    Store slides at 4°C in the dark

Fluorescence Microscopy

Visualize signal with a standard fluorescent microscope. The light source must be of the proper wavelength for imaging the particular chromophobe.

ACKNOWLEDGMENTS

The author is especially grateful to Peter Lichter, Ph.D., Ann Boyle, and David C. Ward, Ph.D., for teaching him methods for in situ hybridization.

REFERENCES

1. Watson JD, Crick FHC. Molecular structure of nucleic acids. *Nature* 1953;171:737–738.
2. Saiki RK, Scharf S, Faloona F, et al. Enzymatic amplification of β-globin genomic sequences and restriction site analysis for diagnosis of sickle cell anemia. *Science* 1985;230:1350–1354.
3. Saiki RK, Gelfand DH, Stuffel S, et al. Primer directed enzymatic amplification of DNA with a thermostable DNA polymerase. *Science* 1988;239:487–491.
4. Grifo JA, Boyle A, Lavy G, DeCherney AH, Ward DC, Sanyal MK. Preembryo biopsy and analysis of blastomeres by in situ hybridization. *Am J Obstet Gynecol* 1990;163:2013–2019.

5. Gardner RL, Edwards RG. Control of sex ratio at full term in the rabbit by transferring sexed blastocysts. *Nature* 1968;218:346–348.
6. Bondioli KR, Ellis SB, Pryor JH, Williams MW, Harpold MM. The use of male specific chromosomal DNA fragments to determine the sex of bovine preimplantation embryos. *Theriogenology* 1989;31:95–104.
7. Croxatto HB, Fuentealba B, Diaz S, Pastene L, Tatum H. A simple nonsurgical technique to obtain unimplanted eggs from human uteri. *Am J Obstet Gynecol* 1972;112:662–665.
8. Buster JE, Bustillo M, Rodi IA, et al. Biological and morphologic development of donated human ova recovered by non-surgical uterine lavage. *Am J Obstet Gynecol* 1985;153:211–217.
9. Verlinsky Y, Ginsberg N, Lifchez A, Valle J, Moise J, Strom CM. Analysis of the first polar body: preconceptual genetic diagnosis. *Hum Reprod* 1990;5:826–829.
10. Monk M, Handyside AH, Hardy K, Whittingham D. Preimplantation diagnosis of deficiency of hypoxanthine phosphoribosyl transferase in a mouse model for Lesch–Nyhan syndrome. *Lancet* 1987;2:423–425.
11. Monk M, Muggleton-Harris AL, Rawlings E, Whittingham DG. Preimplantation diagnosis of HPRT-deficient male and carrier female mouse embryos by trophectoderm biopsy. *Hum Reprod* 1988;3:377–381.
12. Summers PM, Campbell JM, Miller MW. Normal in vivo development of marmoset monkey embryos after trophectoderm biopsy. *Hum Reprod* 1989;3:389–393.
13. Wilton LJ, Trounson AO. Biopsy of preimplantation mouse embryos: development of micromanipulated embryos and proliferation of single blastomeres in vitro. *Biol Reprod* 1989;40:145–152.
14. Wilton LJ, Shaw JM, Trounson AO. Successful single cell biopsy and cryopreservation of preimplantation mouse embryos. *Fertil Steril* 1989;51:513–517.
15. Handyside AH, Penketh RJA, Winston RML, et al. Biopsy of human preimplantation embryos and sexing by DNA amplification. *Lancet* 1989;1:347–349.
16. Handyside AH, Kontogianni H, Hardy K, Winston RML. Pregnancies from biopsied human preimplantation embryos sexed by Y-specific DNA amplification. *Nature* 1990;344:768–770.
17. Grifo JA, Tang YX, Kogelman L, Pratten MK, Sanyal MK, Fenton W. Characterization of a new Y-chromosome specific primer pair for polymerase chain reaction (PCR). *J In Vitro Fert Embryo Transfer* 1990;7:192.
18. Monk M, Holding C. Amplification of a (beta) hemoglobin sequence in individual human oocytes and polar bodies. *Lancet* 1990;335:985–988.
19. Saiki RK, Bugawan TL, Horn GT, Mullis K, Erlich HA. Analysis of enzymatically amplified (beta)-globin and HLA-DQX DNA with allele-specific oligonucleotide probes. *Nature* 1986;324:163–166.
20. Strom CM, Verlinsky Y, Milayeva S, et al. Preconception genetic diagnosis of cystic fibrosis. *Lancet* 1990;336:306–307.
21. Lichter P, Ward DC. Is noniotopic in situ hybridization finally coming of age? *Nature* 1990;345:93–94.
22. Penketh RJA, Delhanty JDA, Van De Berghe JA, et al. Rapid sexing of human embryos by non-radioactive in situ hybridization: potential for preimplantation diagnosis of X-linked disorders. *Prenat Diagn* 1989;9:489–500.
23. Maniatis T, Fritsch EF, Sambrook J. *Molecular cloning, a laboratory manual.* Cold Spring Harbor, NY: Cold Spring Harbor Laboratory; 1982.
24. Tarkowski AK. An air drying method for chromosome preparation from mouse eggs. *Cytogenetics* 1966;5:394–400.
25. Dyban AP. An improved method for chromosome preparations from preimplantation mammalian embryos, oocytes or isolated blastomeres. *Stain Technol* 1983;58:69–72.
26. Lichter P, Tang CJ, Call K, et al. High resolution mapping of human chromosome 11 by in situ hybridization with cosmid clones. *Science* 1990;247:64–69.

10

Tools and Techniques for Embryological Micromanipulation

Henry E. Malter

To manage the instrument successfully, delicacy of touch and a great deal of patience are required; but it is only the latter, combined with perseverance, energy, and close observations that scientific facts have, or ever will be established.

Dr. H. D. Schmidt,
1859 on the use of his
"microscopic dissector"

There are three basic requirements for success at micromanipulation which I call the three P's. These are Patience, Practice, and Profanity.

Henry Malter, 1989
opening address to the
first workshop on
micromanipulation of
human gametes and
embryos. Emory
University

In this chapter the technical aspects of embryological micromanipulation techniques and the fabrication of microtools are described. First, the outfitting of a modern micromanipulation laboratory is discussed. Then, specific techniques for micromanipulation and microtool fabrication will be described. We will not attempt to describe the gamut of embryological micromanipulation procedures in detail. For this, the reader is directed to the original papers, which have been cited in preceding chapters. We will provide an overview of the basic microtools and their general use. For many procedures, microtools must be fabricated to meet certain specifications; for instance, the different sizes of nuclei or blastomeres from a particular species and developmental stage. No amount of description can substitute for hands-on experience with the micromanipulation apparatus as well as the experimental material.

From the large body of literature discussed in this volume, it should be obvious that current micromanipulation techniques are derivative of an extensive history of research and innovation, spanning almost a century. When possible, credit will be given to the originator of a particular device or technique. It is sometimes difficult to attribute this credit with certainty. Techniques are, no doubt, often reinvented many years after the date of their true inception. Our own experience is derivative of the contributions of perhaps hundreds of fellow researchers who have affected our work in some way. In describing the motion of micromanipulators, we will use the established convention of the X, Y, and Z axes. The X and Y are the two horizontal axes and the Z is the vertical, or focus, axis.

A MODERN MICROMANIPULATION LABORATORY

Equipping a modern laboratory for micromanipulation is a straightforward task. Investigators are no longer required to design and fabricate their own apparatus. There are several excellent commercial systems to choose from that are compatible with a wide selection of microscopes. Entire setups, including the microscope, the micromanipulators, and the microtool fabricating equipment may be purchased through a microscope dealer. Alternatively, individual units may be selected to equip an existing microscope with micromanipulation capability. The following discussion will concern the selection of a micromanipulation microscope, the micromanipulators, the microinjector, and the microtool-making equipment.

Selection of a Microscope For Micromanipulation

The first factor in selecting a microscope is determining the degree of magnification required. Some simple procedures, such as the splitting of embryonic morulae, can be accomplished using a dissecting-type stereomicroscope. Much large-animal work is done with these units. However, for critical work, and certainly for any clinical application, a high-power microscope is required. Microscopes used for embryological micromanipulation should be equipped with a least 4×, 10×, and 20× objectives. Most mammalian embryological micromanipulation is done at 200× magnification. For some procedures and for tool alignment, 100× can be used. A low-power objective is also useful for microtool setup and for locating specimens. For some critical procedures involving nuclear injection or transfer, it may be desirable to have 400× magnification available, although this is usually not necessary.

Micromanipulation requires that the stage supporting the specimen remains stationary. Since many standard microscopes are focused by moving the stage, they are not suitable for micromanipulation. Therefore, either a fixed-stage upright or an inverted tissue culture microscope is required. These are focused by adjusting the tube itself. Inverted microscopes are probably the more versatile option, in that they allow a wide variety of specimen holders to be placed on the stage. Slides, as well as dishes and other containers, can be accommodated. Upright microscopes are limited to hanging-drop chambers, slides, or reasonably shallow containers. This issue of working distance is obviously of great importance in micromanipulation, since the microtools must have unrestricted access to the specimen. Working distance is dependent on the optical components of the microscope. Microscopes used for micromanipulation should have "long" or "ultralong" working-distance condensers or objectives, or both. These optical components have a longer focal length than standard lenses and permit proper focusing at a greater distance between the final lens element and the specimen. For most purposes, the tissue culture dissecting microscope is perhaps the best suited for micromanipulation. The finest fixed-stage upright microscopes may provide a slightly superior optical system. These are selected for situations during which image quality is of primary importance, and the use of a shallow specimen holder is feasible. In general, a microscope used for micromanipulation should be of the highest quality possible and be well maintained. Since long periods are spent at the microscope during micromanipulation procedures, poor image quality can quickly result in eyestrain and fatigue. The design of the apparatus for focusing, stage movement, and other common adjustments should provide comfortable working conditions. An integral video system is of great advantage for teaching and for establishing video tape records of procedures.

A final issue is the selection of a special image-enhancement optical system. Interference contrast optics provide a vastly superior image for embryological micromanipulation. The pseudo–three-dimensional image provided by the Nomarski or Hoffman optical systems is of great value in the intricate positioning of microtools during microsurgical procedures. This type of image is especially desirable in procedures involving the visualization of nuclei. These systems consist of special condenser elements, polarizing filters, prisms, and objectives. The Nomarski system is designed for an optical path through glass only. Therefore, a correct image is not obtained when plastic specimen containers are used. The Hoffman system is designed to compensate for the effect of plastic and gives excellent results with specimen holders such as tissue culture dishes. The Hoffman system provides a monochromatic image, whereas the Nomarski image can be adjusted using a rotating prism to provide a wide range of color combinations that are useful for photography. The Hoffman system seems to be more sensitive than Nomarski to the type of aberrations introduced by a round surface, such as the well of a depression slide. These systems, especially Nomarski, are quite expensive. However, the image they provide is definitely superior to standard phase-contrast or bright-field scopes. This superior image can certainly be a factor in reducing eyestrain and fatigue during micromanipulation. Interference contrast optics are thus highly recommended for any type of critical micromanipulation procedure.

The Micromanipulators

There are currently two main systems used for embryological micromanipulation: Leitz and Narishige. Several other systems are, for various reasons, considered less adequate. These secondary systems will be discussed briefly and a complete description of the Leitz and Narishige systems will follow.

The original de Fonbrune micromanipulator is still being manufactured and sold today. The current system, available from the Technical Products International (TPI) corporation of St. Louis, follows the exact design of the original, utilizing improved modern materials for some components of the mechanism. A new design is also available that incorporates a compact microscope-mounted unit as illustrated in Fig. 10.1

The Carl Zeiss company has a long history of micromanipulation innovation. They first marketed a unique model based on the direct manual positioning of a massive plate, which was connected with the microtool holder (1). The movement of this plate was dampened by a film of grease, so the motions of the operators hands were effectively reduced to the microscopic scale. Zeiss-Eppendorf sells an excellent electronic micromanipulator based on microprocessor-controlled motors. The motion of an electronic joystick is translated into a proportional response by three massive stepper motors that drive the microtool holder. A great advantage of this design is that the micromanipulator can be directly controlled by a microprocessor to provide a variety of convenient control features, in addition to automated operations. A system is available with which objects can be selected from a video image and subsequently injected automatically through the computer-controlled stage, micromanipulator, and microinjection unit. This is of tremendous value in cell culture work, for which large numbers of cells in monolayers can be quickly injected in a repeatable and precise manner. However, this system is expensive and not particularly advantageous for most embryological applications.

Several manufacturers produce high-quality mechanical micromanipulators. Research Instruments sells a complete range of micromanipulation and microtool fabricating equipment. Two basic micromanipulator designs

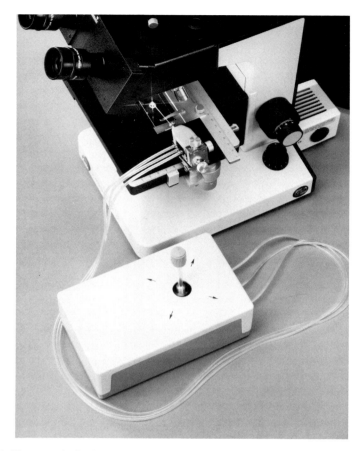

FIG. 10.1. The new de Fonbrune-type micromanipulation system. The joystick unit controls the motion of a compact micromanipulator, mounted on the microscope stage, by a pneumatic mechanism. (Courtesy of TPI Inc., St. Louis, Missouri.)

are available. A simple self-contained unit for work with large-animal embryo splitting and other similar procedures is designed for use with dissecting-type microscopes. A high-precision manual joystick micromanipulator is also available that is suitable for critical high-magnification procedures. The Stoelting company offers a variety of micropositioners manufactured by Prior Instruments and other companies using both simple three-axis and joystick designs. Some of these are suitable for embryological work.

The Leitz Micromanipulator

Since its introduction in the early 1950s, the Leitz micromanipulator has been the most popular device for biological work. It is a purely mechanical design based on the eccentric motion of a spherical component, which forms the apex of a "hanging joystick" (Fig. 10.2). Horizontal motion along the surface of the sphere is translated through a linkage into a reduced proportional X–Y motion of the microtool holder. The reduction ratio is adjustable between 16:1 and 800:1. Vertical motion is provided by a concentric course and fine micrometer drive. With practice, the vertical drive and joystick can be adjusted together to provide simultaneous X–Y–Z motion of the microtool. Coarse positioning in the two horizontal axes is accomplished by two screw drives. The Leitz is a self-contained unit, usually mounted on a massive base plate that can accommodate two micromanipulators and the microscope (Fig. 10.3). Alternatively, individual units can be mounted on adapter columns for support in special situations. The stability, precision, and reliability of the Leitz mechanism have been well

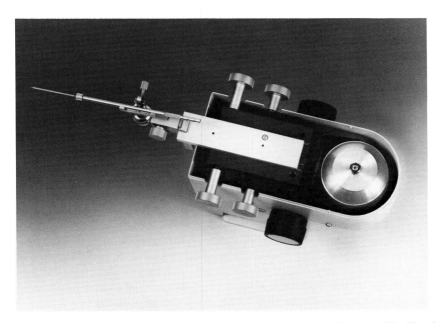

FIG. 10.2. An interior view of the Leitz micromanipulator mechanism. The round "ball" at the *right* forms the top of the hanging joystick. Movement of this ball is translated into a reduced proportional motion in the microtool holder on the *left*. (Courtesy of Leica Inc., Rockleigh, New Jersey.)

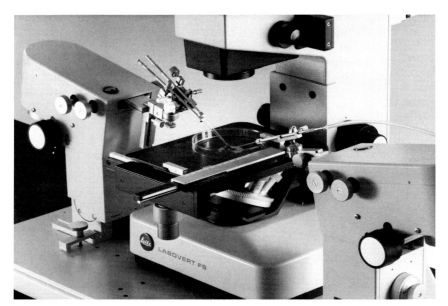

FIG. 10.3. The classic Leitz micromanipulator setup with two units mounted on opposite sides of the microscope, supported on a massive base plate. (Courtesy of Leica Inc., Rockleigh, New Jersey.)

demonstrated over the past 35 years. It remains the micromanipulator of choice for the most critical positioning tasks, such as the placement and maintenance of microelectrodes in electrophysiological procedures. The Leitz micromanipulator has also been quite popular for embryological work, although currently the Narishige system seems to offer the best design for work in this area.

The Narishige Micromanipulator

The Narishige system, available from Nikon, seems to combine some of the best design elements from previous micromanipulators. The unit was developed in the early 1980s, in response to a request from Dr. Y. Hiramoto at the Tokyo Institute of Technology for a new type of manipulator that would allow ultraprecise remote-controlled operation with inverted microscopes (Vratny M, Nikon Inc., personal communication). The use of the older mechanical units, such as the Leitz, with inverted microscopes, required that they be raised up on supports to provide access to the stage, making the joystick difficult to operate. The Nikon-Narishige NT-88 micromanipulator is quite similar, in theory, to the de Fonbrune system in that it relies on three hydraulic cylinders to derive simultaneous three-dimensional remote-controlled positioning. The Narishige cylinders, like those of the earlier Dunn micromanipulator, operate using an incompressible oil (2). Movement of the joystick operates two horizontal cylinders, while a third vertical cylinder is driven by a micrometer drive incorporated into the joystick. These cylinders are connected by flexible tubing to three similar cylinders making up the actual micromanipulator that drives the microtool holder. The fundamental advantage of the Narishige system is that separate high-precision micrometer drives are included on both horizontal joystick cylinders. These provide the most convenient X–Y motion control of any commercial micromanipulator. By adjusting these drives, the microtool can make precise, yet wide-range, linear movements. With practice, the operator can simultaneously operate these drives and easily direct the microtool. In effect, the Narishige system combines the convenient three-dimensional control of the joystick with the precise linear control of

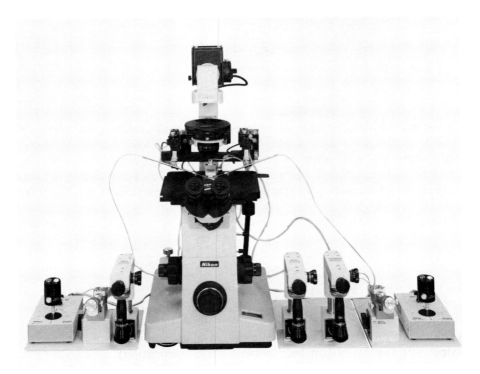

FIG. 10.4. The Nikon–Narishige micromanipulation system. The hanging joystick units control individual microscope-mounted micromanipulators and a micromanipulator stage Electronic joystick controls operate the motor-driven coarse positioners. (Courtesy of Nikon Inc., Instrument Group, Melville, New York.)

separate single-axis units. This wide range of horizontal motion is of great advantage in the general positioning of microtools and for procedures such as needle insertion during zona dissection. The joystick with its integral Z-axis control is convenient for procedures requiring critical simultaneous horizontal and vertical adjustment, such as zona massage.

The hydraulic drive device is mounted to the microscope on a separate micromanipulator that provides three-dimensional coarse positioning. Narishige offers two options for coarse positioning. One is a simple mechanical rack-and-pinion–based unit. The other consists of an electronic joystick remote-control that drives three high-precision electric motors. This provides a very convenient and versatile system wherein all of the controls necessary for both coarse positioning and micromanipulation are at the operator's fingertips, as illustrated in Fig. 10.4. The micromanipulators can be mounted to the body of several types of microscopes by using adapter mounts. Narishige also markets several mechanical micromanipulators that can be used for noncritical or large-animal embryological procedures.

Piezoelectric Micromanipulators

The insertion of micropipettes, especially ultrafine microelectrodes, into living cells can sometimes be difficult owing to the resilience of the extracellular coats or of the cell membrane itself. One innovative solution has been to induce an extremely rapid movement or a high-frequency vibration into the micropipette using a piezoelectric manipulator, as discussed in Chapter 1. By incorporating the piezoelectric mechanism into a micromanipulator either a rapid precise motion, or a continuous vibration, may be obtained through the adjustment of an electronic control. These systems had been used mainly for electrophysiological studies, but recently, they are being put to use in embryological procedures. The penetration of the zona pellucida by large microtools can be enhanced by piezoelectronic vibration (Hosoi Y, personal communication). Piezoelectric microdrives are available from the Stoelting company and from other suppliers.

Microinjector Units

The basic design of microinjector units has changed very little since Chambers' original unit (see Chap. 1). Glass syringes under the control of a variety of microdrives are marketed by all of the major micromanipulator companies including Leitz, Nikon–Narishige, and Stoelting. The Nikon–Narishige microinjector is illustrated in Fig. 10.5. The performance of most units may be enhanced by substituting a high-quality syringe such as a Hamilton gas-tight with a Teflon plunger for the simple glass-plunger syringe with which they are equipped. These syringes are less prone to

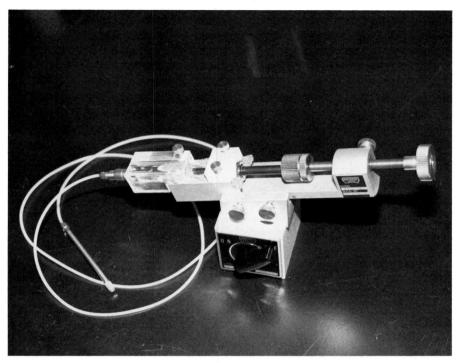

FIG. 10.5. The Nikon–Narishige microsyringe system. The screw mechanism is connected to the syringe plunger. The standard syringe has been replaced with a high-quality Hamilton syringe.

leaking than standard models. For connection to the micropipette holder, flexible plastic tubing with Luer or other airtight fittings is included. The Narishige and Leitz systems use a micropipette holder such as Chambers described, with a resilient rubber "washer" that is tightened against the micropipette with a screw-down cap, providing an airtight seal. Alternatively, the micropipette can be simply inserted into the plastic tubing itself and secured with a standard clamp holder. The outfitting of microinjectors will be discussed in a following section on laboratory arrangement.

Several manufacturers have developed electronically controlled microinjector systems. These provide some advantages over syringe-based setups. The two most popular units are the Zeiss-Eppendorf microinjector and the Nikon–Narishige Picoinjector (Fig. 10.6). These systems use compressed gas and pumps to produce pressure and suction for micropipette operation and provide for pushbutton operation. Very exact and repeatable control of injection volume through both pressure and injection-time adjustment is possible. This arrangement provides a much more reliable, precise, and

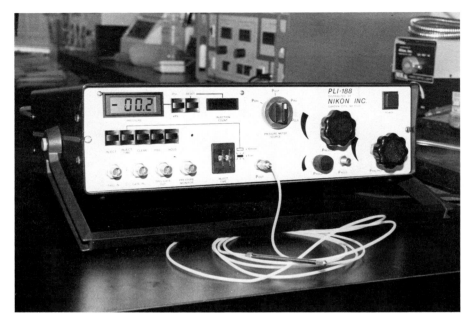

FIG. 10.6. The Nikon–Narishige Picoinjector. A microinstrument holder is connected by plastic tubing to an outlet that provides electronically controlled suction and pressure. Controls permit adjustment of pressure and the timing of injection.

convenient control method than a microsyringe, albeit at a considerable increase in cost. For situations requiring the most critical microinjection and for very labor-intensive injection work such as cell monolayers, electronic microinjectors are of great advantage. As stated previously, the Zeiss-Eppendorf setup may be combined with a computer-controlled system for automated cell injection. The Narishige also has a provision for electronic triggering of the injection process by an external control.

Mouthpiece Control for Micropipettes

The mouthpiece can provide an intuitive and very precise control over the microtool. The use of a mouthpiece also eliminates the need for the extra hand motions needed to control a microinjector drive. Mouthpieces are available from scientific suppliers for use in micropipetting applications. These are modified by adding extra tubing to increase the length. If desired, a sterile filter, such as 0.2-μm syringe filter, can be incorporated into the mouthpiece to provide sterility and ensure that saliva does not foul the micropipette holder. The end of the mouthpiece tubing is simply attached to the back of the pneumatic micropipette holder. Figure 10.7 illustrates the mouthpiece system used in our clinical laboratory.

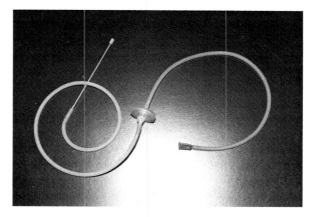

FIG. 10.7. A typical mouthpiece for the operation of microtools. The end of the tubing is connected directly to the microinstrument holder. A 0.2-μm syringe-filter is used to protect the microtool from contamination.

The Arrangement of a Micromanipulation Laboratory

A laboratory intended for micromanipulation should contain a relatively isolated area in which to locate the actual micromanipulation system. The area should be free from excess traffic and other activity and provide enough room for all of the necessary equipment. For embryological micromanipulation, the system should be placed near the incubator and sterile hood. A protected and clean storage area for microtools and other small precision components is also required.

An important factor, mentioned previously in Chapter 6, is the need for temperature control. Ambient temperature is of vital importance, especially for the culture of human eggs. A metallic microscope stage is an excellent conductor of heat. A microdrop on a glass slide would, no doubt, be subject to substantial heat loss when maintained on a cool stage, even for the brief periods required for micromanipulation. Therefore, it is important to fit the microscope stage with some form of temperature control. Dissecting microscopes are often equipped with a flat, transparent, stagelike vessel that is connected to a source of temperature-controlled water. This way, the entire working surface of the microscope is heated uniformly. The wide adjustment of focus depth available on this type of microscope allows compensation for the thicker stage. On higher-power microscopes, this type of warm stage is usually not compatible with proper optical alignment, even with the increased working distance used for micromanipulation. Alternatives are the use of thin membrane-type electric-heating pads, the installation of heaters within the microscope stage itself, or the control of ambient temperature through warm boxes or "hot rooms." We have found that most electrical shops can devise a precise electronic temperature control unit for use

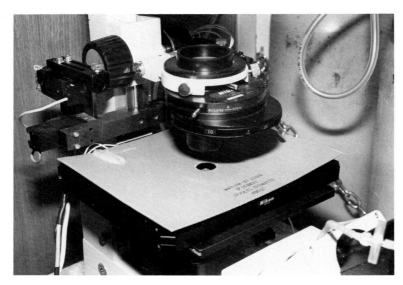

FIG. 10.8. A microscope stage warmer fabricated from flexible silicone rubber heating material. A temperature sensor (attached with silicone glue) and electric leads connect the unit to a digital temperature control.

with thin rubber heating material as illustrated in Fig. 10.8. This can be custom fabricated to fit the required stage and provides a stable, relatively uniform temperature-control surface, that permits proper optical focus on high-power microscopes. The supplier of this material is listed in the Appendix.

Vibration in the Micromanipulation Laboratory

The micromanipulation system can be placed on a variety of supports; however, vibration must be considered. Microtools are very sensitive to ambient vibration. Usually, a rigid bench-top or table is satisfactory. The best support for a micromanipulation setup is probably a heavy microscope or balance table. In some cases, severe vibration may be present owing to adjacent building equipment, such as elevators or air-conditioning systems. If this is the case, some method of vibration control must be applied. Bolting the table to the floor or wall or using a massive support, such as a granite balance table, may be sufficient. Otherwise, more drastic measures may be required. One solution is to attach the microscope and micromanipulator to a heavy metal plate that is supported by a resilient material, such as foam or partially inflated pneumatic cushions (bicycle inner-tubes are useful for this purpose). If severe, constant vibration is present and the system cannot be moved to another location, a commercial vibration control system will be required. These are tables or supports that use pneumatic or electronic mechanisms to isolate the micromanipulation system from ambient vibration. These units can be very expensive. It is sometimes difficult to assess a vibration problem in advance of setting up the micromanipulation system. If specimens under high-power magnification show noticeable constant vibration, there most likely will be a problem when micromanipulation equipment is used. However, microtools can also be sensitive to transient vibration, such as footsteps within the laboratory or the traffic of carts or gurneys in an adjacent hallway. It is probably best to set up the micromanipulation system in the most stable manner possible and then resolve any vibration problems as they occur.

Microinjector Operation and Maintenance

The proper setup of the microinjector system is critical to success. Usually, the entire system is filled with an incompressible liquid such as silicone, paraffin oil, or Fluorinert. Fluorinert has the advantage that it is highly incompressible yet not viscous like oil and, therefore, does not result in a greasy mess if it leaks or spills. However, Fluorinert is volatile and, accordingly, must be replenished frequently. It is also a somewhat toxic compound and is quite expensive relative to oil. As stated previously, the system can be set up with the micropipette simply inserted into the end of the plastic tubing. For microtools fabricated from 1-mm capillary tubing, the correct size of tubing is PE-60. Some workers ensure that the entire system, from syringe to the micropipette itself, is filled completely with the fluid—free of any air bubbles. This is probably necessary for the most critical procedures, especially those involving the intracellular aspiration of material. However, adequate control is possible, especially for continuous injection flow or holding pipette operation, with the back of the micropipette and even the pipette holder filled with air. In operation, the microinjector unit is often placed on the side opposite the appropriate micromanipulator. In this way, one hand can be used to control the movement of the microtool while the other hand operates the microinjector.

The maintenance of microinjectors can be a difficult and time-consuming activity. Tremendous pressure is developed during the operation of micropipettes, especially with fine needles for intracellular or nuclear injection. Even the most finely machined syringe and the tightest tubing and pipette holder fittings will inevitably leak at some point. Air enters the system and eventually results in the loss of control. The syringe and tubing should be checked before every use and refilled if necessary. The fittings can develop leaks, especially at the plastic tubing connections and the micropipette "chuck." To ensure proper operation, these connections must be periodically replaced.

EQUIPMENT FOR THE FABRICATION OF MICROTOOLS

Micropipette Pullers

There are a wide variety of micropipette pullers available to the modern microtool maker. Designs range from simple systems operating by gravity, allowing little control over the needle form, to complex microprocessor pullers that permit the precise, repeatable control of every phase of the needle-pulling procedure. Rather than discuss every design, we will describe representative simple and complex units. Pipette pullers basically offer a source of adjustable heat and pulling force. The more complex models offer greater flexibility and control in regulating these factors. Many of the complex mechanisms and features of the more-advanced pullers are of particular importance in the fabrication of electrophysiological instruments, such as submicron-tipped needles and short, patch clamp pipettes. However, the precision and control of these units can be put to good use in the fabrication of embryological tools as well. For instance, the adjustment of needle-tip length to obtain the optimum diameter and taper characteristics for a particular sperm-injection needle would be accomplished much more easily and repeatably with a sophisticated programmable puller. The theory of microtool fabrication will be discussed only as it pertains to particular puller design elements in this section. Later sections will deal with this in more detail.

The simple pipette puller illustrated in Fig. 10.9 is the Narishige PB-1. The strength of the pull is controlled by the amount of mass suspended from the lower pipette carriage. Four weights, two "light" and two "heavy," can be combined to obtain the desired amount of pulling strength. This is a crude method that does not provide the ability to alter needle form with any precision. Also, the maximum force available does not provide the acceleration required for producing the finest needle tips. Heat is provided by an electric filament that is under the control of a simple electrical circuit. By modifying the filament temperature and the pulling weight, needle length can be adjusted. This unit also offers a simple two-stage pull feature for creating patch clamp pipettes. This puller is suitable for pulling basic needles for embryological micromanipulation. It is a rugged mechanism that does not require much attention or maintenance. Research Instruments markets a simple micropipette puller that is similar to the original du Bois puller in that it uses spring tension for the pulling force. The Stoelting company offers a basic vertical-design electromagnetic puller.

The complex puller illustrated in Fig. 10.10 is the Sachs–Flaming PC-84 from Sutter Instruments. This puller represents one of the more versatile units available. Pull strength is derived from an electrical solenoid, as in the original Alexander and Nastuk puller (2). In this design, however, the solenoid voltage is under the control of a sophisticated microprocessor that

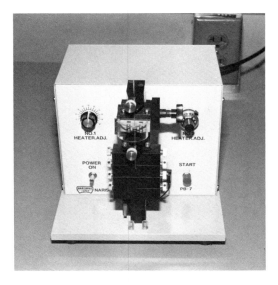

FIG. 10.9. The Nikon–Narishige PB-1 pipette puller. The bottom carriage accommodates four weights for use in adjusting pulling force.

allows programmed cycles of pulling. A sensor determines the position of the carriages during a pull, and by setting parameters, such as distance traveled and time, along with the force, very precise and repeatable control over the pulling process is obtained. The position of the filament and the filament temperature are controlled by the same microprocessor. Program lines including filament voltage, pull strength, and control parameters are entered into the machine and stored in memory slots. Programs for particular tools or glass types can be retained in memory and selected for later use. A related instrument, the Brown–Flaming PC-87, offers a computer-controlled gas jet for cooling the filament during the pulling process and during extremely rapid pull acceleration for the creation of the finest needle tips.

The Cambridge 763 puller available from Stoelting also offers microprocessor control and program storage of heat and pulling parameters with the added feature of a temperature sensor to provide even more precise control of needle formation. With the added precision of these sophisticated models comes a requirement for greater care in their operation and maintenance. The fine platinum filaments on the Sutter units are easily damaged. The alignment of the pulling components is adjustable and, therefore, subject to misalignment. As with any piece of sophisticated and delicate equipment, thorough operative knowledge and care is required for successful use. The selection of a pipette puller is based on the type of work

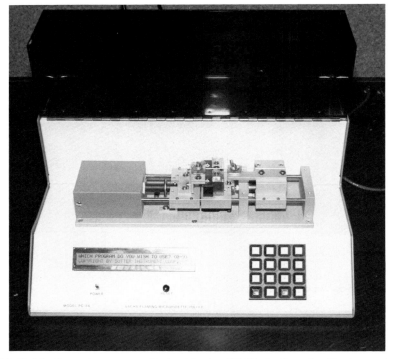

FIG. 10.10. The Sutter Instruments Sachs–Flaming PC-84 pipette puller. The key-pad allows the input of pulling parameters, which are indicated on the LCD readout. Pulling force comes from the solenoid unit at left.

to be done and the cost. The microprocessor-controlled units are considerably more expensive than the simple pullers. For critical research applications, the power, flexibility, and repeatability offered by the more complex systems are preferable.

The Microforge

The original model devised by de Fonbrune is still being manufactured and is available from the TPI corporation as illustrated in Fig. 10.11. Narishige, Prior Instruments, and the Stoelting company sell similar systems, which are often referred to as the "de Fonbrune type." The de Fonbrune unit offers the most versatile features, such as the built-in cooling jet system and the ability to easily change the filament orientation. This is also the most well-built instrument in our experience; it contains a rugged, heavy-gauge filament, and it is easily maintained. However, many of the

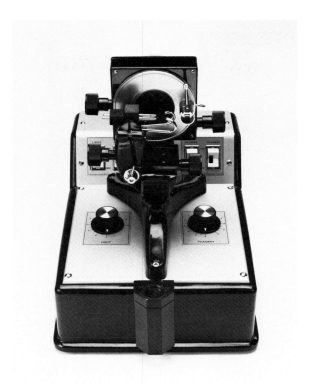

FIG. 10.11. The de Fonbrune microforge. During use, a microscope would be mounted in the *front* adapter hole. The filament is mounted to the massive micromanipulator unit at the *left*. The microtool is placed in the rotating holder surrounding the light source at the *rear.* (Courtesy of TPI Inc., St. Louis, Missouri.)

design features, such as the separate mounting of the filament on its own micromanipulator, are no longer necessary for modern embryological microtool techniques and can make the unit cumbersome for this use. The Stoelting unit is similar to the de Fonbrune. The Prior microforge has the micropipette mounted on the most sophisticated micromanipulator of any unit and seems to be well designed and constructed. One of the most convenient designs for embryological microtool procedures is the Nikon–Narishige MF-9, which is illustrated in Fig. 10.12. This model comes complete with a 100× high-power microscope. This level of magnification is essential for the fabrication of relatively small tools, such as sperm injection or enucleation pipettes. The key feature of the Narishige microforge is that the microscope is mounted on an integral micromanipulator, with the heating filament attached to the objective. Therefore, the filament and the

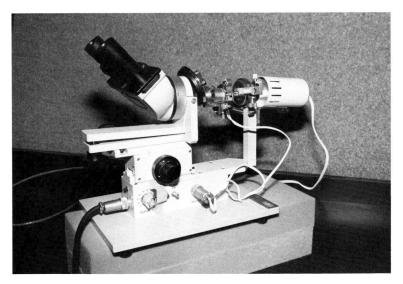

FIG. 10.12. The Nikon–Narishige MF-9 microforge. The integral microscope is mounted in a micromanipulator with the filament attached to the microscope objective. The microtool is placed in a smaller micromanipulator attached to the light source at the *right.*

microscope move as one unit, while the microtool is mounted on a separate coarse micromanipulator. As the microscope is focused on the tool, proper placement with relation to the filament is guaranteed. This is an extremely convenient design that permits quick and precise positioning of the microtool for forging procedures. A single metal jet is provided for the attachment of an air supply for cooling. However, this is not necessary for successful embryological microtool fabrication. The construction of this setup is poor, and the filament is a thin platinum wire that is subject to frequent burnout (an expensive and difficult replacement). However, the ease of use of the Narishige design is definitely superior.

The Microgrinder

Microgrinders for beveling micropipettes are offered by Nikon–Narishige, Research Instruments, Sutter, Stoelting, and other companies. The Sutter Instruments Brown–Flaming pipette beveler was designed for the creation of submicron bevels on the tips of microeletrodes. This level of precision, however, is unnecessary and, in fact, is inappropriate for general embryological work. The Narishige MG-4 (Fig. 10.13) consists of an abrasive wheel that is mounted directly on a motor drive. A concentric, coarse and fine micrometer drive is provided to advance the micropipette onto the

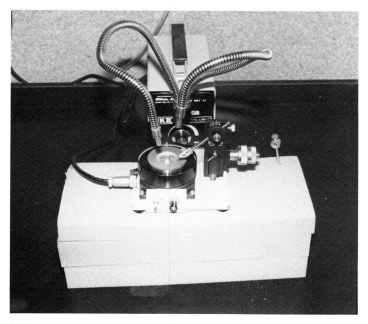

FIG. 10.13. The Nikon–Narishige MG-4 microgrinder. The microtool is mounted into the vertical micromanipulator at the *right*. The entire unit is placed on a pad of resilient foam to isolate it from vibration of the fiberoptic light source (at *rear*).

grinding wheel. This is a very simple unit that is well-suited for convenient and rapid beveling of the 10- to 50-μm–sized tools used for embryological work. It does not produce consistent ultrafine bevels in our experience. The Research Instruments MB-1 beveler uses the unique design of a horizontally mounted abrasive wheel that allows one to mount an integral light source and microscope for observing the beveling process. This unit is apparently suitable for beveling to the 10-μm range.

The Microtool Workshop

Like the micromanipulation system itself, the instruments used for the fabrication of microtools require a stable, quiet work space. Vibration may be a problem with the operation of the needle puller and microforge, but this is less critical than for actual microsurgical procedures. The individual units can be isolated on foam pads or other resilient material if necessary (Fig. 10.14). Ideally, the microforge should be placed in a location that will allow comfortable operation, such as a desk. The best source of heat for hand pulling is a microburner, so a gas supply should be available. Otherwise, a

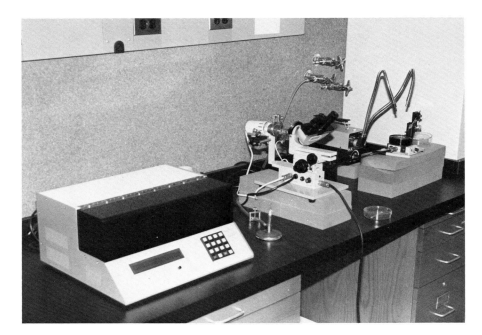

FIG. 10.14. A typical laboratory for the fabrication of microtools.

small alcohol burner can be used. The area should be free of drafts, which could disturb the burner flame. A supply of compressed-air may also be desired for attachment to the cooling elements on the microforge or the pipette puller, or for use in cleaning pipettes. Adequate lighting is also important. Some microgrinders are equipped with a light. Otherwise, the microgrinder is perhaps best arranged with a source of strong directional lighting, such as a fiberoptic illuminator. Proper illumination is critical to the placement of the pipette tip onto the grinding surface. Secure storage are required for the capillary tubing and for the requisite tools and peripheral equipment for microtool fabrication.

Types of Microtools

Embryological micromanipulation requires basically two types of micro-tools; the holding pipette and some type of needle or suction/injection pipette. The holding pipette, as its name suggests, is used to hold the egg or embryo during a procedure. The holding pipette is a blunt-ended tube, with a constricted lumen. During use, a partial vacuum is pulled through the pipette causing the cell to be pulled up and clamped tightly against its face.

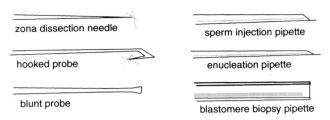

FIG. 10.15. A selection of microneedles. On the *left* are various needles and probes. On the *right* are pipettes for aspiration and injection.

Design is based on size and shape of the cell that is being held. For instance, holding pipettes for mouse embryos would be smaller than those for human embryos.

There are two basic types of "needles" used for embryological micromanipulation; the simple probe or spear and the injection–aspiration pipette. A sharp probe may be used for tasks such as piercing and cutting the zona pellucida, or may be modified into a hook or blunted probe for other manipulative tasks. The injection–aspiration pipette has an open lumen that can be used to inject fluids or cells, such as spermatozoa, or to aspirate cellular components, such as nuclei or polar bodies and blastomeres. Simple glass needles pulled from capillary tubing may be sufficient for the intracellular or nuclear injection of fluids; but for tasks, such as sperm injection or blastomere biopsy, more complicated pipettes must be constructed. A selection of microneedles is illustrated in Fig. 10.15.

Glass for Microtools

Microtools are fabricated from glass capillary tubing. Capillary tubing is manufactured in various formulations and sizes intended for a variety of uses. Many types of commercial capillary tubing are suitable for use in microtool fabrication.

Capillary Tubing

A primary consideration for selection of capillary tubing is the outer diameter. Most microtool holders are designed to accept tubing of a specified diameter. One millimeter is probably the most common size. This constitutes an upper limit on the size of capillary tubing that can be used. Usually, tubing of a smaller outer diameter can be used, as long as a tight fit is still possible with injection–aspiration needles. Some simple clamp-type microtool holders will accommodate a wide variety of tubing sizes.

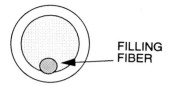

FILLING FIBER

FIG. 10.16. A cross section of filling-fiber tubing. The presence of this fiber permits increased capillary attraction and greatly facilitates the filling of fine-tipped needles.

When a lumen is desired in the microtool, a second important consideration is the inner diameter and wall thickness. Tubing with a thin wall is desirable to maintain a large lumen with the smallest overall tip diameter possible. The relationship between inner and outer diameter is, for the most part, maintained during microtool fabrication steps such as pulling. In some cases, a thicker-walled tubing may be more appropriate, such as for holding-pipettes or the finest needle points. Tubing is available in a variety of wall thicknesses so that the correct tubing can be selected for the desired task.

Another characteristic is the presence of a fiber within the lumen of the capillary tubing. A "filling fiber" is placed in the lumen to provide capillary attraction and thus increase the speed and ease with which a liquid will flow into the tubing as illustrated in Fig. 10.16. This can be of great advantage in filling very finely tipped intracellular or nuclear injection needles.

A final characteristic of capillary tubing is the glass formulation. The most common type of glass used for capillary tubing is probably borosilicate. This is a relatively hard glass with good strength and workability for microtool use. Aluminosilicate glass has a higher-melting point than borosilicate glass, and may be more appropriate for pulling ultrafine-tipped needles (4). Microtools can be made from inexpensive general-use capillary tubing of unspecified formulation. It must be kept in mind, however, that each glass formulation will react differently during microtool fabrication, and adjustments will have to be made to account for this.

Sources for Capillary Tubing

Most companies that deal in micromanipulation equipment sell special capillary tubing, in appropriate lengths, that is designed for fabricating microtools for their equipment. This tubing is convenient, but it can be rather costly. If special characteristics, such as very thin wall or a filling fiber, are desired, these types are also available. However, for simple tools, there are a number of alternative sources of tubing.

Bulk borosilicate tubing is available from Kimble, which is satisfactory for most microtool fabrication (listed in the Appendix). Another source of tubing is capillary microliter pipettes. These are already cut to a suitable length and come in convenient boxes, and since they have been largely replaced by adjustable pipettors, many laboratories have an unused supply of them laying around.

It is probably best to start out making microtools with the specialty tubing from the micromanipulator company and then experiment with the different types of tubing once you have gained some experience. Often, a slightly different type of tubing can result in an improved version of a particular tool.

MICROTOOL FABRICATION

Basic Principles

Microtools are made through the application of heat and force to the capillary tubing. In general, heat is applied until the glass reaches a plastic, semimelted state, at which point, force is applied to stretch, bend, or break the tubing. Heat is applied either through a small flame or through an electrical resistance device, such as the filament in a pipette puller or microforge. Force is applied by hand movements, gravity, or electromagnetic means.

Tubing is sometimes simply broken in various ways to yield straight broken surfaces. Microtools may also be modified using abrasive surfaces such as a grinding wheel. Hydrofluoric acid can also be used to "cut" and thin glass microtools.

In the next sections, we will discuss the various instruments used in the construction of microtools. Later, the fabrication of specific tools will be discussed.

The Pipette Puller

The first step in manufacturing most microtools is the formation of a tapered, needlelike pipette, using the pipette puller. Needles can theoretically be pulled by hand. The pipette puller, however, provides a very precise, consistent method for generating needles of the desired size and shape.

As stated previously, pipette pullers consist basically of an electric filament that heats the glass and some type of linear force that pulls the heated glass apart to produce two separate tapered pipettes, as illustrated in Fig. 10.17. If the conditions are correct, the tapered ends of these pipettes will end in sharp points. It is also possible to form the pipettes so that the tips break during the pull to form blunt ends. The two main adjustments used to determine the characteristics of the pulled pipettes are the glass temperature and the strength of the pulling force.

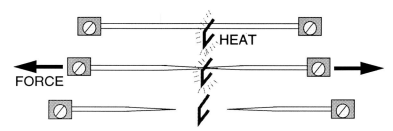

FIG. 10.17. The basic operation of the pipette puller. The filament provides a source of heat which partially melts the glass. Pulling force is applied to draw the tubing apart producing two sharp needles.

Glass Temperature

By controlling the temperature of the glass during pulling, the desired degree of plasticity is obtained. In general, higher temperature produces greater plasticity, resulting in finer-tipped needles, with longer tapered sections. At very high temperatures, however, the glass will become too plastic and pulling will result in long wisps of glass. Pipette pullers are, of course, designed to provide a practical range of glass temperatures. Glass temperature is controlled principally by the filament temperature, which is a result of the voltage applied. Pipette pullers usually have a knob or other control to regulate voltage. More sophisticated pullers have more precise and stable voltage regulation, resulting in greater flexibility and repeatability in temperature adjustment.

Glass temperature can be controlled in other ways. Some pullers offer programmable "waiting" periods. The filament is heated to the desired temperature and then voltage is turned off (or reduced) and a user-specified waiting period is initiated before the pulling force is applied. In this way, the glass can cool slightly before pulling occurs. Also, some pullers offer a gas jet that can instantaneously cool the filament and glass at specified times during the pull cycle. This cooling feature can result in fine-tipped needles with very short tapered sections.

Different filament shapes are available. Perhaps the most common is a simple loop. Box and round filaments completely enclose the capillary tubing, whereas trough filaments surround the glass on three sides. Box and round filaments deliver relatively more heat to the glass than trough filaments. In general, longer filaments, which expose a greater length of glass to the heat, produce smaller needle tips with longer tapers. It is very important to note that the physical positioning of the filament can be crucial to the actual heating of the glass. Very slight alterations in filament position can have profound effects on the needles. If the filament is not centered around the capillary, bent or skewed needles will result. Small changes in the proximity of the filament to the capillary can produce large differences in the voltage setting required to heat the glass.

For most general embryological microtool making, critical adjustment of glass temperature is not necessary. Fine-tipped needles, like those used for zona dissection, are easily pulled over a range of temperature. However, it is often desirable to be able to adjust the tip size and taper length of needles; accordingly, embryologists should familiarize themselves with temperature adjustment on their puller. As with aspects of microtool making, there is no substitute for personal experimentation with your own equipment. Individual instruments of the same puller model will often exhibit a wide variation in response to temperature and other settings.

Pulling Force

Pipette pullers generate pulling force by a variety of methods. Gravity is commonly used in vertical pullers. An electromagnetic device such as a solenoid is used in various ways to generate force in horizontal and in some vertical pullers. Pulling force must be considered in the context of glass temperature. Obviously, if the glass is not heated to a plastic condition, no amount of pulling force will be able to draw it out.

In gravity-based pullers, pulling force is adjusted by the addition or subtraction of mass from the lower capillary clamp. As the glass is heated, it is pulled down with a force relative to the weight suspended from it. More mass equals a stronger pull. This is a simple method that works well for simple needles.

Electromagnetic force can be adjusted in a much more precise manner; with pull strength related to the current applied to the solenoid. This current can be controlled by a simple knob or by a more complex microprocessor system.

In general, the greater the pulling force, the smaller the needle tip. The production of sharp needles generally requires a strong pulling force. This would probably necessitate the use of the maximum weight on gravity-driven pullers or a high pull setting on solenoid pullers.

When pulling force is reduced, two general effects are possible, as illustrated in Fig. 10.18. The capillary can be simply drawn out, producing a tapered section (without separating the glass or forming points). Also, by adjusting pull strength and lowering glass temperature, a pull can be initiated that draws out the capillary beyond the plastic limit of the glass, causing a break to occur at a desired point in the tapered section. In this way, pipettes with cylindrical tips, rather than sharp points, can be formed. It can be difficult to "fine-tune" the pulling parameters in creating cylindrical-tip pipettes. These weak-pulling force effects are involved with performing "two-stage" or multiple-stage pulls (see Fig. 10.18). Most pullers allow two-stage pulls. During a two-stage pull, the movement of the capillary is

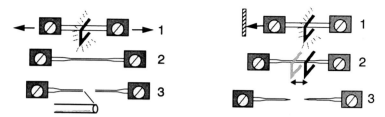

FIG. 10.18. Weak pulling protocols. On the left—a weak pull *(1)* can result in drawing out the glass into an unbroken section *(2)* or separation to produce two pipettes, with straight, blunt tips *(3)*. On the right—during a two-stage pull, the movement of the carriage is restricted so that the glass is drawn out only a selected distance *(1)*. This is followed by recentering the filament *(2)* and a second or multiple pulls to produce two pipettes with the desired form *(3)*.

restricted during the pulling process. Simple pullers use an adjustable stop or spacers of variable thickness to block the pulling movement. More sophisticated pullers monitor the position of the capillary and control its movement through a programmable microprocessor. With use of a low pulling force the capillary is first drawn out a specified distance, and the pull is terminated, creating a tapered section of the desired length. At this stage, the filament must be repositioned so that it is centered along the tapered section. Some pullers do this automatically. Then, a second pull is initiated. This second pull can be used to form sharp or cylindrical points or as a second nonbreaking pull as part of a multiple-stage pull protocol. In this way, pipettes can be pulled that have extremely short tapers, such as are used as "patch-clamp" electrodes. Multiple-stage pulls are not of great importance in making tools for general embryological work. Pulling large-bore pipettes (70 to 100 µm, for holding pipettes) can be attempted using a weak pulling force and possibly multiple-stage protocols. This is one of the most problematic pipette puller techniques, especially with the more simple vertical units. However, by careful experimentation, a holding pipette protocol can be developed. Holding pipettes are also easily pulled, by hand as discussed in a later section on their fabrication.

Pulling Pipettes

In practice, a worker must experiment with his or her own puller and capillary tubing to develop protocols for the desired micropipettes. A protocol will involve the type of glass used and the settings for filament temperature and pull strength. Highly sophisticated pullers, such as the Sutter horizontal models, offer a plethora of variables that can be adjusted to control glass temperature and the power, acceleration, and timing of the pulling force.

Sharp needles are probably the most "forgiving" microtool to create. Beginners will find that sharp-pointed needles can be pulled over a range of

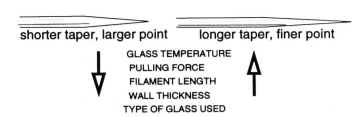

shorter taper, larger point   longer taper, finer point

GLASS TEMPERATURE
PULLING FORCE
FILAMENT LENGTH
WALL THICKNESS
TYPE OF GLASS USED

FIG. 10.19. Various factors that affect the formation of needle tips during pipette pulling.

temperature and pull settings. Once the settings that produce a sharp needle are elucidated, tip size, taper length, and shape can be altered by fine adjustment of heat and pull or the use of a different type glass as summarized in Fig. 10.19.

A discussion of the pulling protocols for specific tools will follow the next section, which deals with the second important piece of microtool fabricating equipment, the microforge.

The Microforge

During microtool fabrication, it is often necessary to alter the pulled section of the capillary in various ways. To perform these delicate procedures, the microforge was developed. With the microforge, the tapered sections of a micropipette can be cut, bent, constricted, or pulled.

The microforge basically consists of a heating filament (such as in the pipette puller) and micromanipulators to precisely position the filament and microtool during use, as illustrated in Fig. 10.20. The temperature of the filament is controlled by an electronic system, with an adjustment knob and usually a foot pedal for hands-free control of on–off switching. A magnification system (50 to 100×), with an eyepiece micron scale, is arranged to focus on the filament and tool during forging procedures. Often, a "cooling" air jet of some kind is provided—directed at the filament. Some workers construct their own microforge from an old microscope or dissecting scope and the requisite electronics and micropositioners. Otherwise, several good commercial models are available as discussed previously.

Microforge Setup

The microforge is arranged so that an image of the filament is centered and focused through the optics. An important aspect of many microforge procedures is the use of a glass ball on the filament.

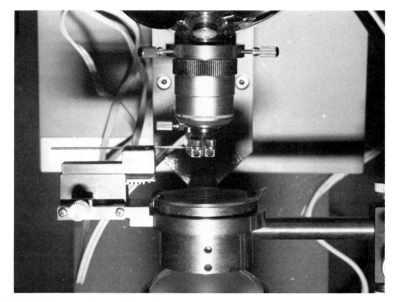

FIG. 10.20. A closeup view of the microtool in relation to the filament for microforging techniques. The filament is mounted at the end of the objective (between the two small metal blocks at the *center* of the photo). The pulled section of the microtool is positioned above the filament, with the shank extending to the *left* from the micromanipulator.

A sharp needle is first pulled on the pipette puller and clamped into position in the microforge, with the tip facing the filament. The filament is turned on and the heat adjusted such that the glass is easily melted. The needle tip is brought into contact with the hot filament so that a ball of glass melts on its surface. The needle is drawn away and the heat turned off, leaving a ball of glass adhering to the filament. In practice, this may require several steps of moving the needle into and away from the hot filament. Once a glass ball is set up it can be used for a long period. As the forge is used and small sections of glass tubing melt into the glass ball, it will grow in size. Eventually, it will be too large for easy use and must be removed by breaking it off of the filament with a pair of forceps. For critical procedures with the glass ball, it can be important that the ball is formed of the exact same glass formulation as the microtool that is to be forged.

The Microforge Filament

The filament will occasionally burn out and require replacement. Extra filaments or a length of filament wire is usually included with the forge for this purpose. A new filament's heat response (to the voltage applied) will probably vary from that of the old filament. In general, at the level of precision present in microforge techniques, every filament is unique. Changes to the filament, such as glass ball size and even the surrounding airflow, can also affect the heat/voltage response.

As the filament heats up, it expands in size. This expansion will also vary from filament to filament. Filament expansion, if not monitored, can drive the hot filament directly into a microtool during forging with disastrous results. During microforging procedures it is usually best to turn on the filament at a low-voltage setting and then slowly raise the voltage up to the desired level.

Microforge Techniques

There are four major toolmaking techniques performed on the microforge: heat polishing and constricting, bending, breaking, and pulling. These were first described by de Fonbrune (5)

Heat Polishing

The hot filament of the microforge can easily be used to "polish" the sharp edges of microtool tips as illustrated in Fig. 10.21. The tool is placed in the micromanipulator and positioned with its tip facing the filament. Filament voltage is turned on and adjusted until heat output is sufficient. The tip of the tool will slowly become plastic and flow resulting in a softening of the sharp edges. When the desired effect has been achieved, the filament is turned off. By extending the polishing time, the lumen of a tool can be constricted as the tubing walls flow and thicken. This is the last step in the fabrication of a holding pipette.

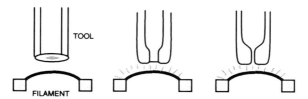

FIG. 10.21. Heat polishing on the microforge. The tip of a microtool is positioned facing the filament. The filament is activated, and the heat softens and constricts the lumen of the microtool.

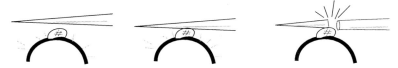

FIG. 10.22. Breaking on the microforge. The filament is set up with a ball of glass. The microtool is positioned with the area where a break is desired above the glass ball. The filament is carefully activated and the temperature adjusted so that when the microtool is brought into contact with the warm filament adhesion occurs. When the filament is turned off the microtool is pulled away, and a straight break forms at the point of attachment to the glass ball.

Breaking

By using the glass ball, a needle or holding pipette tip can be broken in a very precise manner. This technique relies on the property of adhesion. When the glass ball and microtool are heated to a certain temperature, they will partially melt and adhere to each other. This can be used to stabilize the tip of a tool against the filament.

Breaking is illustrated in Fig. 10.22. The tool is positioned tangentially to the surface of the glass ball, at the area along the tip where a break is desired. The filament is turned and slowly warmed up while the tool is brought carefully into contact with the glass ball. A back-and-forth motion of the tool is helpful at this point. The temperature is slowly turned up until the tool is seen to adhere to the glass ball, at which point, the filament is turned off. For small-diameter breaks, the slight movement of the filament that occurs during cooling is enough to cause the pipette to snap off at the point of attachment to the glass ball. For larger pipettes, a slight movement of the micromanipulator or a tap on the side of the forge may be necessary to cause the break. The break will usually be straight, especially for small-diameter tips. However, jagged or angled breaks can occur. The angle between the tool and the glass ball should be as straight as possible to avoid angled or jagged breaks. If the wall of the tubing is very thick, it can be quite difficult or impossible to break. The breaking of very small-diameter tips may require a new, very small glass ball.

Pulling

By adhering the very tip of the microtool to the glass ball, a point of glass can be pulled away from the tip, creating an ultrasharp point (Fig. 10.23). During pulling, the tool is positioned so that its tip can be brought into contact with the glass ball. The filament is activated, and its temperature slowly increased while the tip of the tool is advanced carefully against the glass ball. At some point, the temperature will be sufficient to cause adhe-

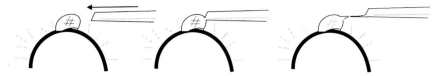

FIG. 10.23. Pulling on the microforge. The microtool is positioned with its point adjacent to the glass ball. The filament is activated, and its temperature is carefully adjusted so that, as the point of the tool is brought into contact with the glass ball, partial melting occurs between the tool and the ball. When the tool is pulled back, a small point of glass is drawn away, forming a sharp point.

sion between the tip and the glass ball, and, upon drawing back the tool, a point of glass will be pulled out from the tip. This can be done with both straight and beveled tips. Once again, for very small tips, a correspondingly small glass ball is appropriate.

Bending

The hot filament can also be used to soften the tapered section of the capillary, causing it to bend (Fig. 10.24). The area where a bend is desired in the tool is positioned above the filament. When the filament is heated, the glass will soften and bend down at that point.

The tip of a pipette can also be bent—for instance, back into a hook shape—by forcing it directly against a warm filament. Here, the filament is heated carefully just to the point at which the glass of the tip is slightly softened. The tip of the tool is carefully pushed against the filament and will curve against it. This technique requires practice in judging the filament temperature. As the bend proceeds, filament temperature may have to be turned up slightly to keep the larger section of glass malleable. If the temperature is too high, the glass will stick to the filament and break or simply melt. This technique works best when done quickly, to avoid any unwanted

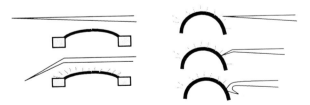

FIG. 10.24. Bending on the microforge. The microforge filament can be used to simply bend the apical section of microtools. On the *left,* a hot filament causes the glass to soften and bend. Also, by carefully adjusting filament temperature, the microtool tip can be bent against the filament itself to form hooks or loops, as shown on the *right.*

distortion of the tool from heating. Therefore, some practice will be a requisite for success. With imagination, this technique can be used in a variety of ways to modify the apical section of microtools.

Chemical Treatment of Microtools

The most common chemical treatment used during the fabrication of microtools is hydrofluoric acid. This acid has the property of dissolving glass and, therefore, can be used to thin and "cut" the tip of microtools. Usually, a 20% to 30% aqueous solution is made up for use, although weaker or stronger solutions can be used as desired. In practice, the microtool is fitted onto a compressed-air source, and the tip is immersed in the solution. If a thinning of the wall is desired—without any effect on the lumen size—a constant flow of air is maintained to prevent acid from entering the lumen. Otherwise, the airflow can be intermittent. With practice, a variety of effects can be achieved, from a slight thinning of the wall to a complete "cutting-back" of the tip. The size of the tip can, with experience, be judged by the size of the bubbles produced. After hydrofluoric acid treatment, the tip is immersed in water or other solvent to wash off any residual acid.

If desired, microtools are occasionally given a water-repellent coating by being immersed in a silicone solution (Dricote, Sigmacote, or other). This is not necessary for general embryological work.

Other Requisites

Some procedures can be done to microtools with a common laboratory burner. Holding pipettes can be easily pulled by hand with use of an alcohol burner or small gas flame. Some workers construct a microburner, using a 16- to 20-g needle as the flame orifice and constricting the gas flow with an adjustable clamp or needle valve as illustrated in Fig. 10.25. The microburner produces a very small flame (5 mm or so high) that is convenient for pulling holding pipettes and works very well for placing bends in the shank of microtools—as are sometimes desired for particular setups.

It is recommended to have several forceps, probes, and such, to assist in working with the capillary tubing, such as for holding hot glass during hand-pulling procedures. Also, it will probably be necessary to have some type of glass-cutting device to aid in cutting the capillary tubing. A diamond marking pencil is easy to use for cutting tubing. A small "rat-tailed" file will also work.

Cans of compressed-air are of great use in working with microtools. They usually come with plastic nozzles that will fit, or can be modified to fit, onto

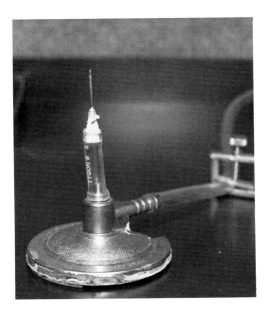

FIG. 10.25. The microburner. A blunted 16-gauge needle has been connected with plastic tubing to the base of a standard burner. The gas supply tubing is constricted with a clamp to control the flow of gas.

the back of a microtool. In this way the tool can be blown out. This is done during the cleaning of some tools after use and in performing certain treatments such as with hydrofluoric acid. An alternative to compressed-air is a syringe setup, with a piece of tubing that fits the microtool. The syringe plunger is compressed, providing a flow of air to clean out the tool. Also, a laboratory compressed-air supply can be used with a length of tubing that terminates with an adapter for the capillary tubing, such as an old syringe with a needle stub of the appropriate size. Once microtools are made, they must be stored. Plastic or glass petri dishes with a thin piece of nontoxic clay spanning the center are the classic method of storing tools. However, a variety of disposable containers often with "locking" lids can be modified for use as storage boxes. A thin piece of dense foam-rubber, such as used for packing material, can be glued inside the box, providing a permanent replacement for the clay (which with time becomes dried out and useless). This foam is then cut with slits all along its length to accommodate the microtools. Both types of microtool boxes are illustrated in Fig. 10.26. Microtools will rapidly become "dirty," picking up dust and particulate matter from the air, if they are not immediately stored in a sealed container.

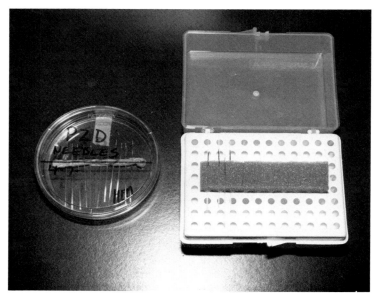

FIG. 10.26. Two methods for storing microtools. On the *left* is a sterile plastic culture dish with a section of plasticine material for holding the tools. On the *right,* a more permanent setup can be devised for research tools, using an old pipette tip box and a section of plastic foam, with slits cut for holding the microtools.

THE CONSTRUCTION OF SPECIFIC MICROTOOLS

The Holding Pipette

Holding pipette construction is considered by some to be close to alchemy. Different workers swear by wildly different methods, often involving secret techniques that, in the end, all result in basically identical tools. There is obviously more than one way to make a holding pipette. Pulling a capillary out to the correct diameter and obtaining a straight break can be quite difficult. Beginners are sometimes taught that the only way to pull a perfect pipette is in one draw, ending with a snap, to produce a straight break. There are several methods for pulling and breaking that will result in excellent holding pipettes.

Pulling

The first step in the construction of a holding pipette is pulling to thin the glass. Just about any type of capillary tubing can be used. What is desired is a pulled section of capillary that is at least a centimeter in length and of the correct diameter in the area of the tip. If the length is too short, the large tapered and shank sections of the tool will contact the slide during micromanipulation, preventing proper alignment. This is why one cannot simply break off a pulled needle at the correct diameter—since this point would be on the taper itself and much too close to the shank. The diameter will vary depending on the cell to be held. For rodent eggs it will be about 75 to 80 μm, and for human eggs, 120 to 170 μm. In general, a diameter of between 60% and 100% of the diameter of the cell to be held will be appropriate. For some techniques, such as partial zonal dissection, for which the holding pipette might block the passage of the needle, a smaller size is desired. For other techniques, such as intracellular injection for which stability is of utmost importance, a larger size would be appropriate.

In practice, a section of capillary tubing is held and heated in, or adjacent to, the flame of a microburner or alcohol lamp. When the glass has been heated sufficiently and is plastic, the hands are carefully moved apart, drawing the glass out into a straight pulled section several centimeters in length. This pulled section is broken in the center, to produce two putative holding pipettes. The correct degree of pulling relative to the diameter of the pulled section can be judged only with experience. However, if the pulled section is too large; it can be repulled to reduce its diameter further. The pulled section is reoriented near the flame and carefully pulled again. If the pulled portion is too short, a pair of forceps can be used. Usually, the pulled section will be tapered so that at some point along its length the diameter will be suitable for the desired holding pipette. The diameter of the pulled section is determined with the microforge micrometer.

An alternative to hand pulling is the use of a pipette puller. The pulling of large, long pipettes, suitable for holding, is one of the most problematic pipette puller techniques. Generally, a weak pull is used to draw the glass out, without breaking. This may also involve cooling the glass during the pull or using a multistage pull. The main problem is getting a pipette that is long enough for use as a holding pipette with the correct diameter. Automated pulling of holding pipettes is probably as variable as the hand-pulling method.

Breaking and Polishing

The next step in holding pipette construction is breaking the tip. Actually, the tip can be broken during the pulling step, simply by controlling the pulling motion and giving the glass a sudden pull just as it cools. However, this is a difficult and unreliable method for producing tools of the correct length and diameter. Breaking is probably most easily done using the microforge as described in the previous section of general microforge techniques.

The breaking of holding pipettes usually requires a final twist of the micro-manipulator to snap the tool. Maintaining a parallel orientation between the pipette and the glass ball is important in creating a straight break. Often the break will have a slight angle or imperfection. This may not matter, as the final polishing step will "melt down" small bumps. However, if the deviation of the tip is more substantial, it will have to be rebroken. An alternative to microforge breaking is the use of a glass-cutting tool such as a diamond pencil, microfile, or even another piece of glass, to score the pulled section at the desired point for breaking. The microforge allows the procedure to be observed, so that the correct diameter is easily obtained.

Once the pipette has been broken to yield a straight tip of the desired size, it must be heat polished to soften the edges and constrict the lumen. This was discussed in the previous section on microforge techniques.

Pipettes for Injection and Aspiration

Pipettes with open lumens of a defined size are required for the tasks such as enucleation or sperm injection. These are made by breaking the tip of a sharp needle at the desired point, to produce the required tip and lumen size. Further modifications, such as the creation of a bevel or sharp point, are also possible. Most of the techniques for the fabrication of these tools were first described by de Fonbrune. McGrath and Solter (6) published perhaps the best recent description of micropipette formation, including the use of grinding to produce beveled pipettes.

The fabrication of microtools for injection and aspiration begins with the pulling of a sharp needle on the pipette puller. The wall thickness of the capillary tubing should be as thin as possible. Glass temperature and pull strength should be high to produce a long, thin-tapered section. Some needle pullers may allow precise glass temperature adjustment during pulling, to create broken-tipped needles of the requisite size. Otherwise, sharp-pointed needles are easily modified with the microforge. The needle is fitted into the microforge and positioned for breaking the tip, as discussed in the section on microforge techniques.

Figure 10.27 illustrates the initial breaking diameter of several different injection or aspiration pipettes. Some microtools, such as small-injection pipettes or blastomere-transfer pipettes, are completed once broken to the correct size. Other pipettes, such as enucleation or sperm-injection pipettes, require further steps.

If a large lumen is not absolutely necessary or desired, a sharp point can be simply pulled from the straight broken tip of the micropipette. If desired, the wall can be thinned with hydrofluoric acid before tip pulling. This method is sufficient to produce sharp aspiration pipettes for human enucleation.

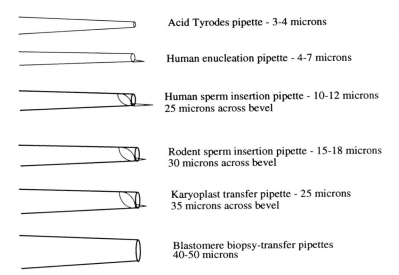

Acid Tyrodes pipette - 3-4 microns

Human enucleation pipette - 4-7 microns

Human sperm insertion pipette - 10-12 microns
25 microns across bevel

Rodent sperm insertion pipette - 15-18 microns
30 microns across bevel

Karyoplast transfer pipette - 25 microns
35 microns across bevel

Blastomere biopsy-transfer pipettes
40-50 microns

FIG. 10.27. The initial breaking diameters and dimensions for several common micropipettes.

Some pipettes, such as for sperm injection or karyoplast removal, require a large, open lumen with a sharp point. This requires the use of a microgrinder to cut a bevel on the tip. If a pipette is to be beveled, this must be taken into account during the original breaking step, since the beveling process will increase the size of the lumen. It might be considered that, in making beveled pipettes, the breaking step could be eliminated by simply grinding the tip of the pulled needle to the correct size. However, breaking the tip to the approximate size before beveling provides a much quicker, easier, and cleaner procedure overall.

The pipette is clamped in the micromanipulator on the beveler. The bevel angle is adjusted as desired. For most beveled tools, an angle of 45° is used. If the angle is too shallow, the lumen will be too "long," making some procedures more difficult. On some models, the speed of the wheel is adjustable. The fastest speed can be used for large pipettes and a reduced speed for smaller tools. For the beveling of sperm-injection pipettes on the Narishige microgrinder, a speed of 50% of maximum works well. Once the speed is selected, the pipette is carefully advanced down onto the grinding surface. As mentioned earlier, some models feature a microscope for monitoring the beveling procedure, but this is not necessary. The microgrinder should be positioned at a level that will provide comfortable observation from the side. A bright, directional light, such as a fiberoptic illuminator, should be directed onto the grinding wheel from above. It is advantageous to place a matte black surface behind the grinder, to provide a high-contrast background for observing the microtool. As the tool is lowered onto the surface of the wheel, using the coarse and then the fine control, it is carefully observed from the side as illustrated in Fig. 10.28. As the tip of the tool touches the wheel a slight bow will be introduced into the tool. This is easily observed and is a definite indication of contact between the microtool tip and the grinder.

The time of grinding obviously depends on the desired degree of beveling. If the particular pipette was broken off slightly smaller than desired, grinding time can be extended. For human sperm-injection pipettes with a 25-μm bevel length, grinding time (with a 15-μm starting tip) can be as short as 10 seconds (Narishige microgrinder, speed:50, thin walled tubing). If the tip was smaller to begin with, grinding times of 20 seconds to 1 minute can be typical. For the beveling of larger tools, such as large, cell injection pipettes, longer grinding times, up to a few minutes, may be required. Some period of trial-and-error will probably be required in developing a successful grinding protocol.

Once grinding is finished and the tool is raised from the wheel, the next step is washing. Before removal, the shank of the tool is marked with a magic marker to indicate the position of the bevel as shown in Fig. 10.29. The tool is then removed and quickly washed as follows: Small (plastic)

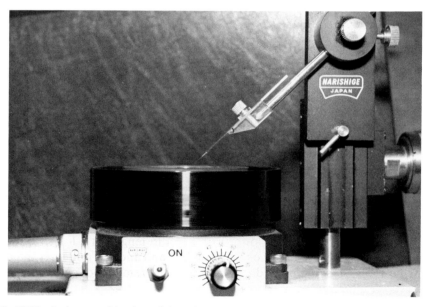

FIG. 10.28. A closeup side view of the microtool in contact with the abrasive wheel of the microgrinder. Contact can be easily determined from simple observation, without the use of a microscope.

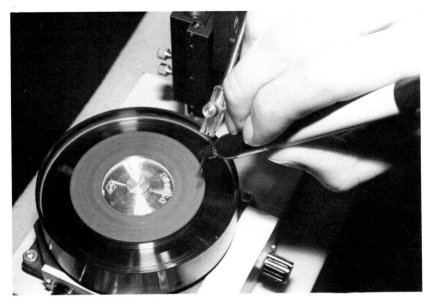

FIG. 10.29. After the grinding procedure, the tool is marked to indicate the position of the bevel.

containers of hydrofluoric acid and deionized water are set up on the bench top. The microtool is inserted into a source of compressed-gas, such as described in the equipment section. The tip of the microtool is placed in the hydrofluoric acid for approximately 10 to 20 seconds (depending on the strength of the acid) while intermittent bursts of gas are given. Bubbles should flow from the tip during these bursts. The tool is then rinsed in the water with a similar treatment. This should produce a clean tool with a slightly thinned tip.

The tool is then placed in the microforge for the final pulling step. The tip of the microtool is positioned so that the very apex of the bevel can be brought into contact with the glass ball. The mark on the tool shank is a convenient guide for placing the tool in the microforge. The filament is heated and the tip is brought into contact with the glass ball and a point pulled, as described in the section on microforge techniques. The point should ideally be very small, only 1 or 2 μm in length. If a longer point is obtained, it can be broken off on the glass ball and another pull attempted.

Microtools for some procedures involving the removal of cells or cellular material can be treated with a repellent silicon coating. This was suggested by Kopac (7) during the development of his microcytochemical work. The capillary tubing itself can be coated before pulling; but usually the apical section of a complete pulled pipette is treated in a fashion identical with the hydrofluoric acidic-washing method. The pipette is connected to a source of compressed-gas, and its tip is immersed in the siliconizing solution. The pipette is blown out and allowed to air-dry or is heated in a warm oven.

Techniques with Aspiration or Injection Pipettes

During use, large aspiration and injection pipettes are placed under the control of the desired microinjection device. Many procedures, including acidic Tyrode's drilling, sperm injection, and blastomere biopsy, can be done using a mouthpiece. These techniques have been described in previous chapters. Cell and nuclear transfer has been discussed briefly also. Cell transfer is basically identical with blastomere biopsy, except that the blastomere is transferred under the zona pellucida of another embryo or enucleated egg. Openings to accommodate the insertion of the large cell-transfer pipettes are made in the zonae pellucidae using mechanical or acidic Tyrode's drilling. There are two basic techniques for dealing with cell nuclei: In one method, a sharp beveled pipette of the requisite size is introduced directly into the vitellus and the nucleus is aspirated. This invasive technique can be used for the actual transfer of nuclei, but it is probably best suited for the simple removal of nuclei or metaphase plates, either for polyspermy correction or to create enucleated eggs for use in genome extension. Human zygotes survive this procedure quite well, whereas rodent zygotes do not. In the ingenious method developed by McGrath and Solter (8), an enucleation pipette is used to draw up a membrane-bound karyoplast that contains the desired nucleus. The removal of a karyoplast requires that the embryo be incubated in a cytoskeletal relaxant solution. The aspiration and, especially, the expulsion of a nuclear karyoplast requires very precise control. This work is usually done using an oil-filled system, a micropipette, and a high-precision microsyringe. For transfer, the micropipette is inserted into the perivitelline space of the requisite embryo and the karyoplast is carefully expelled. A final consideration for nuclear and cell transfer is the process of fusing the karyoplast or blastomere to the egg or embryo. This is a complex subject and will not be discussed in detail. Early experiments used the membrane fusion properties of the Sendai virus. The current method of choice is the use of an electrofusion apparatus. This is an electronic device that provides a pulse of electrical energy across a microscope specimen container. Apparently, this electrical field partially disrupts the membranes of the two cells and, if they are in close contact, the membranes can re-fuse together. Currently, the most popular commercial device for electrofusion is the BTX ECM-200, illustrated in Fig. 10.30. The electric pulse is delivered across two electrodes, which are incorporated into a slide-based specimen holder shown in Fig. 10.31. Electrofusion is usually performed in a nonionic medium, such as an isotonic sugar solution. One of the most critical factors

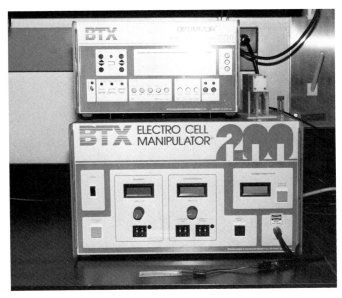

FIG. 10.30. The BTX ECM-200 Electrocell Manipulator. The top unit provides a readout of the actual parameters of electrofusion events. Electrical leads (in *front*) are connected to the electrofusion chamber.

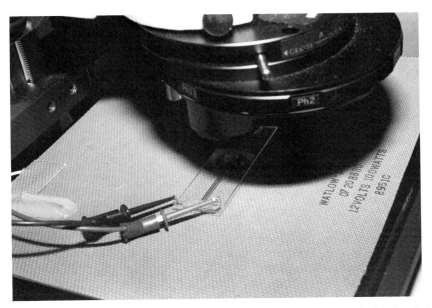

FIG. 10.31. The BTX slide chamber. The two wire electrodes are connected with the electrofusion unit. Specimens are placed between the electrodes and can be observed under the microscope during the procedure.

is the adjustment of the electrical parameters during the application of a pulse. The voltage supplied by the system is set to a certain value, but the actual voltage delivered across the specimen will depend on the complex interaction of a variety of factors, including the actual ionic makeup of the surrounding solution and the physical geometry of the chamber. The BTX model is available with a peripheral device that provides real-time analysis of the actual pulse delivered across the chamber. Basically, the two cells are positioned so that the desired plane of fusion is parallel with the electrodes. A preliminary alternating current can be applied, which causes an attraction between the cells, increasing membrane contact. Then, a single pulse or multiple pulses of direct current are applied across the electrodes. Electrofusion works best when the cells are similar in size.

Stem cell transfer is essentially similar to karyoplast transfer. Stem cells are aspirated into the lumen of a sharp, beveled pipette of the appropriate size. This pipette is introduced into the blastocoele of an embryo, and the cells are expelled. Here, less precision is required than for nuclear transfer.

Intracellular and Nuclear Injection Needles and Procedures

Needles for cell injection are usually made by simple pulling. The tip size should be as fine as possible, with a long gradual taper, so that the relative diameter of the apical section is as small as possible. Capillary tubing with a filling fiber is used for these tools. Usually, needle tips are open; however, closed needles can be opened by touching against the holding pipette. The problem with the use of fine-tipped needles for injection is that they become clogged with debris from the injectant or with cellular material. Microbevels can be placed on the tips of injection pipettes, but this is a problematic and time-consuming process. The usual procedure for gene injection is that a simple pulling protocol is developed for pulling satisfactory needles that are fine-tipped, but have a reasonable rate of clogging. Before each experiment, an appropriate number of needles are pulled, so that as clogging occurs, quick replacement is possible. Sometimes extra pressure from the microinjector can be used to open a clogged tip. Also, rubbing on the holding pipette can sometimes release a clog.

Fine-tipped needles can be filled in a variety of ways. A pulled glass Pasteur pipette of suitable size or a spinal needle on a small syringe filled with the solution can be inserted into the back of the pipette. Alternatively, the pipette can be filled from the front by immersing its tip in the desired solution and applying suction. This second method works best for needles with a larger lumen.

For the actual cell or nuclear injection, two basic methods can be used. In the continuous-flow method, a constant flow is obtained from the lumen of the microneedle. This is done by applying constant pressure from a microsyringe or compressed-gas system. Electronic units that use compressed-gas or pumps have been described. A basic system can also be arranged, using a compressed-gas tank, simple valves, and the appropriate tubing for connection to the pipette holder. Flow rate from the tip can be judged by dragging the tip into the adjacent oil and observing the formation of spherical drops of the aqueous injection solution. The micropipette is simply introduced into the cell or nucleus, and injection is controlled through timing and observation of swelling. Alternatively, individual injection is possible by the application of a controlled transient increase in the microinjection system pressure. This can be easily accomplished with an electronic microinjector unit or with a carefully set up and maintained microsyringe unit. In their excellent book on murine micromanipulation, Hogan and coauthors (9) describe another common system used for gene injection. The microsyringe system is replaced by a large 50-mL glass syringe. The syringe, connecting tubing, and pipette holder remain filled with air. When a flow of material from the micropipette is desired, the large plunger is simply compressed by hand to provide the necessary pressure.

An important consideration during injection is that the needle is actually inserted into the cell or nucleus. The cell and the nuclear membrane, in particular, are extremely resilient. During the insertion of even the sharpest needle, the membrane can simply deform around the tip and penetration will not occur. The needle must be forced even farther "into" the cell or nucleus, sometimes even to the point that the needle appears to have completely traversed the cell, before actual penetration occurs. Sometimes a sharp motion or "tap" against the microtool can aid in penetration. Piezo-electric devices could possibly be used to advantage for this purpose, but no reports of their use in gene-injection experiments have been put forth. If injection is attempted following unsuccessful penetration, the membrane will often balloon out, away from the needle tip with the flow of solution. If difficulty with needle penetration persists, this probably indicates that the tip has been fouled and needle replacement is required.

METHODS FOR SPECIMEN HANDLING

There are two basic methods for handling specimens for micromanipulation: the hanging-drop method and the standard slide or dish method. Barber (10) developed the hanging-drop method for use in micromanipulation, since this was the only way to achieve acceptable optical performance with the crude microscopes of his day. The great advantage of this method is that it allows the easy application of very high-power oil immersion objectives—since the specimen is, in effect, placed in the proper orientation for viewing with the standard optical system of an upright microscope. The specimen is placed in a drop of culture medium, which hangs from a coverslip. As illustrated in Fig. 10.32, the coverslip forms the "roof" of a glass chamber, which is placed on the microscope stage in a way such as to allow proper focusing of the optical system on the specimen. The chamber is open on one side to permit the insertion of the microtools, which approach the specimen from below. The tools can be introduced from either side or from the front. For some configurations, the use of a hanging-drop chamber requires that the microtools have bent shanks or tips to allow proper tip orientation. To control evaporation of the microdrop during use, a variety of techniques have been developed over the years, including sealing the chamber in various ways and filling the chamber with a hydrocarbon fluid (11). The hanging-drop method is still in use for the most critical procedures requiring high-power visualization. However, for most routine work, it has been replaced by the more convenient slide or dish method.

The most common method of specimen handling for embryological work involves the use of a standard slide or dish that contains culture medium or a drop of medium under a protective layer of oil. This is much more convenient than dealing with the preparation of a hanging-drop chamber. Especially with the use of a modern tissue culture inverted microscope, this method works well. In general, a dish or slide is prepared with a volume of culture medium in which the specimen is placed; 35- to 100-mm culture dishes or their tops can simply be filled with a volume of medium. Alternatively, a drop or multiple drops of medium can be placed in a dish, dish top, or slide and covered with a layer of oil. The latter is probably the most versatile method, in that multiple drops can be arranged containing different specimens; for instance, eggs and sperm. Drops can be oriented in certain ways to help keep track of specimens during a micromanipulation procedure. Long linear drops can be set up with the specimens placed at one end. As each specimen is subjected to a procedure, it can be moved to the other end of the drop. For handling large drops or multiple drops, the larger-sized dish top is probably the most suitable vessel. Several large drops can be made with plenty of spacing, to avoid mixing. However, it must be recalled

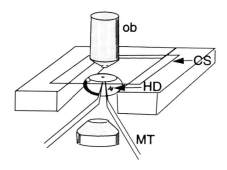

FIG. 10.32. The hanging-drop system. The drop *(HD)*, containing the specimen, hangs from the bottom of a coverslip *(CS)* suspended from a glass chamber placed on the microscope stage. The objective *(Ob)* can thus be placed in proper orientation (even using oil-immersion) with relation to the specimen being manipulated.

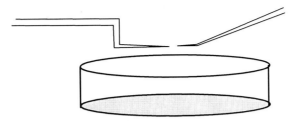

FIG. 10.33. Two ways of bending microtools to accommodate placement in a culture dish.

that the sides of the dish will interfere with the operation of the microtools; hence, the drops must be placed near the center of the dish.

Slides are probably the most convenient specimen-handling method if small drops are satisfactory. The classic method is to use a simple glass depression slide. The central depression provides enough volume for a drop and the oil covering. Alternatively, standard slides can be modified by the addition of shallow walls to create a small holding area. This can be done either in a permanent fashion by cementing small pieces of glass or plastic; or with a temporary system, using petroleum jelly or some such material to enclose a small area. Also, there are several new slide-based cell culture-type products available that can be used as specimen containers, such as the Tissue-tek line from Nunc. These are designed for the microscopic observation of cell cultures and, usually, consist of an optical glass or plastic slide surmounted by some type of culture vessel. This vessel can be modified or removed, leaving a slide that has a built-in holding area for medium and oil.

During use, the holding vessel is simply placed on the stage and the microtools are introduced. With slides, the microtools can usually be oriented into the drop at a slight angle, as described in the chapter on clinical micromanipulation. If necessary, a small bend can be placed in the apical section of the microtool to provide strictly horizontal tools (see Fig. 10.24). With dish-type vessels, some type of bends must be placed into the shank or tip section of the microtools to permit proper clearance and operation around the steep sides of the dish. Figure 10.33 illustrates some of the common methods of tool bending for use with dishes. The shanks of the microtools are easily bent with a microburner and a pair of forceps or probe. The apical sections are bent using the microforge. Careful consideration must be given to the proper specimen-handling method, as this is often of great importance in developing a successful and convenient protocol. In general, it is probably best to start with the simplest technique, such a well-slide, and progress to the other methods if required. Some techniques, such as embryo biopsy or cell transfer, require that specimens are individually accounted for. To perform the procedure on multiple embryos, a method that permits the handling of several individual drops will be necessary.

REFERENCES

1. El Badry HM. *Micromanipulators and micromanipulation.* New York: Academic Press; 1963.
2. Dunn FL. The use of hydraulic devices for obtaining micromanipulation. *J Infect Dis* 1928;40:383–398.
3. Alexander JT, Nastuck WL. An instrument for the production of microelectrodes used in electrophysiological studies. *Rev Sci Inst* 1953;24:528–531.
4. Brown KT, Flaming DG. *Advanced micropipette techniques for cell physiology.* New York: John Wiley & Sons; 1986.
5. de Fonbrune P. Demonstration d'un micromanipulateur pneumatique et d'un appareil pour la fabrication des microinstruments. *Ann Physiol Physiochem* 1934;10:4.
6. McGrath J, Solter D. Nuclear and cytoplasmic transfer in mammalian embryos. In: Gwatkin RBL, ed. *Manipulation of mammalian development.* New York: Plenum Press; 1985.
7. Kopac MJ. Submicro methods in enzymatic cytochemistry. *Trans NY Acad Sci* 1953; 15:290–297.
8. McGrath J, Solter D. Nuclear transplantation in the mouse embryo by microsurgery and cell fusion. *Science* 1983;200:1300.
9. Hogan B, Constantini F, Lacy E. *Manipulating the mouse embryo: a laboratory manual.* Cold Spring Harbor, NY: Cold Spring Harbor Laboratory; 1986.
10. Barber, MA. A new method of isolating micro-organisms. *J Kan Med Soc* 1904;4:487.
11. Kopac MJ. Recent developments in cellular microsurgery. *Trans NY Acad Sci* 1955;17: 257–265.

Appendix: List of Suppliers of Micromanipulation Equipment

MICROMANIPULATORS AND MICROTOOL FABRICATION EQUIPMENT

De Fonbrune micromanipulators and microforge
  Technical Products International, 5918 Evergreen, St. Louis, MO 63134
  (314)522-8671
Leitz micromanipulators
  Leica Inc., 24 Link Drive, Rockleigh, NJ 07647
  (201)767-1100
Nikon–Narishige micromanipulators and microtool equipment
  Nikon Inc., 1300 Walt Whitman Rd, Melville, NY 11747–3064
  (516)547-4200
Prior, Stoelting, and other type micromanipulators, microtool equipment, glass capillary tubing, and accessories
  Stoelting Inc., 620 Wheat Lane, Wood Dale, IL 60191
  (708)860-9700
Research Instruments Ltd. micromanipulators and microtool equipment available in the USA through:
  Energy Beam Sciences, PO Box 468, Agawam, MS 01001
  (413)786-9322

Micropositioners, microtool fabricating equipment, and glass capillary
  tubing
  Sutter Instruments Co., PO Box 6039, Novato, CA 94948
  (415)883-0128
Zeiss/Eppendorf micromanipulators and automated cell injection systems
  Carl Zeiss Inc., One Zeiss Drive, Thornwood, NY 10594
  (914)747-1800

MISCELLANEOUS EQUIPMENT

Electrofusion equipment
  Biotechnologies & Experimental Research Inc., 3742 Jewell St., San
  Diego, CA 92109
  (619)270-0861
Bulk glass capillary tubing
Kimble no. 46485 0.7–1.0-mm od–borosilicate tubing
  Thomas Scientific, PO Box 99, Swedesboro, NJ 08085-0099
  (609)467-2000
  Catalog no. 5698-G12.
Flexible silicone rubber heating fabric for stage warmers
  Watlow Inc., 12001 Lackland Rd, St. Louis, MO 63146
  (314)878-4600
  (Note: This material must be custom fabricated by an electronics shop to
  the requisite shape for the microscope stage or other surface. It cannot
  simply be cut to the desired shape.)

11

The Future of Micromanipulation in Assisted Reproduction

Henry E. Malter and Jacques Cohen

The future of embryological micromanipulation would seem to be limited only by the imagination and perseverance of the scientists involved. As experience is gained both in the large-animal and human clinical fields, existing techniques will be optimized and new techniques developed. Advances in instrumentation, particularly involving the use of the laser, may provide elegant solutions to existing problems and suggest new challenges to be solved. This chapter will briefly examine some of what can be expected in the next decade.

THE DEVELOPMENT OF LASER MICROMANIPULATION TECHNIQUES

Since the use of lasers will be important in several areas of micromanipulation work, we will begin with a brief overview of current laser techniques. As with other methodologies that have become incorporated into the micromanipulation repertoire, laser energy was first used to perform dissection at the tissue level (1). A laser produces a beam of coherent radiation that can be directed and focused to derive an extremely powerful and precise source of energy. This combination of power and precision make the laser beam a perfect "scalpel" for the cutting or targeted destruction of tissue. Advances in design and optics have permitted the reduction of the laser beam to the microscopic scale. For almost 30 years, the laser has been used for cellular micromanipulation (2). Several early experiments using the laser were discussed in Chapters 1 and 5.

In the near future, laser micromanipulation will probably become increasingly important in embryological micromanipulation. The precision

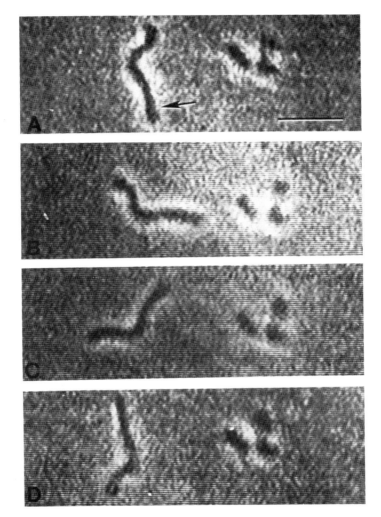

FIG. 11.1. Chromosome movement using an optical trap. **A:** A chromosome of a lysed tissue culture cell *(arrow)* is positioned in the beam of a laser-generated optical trap. **B–D:** The chromosome is rotated 180° by manipulation with the trap. (From Berns MW, et al. Use of a laser-induced optical trap to study chromosome movement on the mitotic spindle. *Proc Natl Acad Sci USA* 1989;86:4539–4543, with permission.)

and ease with which the laser can be controlled will provide improved techniques in microsurgery, gene transfer, cell fusion, and other areas. Basically, the laser is directed into the microscope through an optical port. The beam is transmitted through the standard optical system of the microscope, focused in the plane of the specimen, and positioned in relation to a reference point such as a cross hair. For cutting or ablation, a specimen is positioned using the cross hair, and the laser is activated to produce a pulse of energy that disrupts the target area. The beam can be focused to produce a lesion as small as 0.25 μm in diameter (3).

A second use of the laser for cellular manipulation has involved the "optical trap." Ashikin (4) discovered that the radiation pressure of two focused laser beams could produce a type of "force field," which could be used like miniature forceps to hold small objects, such as cells and cellular

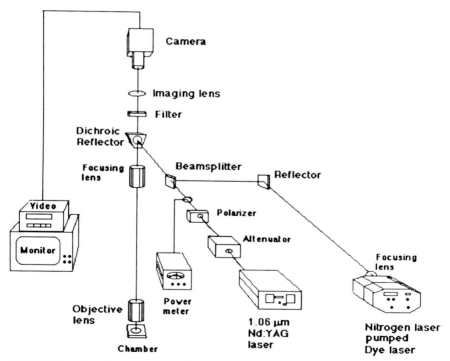

FIG. 11.2. A schematic diagram of a laser micromanipulation system. Two lasers: a Nd:YAG laser for the generation of an optical trap, and a nitrogen-pumped dye laser for cell microsurgery are introduced into a microscope (indicated by the *focusing lens* and *objective lens*). A dichroic reflector allows the laser light to pass into the microscope, while the visible light image of the specimen passes out through an imaging lens into a video camera for observation. (From Steubing RW, et al. Single beam optical trapping and micromanipulation of mammalian cells. *SPIE Laser–Tissue Interactions* 1990;1202:273-280, with permission.)

organelles. Later work showed that a single beam could also be used to generate an optical trap (5). Optical trapping has been used to stabilize and move cells, bacteria, viruses, sperm cells, and even individual chromosomes (6–8). Figure 11.1 shows a single chromosome being rotated by the optical trap. Movement can be accomplished by holding the object with the laser trap and then changing its relative position through movement of the microscope stage (using very precise computer-controlled motor drives). Figure 11.2 illustrates a typical laser micromanipulation setup, developed at the Beckman Laser Institute (9). In this system, two lasers are introduced into the optical path of a standard microscope. A neodymium:yttrium-aluminum-garnet (Nd:YAG) laser is used for generating the optical trap, while a dye laser is used for microsurgical procedures.

As with the early experiments in micromanipulation, this preliminary laser work has been accomplished using complex purpose-built apparatus. However, as this technology matures and becomes incorporated into valuable cell biology techniques, there is no reason why commercial laser micromanipulation equipment could not be developed. This will no doubt take place during the next decade.

RESEARCH AND LARGE-ANIMAL MICROMANIPULATION

Micromanipulation will continue to play a key role in genetic transformation for basic research or the improvement of livestock. The gene-injection technique is likely to remain the method of choice for the near future. However, stem cell-mediated gene transfer, providing the ability for homologous gene replacement or inactivation and genetic selection, is rapidly becoming an important technique for mammalian genetic manipulation. The expected development of embryonic stem cell lines from superior large domestic animals will be one of the most important achievements in the history of animal breeding. Animals with optimized production characteristics, disease resistance, and improved meat and milk quality could be produced. As knowledge of large-animal genomes is gained, desirable genes will be identified. Also, genes involved with survival in arid or high-altitude environments may be identified from exotic species. The transfer of these genes would make possible the development of animal varieties with improved performance under poor conditions. This could be of vital importance, considering the increased erosion, desertification, and potential "greenhouse" effects that the future may bring.

Great advances have been made in the 5 short years since the first report of embryonic cloning in large animals (10). The first dairy cow clones are now valuable production animals (11). Clonal transgenic lines could be developed from stem cells, providing animal breeders with the ability to quickly produce new optimum domestic varieties. Also, the future may bring methods for using other cells as genome source material. As our understanding of developmental genomic alteration (such as methylation) expands, it may be possible to reverse this process and restore the mature somatic genome to an embryonic state so that development can be directed through nuclear transfer, using a wide variety of source material. This would permit true cloning and greatly expand the research and animal improvement strategies available. Seidel (12) briefly discusses this possibility and other future prospects, such as the development of genetic engineering through artificial chromosomes, in a recent article on the next 100 years of embryo transfer research.

The laser may provide improved methods for gene transfer and cell fusion. Laser energy has been used to disrupt cell membranes and permit the entrance of DNA molecules. In this way, transgenic cells can be created (13). This method may find use in the transfer of DNA to gametes and embryos. Laser-mediated disruption of cell membranes has also been used to promote cell fusion. This was first reported by Schierenberg (14) in cells of the developing nematode embryo. For laser fusion to work, cell–cell contact is apparently very important. In the nematode work, the cells were already held in close proximity by the outer shell. In later work, the use of an avidin–biotin bridge allowed laser-mediated fusion between B lymphocytes and myeloma cells (15). Recently, Steubing and coworkers (9) reported on the application of laser energy both to stabilize the cells, using an optical trap, and to obtain cell fusion. Two myeloma cells were held in close contact by the optical trap while high-energy pulses from a second dye laser were used to initiate fusion. A schematic of the laser setup used in these experiments was illustrated in Fig. 11.2. The actual fusion of two cells is shown in Fig. 11.3. Important observations included the improvement of fusion efficiency through the addition of polyethylene glycol to the fusion medium and increasing the temperature to 37°C. This technique could be very important, especially for the situation in which two cells of unequal size are fused. The fusion of very small cells with larger cells has proved to be quite difficult by electrofusion, since the voltage level necessary for fusion is detrimental to the integrity of the smaller cell. Laser cell fusion might facilitate nuclear transfer with stem cells.

Another area in which embryological micromanipulation will be of importance in animal science is in the development of interspecies gestation through inner cell mass transfer. This concept of one species acting as a surrogate mother for the offspring of another species is an important goal for the maintenance and husbandry of exotic and endangered species. Common and hardy species could be used as surrogate mothers for the embryos of exotic or weaker species. Hybrid embryos would be reconstituted through micromanipulation with the inner cell mass (ICM) of the exotic species linked with the trophoblast of the surrogate species. This would theoretically permit an interspecific pregnancy to proceed. Micro-

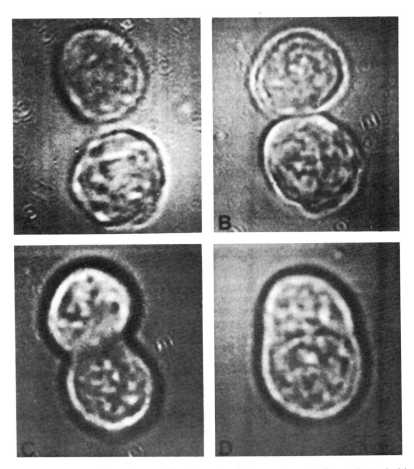

FIG. 11.3. Cell fusion using a laser optical trapping–fusion system. **A:** Two cells are held positioned for optical trapping. **B:** The optical trap is activated holding the cells in close proximity. **C:** Following the application of laser pulses to disrupt the membranes at the point of attachment between the two cells, the cell membranes begin to fuse together. **D:** Five minutes later, the cells have successfully fused. (From Steubing RW, et al. Single beam optical trapping and micromanipulation of mammalian cells. *SPIE Laser–Tissue Interactions* 1990;1202:273–280, with permission.)

manipulation techniques developed for experimental chimera formation, as discussed in Chapters 2 and 3 could be modified to perform this type of microsurgery. Recently, Rorie and coworkers (16) reported a simple micromanipulation procedure for ICM transfer that was used to combine sheep ICM with the trophoblast of goat embryos. Transfer of these hybrid embryos to a goat recipient resulted in the birth of healthy lambs, which were nursed and accepted by the surrogate mother.

LASER MICROMANIPULATION FOR IMPROVED GAMETE INTERACTION

The optical trap–laser microsurgery system may play an important role in research and clinical applications involving gamete interaction. Human sperm have been successfully manipulated in the optical trap (7). Individual sperm could be trapped and held for up to 30 seconds without any apparent effect on viability or motility. Moreover, using the motorized stage, sperm in the trap could be effectively moved around the slide. Preliminary reports have also been published concerning the opening of the zona pellucida by laser microbeams (also discussed briefly in Chap. 6; Berns MW, personal communication; 17). Perhaps, in the future, laser micromanipulation systems, similar to the cell fusion system outlined earlier, will be used for clinical microsurgical fertilization. Laser microbeams will "drill" precise holes in the zona pellucida to permit the entry of an optical trap-directed single sperm cell that could be stabilized and fused with the oocyte using a third application of laser energy. Such a system might make possible routine fertilization using immotile and possibly even acrosome-defective sperm.

GENE TRANSFER IN THE HUMAN

The first step in any attempt at gene transfer is the identification, isolation, and characterization of the desired gene. This is a far from trivial matter. However, many genes of potentially "clinical" interest are already available and, in the future, an exponential expansion in gene characterization can be expected. Once a gene is available, a genetic construct must be devised and created for use in gene transfer. To obtain a satisfactory level of expression with the desired tissue or temporal specificity would probably require the creation of a complex fusion construct, as outlined in Chapter 3. This can be a painstaking and laborious process, involving the precise placement of the transgene in relation to regulatory DNA sequences. It must be recalled that our understanding of gene expression (certainly one of the most complex regulatory systems in biology) is in its infancy. There have been several cases of incorrect and unexplained transgene expression patterns (18,19)

Once a construct is devised and created, pronuclear injection should be a relatively straightforward procedure in the human. In fact, recent experiments involving the microsurgical removal of pronuclei from polyspermic human zygotes indicate that pronuclear injection may be applied efficiently in the human (20). Mouse zygotes are easily killed by the cytoplasmic insertion of a relatively large enucleation pipette, whereas human zygotes survive the procedure quite well (Malter H, personal observation). Also, the pronuclei of human zygotes are readily visualized by light microscopy.

The injection procedure would entail the use of a standard embryological micromanipulation setup. The zygote would be held by a suction holding pipette while a fine-pointed injection needle (preloaded with an aqueous solution of the DNA construct) was introduced into the target pronucleus until pronuclear expansion (perhaps double) was observed, as described in Chapter 3. A percentage of zygotes would be damaged by the procedure. On the basis of murine pronuclear injection, once the injection conditions (timing, size of needle, DNA concentration, and other) were optimized, a success rate of 70% or more could be expected. Certainly there would be some embryonic loss from the injection technique itself, and this would have to be taken into account in its clinical application. Successfully injected zygotes would be cultured and then biopsied before transfer, to determine their genetic component, as discussed in Chapter 3.

STRATEGIES FOR GERMLINE GENE THERAPY

It is unlikely that any attempts will be made to actively incorporate germline therapy into assisted reproductive human technology in the next decade; too many important steps needed for reliable "gene correction" are still missing. Nevertheless, a short discussion of a possible scenario is provided here, especially since such forms of gene manipulation could potentially be far-reaching. Obviously, the ethical, social, and political dilemmas exceed those of already complicated issues, such as the legal status of the four-cell embryo and the definition of motherhood. In a pluralistic society, unanimity on such a major issue as germline therapy, may be beyond the ability of any secular authority.

One great advantage of germline therapy should be that, if successful, it would terminate the heredity of the genetic lesion. A transgenically corrected genome would theoretically be passed on to any future generations (although animal experiments have demonstrated some exceptions to this; 21,22).

any single-gene defect could be corrected by the transfer of a functional transgene with the correct expression pattern and control. Germline therapy would be particularly indicated in treating genetic lesions associated with the central nervous system, since in this case the blood–brain barrier would probably preclude somatic cell gene therapy (23). Several successful mouse models exist for using transgenes to circumvent deficiencies caused by genetic lesions (24,25).

Recently, Gordon (26) suggested several novel treatment strategies for individuals with heritable cancers. Chemotherapy efficacy might be greatly improved if multiple-drug–resistance genes, providing protection from the toxic effects of chemotherapeutic agents, could be transferred through the germlines of affected individuals. Expression could even be targeted, using the appropriate tissue-specific promoters, to organs that are particularly susceptible to chemotherapeutic toxicity. Preliminary mouse experiments have shown that this methodology can work (27). Alternatively, genes for tumor-killing agents could be linked to promoters involved with atavistic expression in malignant cells to create an automatic "magic bullet" for curbing tumor growth (26). Certainly as our knowledge of human genetics expands, new treatment strategies, as well as new treatment challenges, will be defined that will be amenable to germline genetic manipulation.

Considering the present state of knowledge about germline gene transfer and gene regulation, it would be highly premature to proceed with human germline alteration. There is a tremendous amount of research that must be undertaken before we can open this Pandora's box. New methods must be devised to drastically improve the efficiency and control of transgene integration. New strategies for the manipulation of gene expression in the human system will be required. Eventually, direct experience with human embryos must be gained and evaluated.

The ability to alter the human genome will be attended by tremendous responsibility. Negative aspects, such as abusive uses of this technology for eugenic reasons, will have to be dealt with by society. However, the potential to reverse the multitude of genetic lesions that plague the health of millions would seem reason enough to pursue aggressively the goal of human germline therapy.

NUCLEAR TRANSPLANTATION AND ARTIFICIAL TWINNING

Presently, the relevance of techniques involving blastomere separation and nuclear transplantation in the human seems remote (Chaps. 2 and 3). However, it is not the current lack of knowledge of human embryo physiology, but the complex ethical, social, and legal issues involved, that have prevented researchers in this field from applying it to humans. In addition to applications of nuclear transplantation techniques in animals, humans could conceivably also benefit directly. Although ethically, the delivery of more than the occasional twin following scientifically assisted human reproduction would be questionable, there may be some acceptable application both for the treatment of infertile couples and for those whose offspring may be at risk of hereditary disease.

Couples whose infertility leads them to in vitro fertilization (IVF) and who have limited numbers of gametes may, at any IVF attempt, have only one or a few embryos for transfer. If this is due to a severe male factor infertility, it could be feasible to grow the embryo to a later stage and either cryopreserve it or separate its cells (28). The female partner or another oocyte donor could then provide oocytes for enucleation, which could then be used as conception carriers for the diploid nuclei of the original embryo. This would thereby create a limited number of clones with the required genetic background. Cryopreservation of anucleate oocytes would facilitate this approach. Similarly, women with very few oocytes may have their embryos bisected or apply for the enucleation procedure.

In those couples who are otherwise fertile, but who carry inheritable defective genes, preimplantation diagnosis of oocytes or embryos could be followed by bisection of good embryos. Furthermore, healthy embryos could be used for nuclear transplantation into enucleated oocytes, possibly even into those that were shown to be defective by preconception genetic analysis of the first polar body (28). This series of procedures would increase the numbers of transferable and cryopreservable embryos, thereby increasing the possibility of normal pregnancies. Techniques involving nuclear transplantation may also be applied to couples in whom a partner is to receive chemotherapy.

PLACENTA DONATION BY BLASTOCYST RECONSTRUCTION IN THE HUMAN

Surgical replacement of a diseased placenta seems currently beyond the scope of obstetric medicine. However, several experimental embryology techniques can potentially be applied to women who suffer from recurrent idiopathic miscarriage of genetically normal fetuses. Both placental and fetal tissues originate in the preimplantation embryo. Some ICM cells will develop into the fetus, whereas the trophectoderm provides most of the placental material. The two types of tissue can effectively be separated and recombined using two different embryos of the same or closely related species (see Chap. 2 for review). This was mentioned previously in relation to interspecific gestation for exotic animal husbandry. Alternatively, transfer of a blastomere from an eight-cell to a four-cell embryo can yield a chimera in which the four-cell recipient becomes trophectoderm, and the eight-cell blastomere becomes inner cell mass (29,30). Although blastocyst reconstruction and blastomere transfer could directly benefit patients with habitual miscarriage, several ethical and technical issues need to be evaluated.

Removal of the inner cell mass of the donor blastocyst could either be accomplished by immunosurgery or micromanipulation (31,32). Accurate dissection of the donor embryo inner cell mass would be required to avoid construction of a mosaic fetus. Consequently, it would be preferable to develop donor trophectodermal vesicles devoid of inner cell mass. This can possibly be accomplished by combining donor morulae or inhibiting proliferation prior to blastulation. An additional ethical advantage would be that the donor embryo(s) would never develop the potential to form a normal pregnancy on their own.

REFERENCES

1. Nelson JS, Berns MW. Laser applications in biomedicine—Part II: Clinical applications. *J Laser Appl* 1989;1:9–20.
2. Berns MW, Rounds DE. Cell surgery by laser. *Sci Am* 1970;222(2):98–110.
3. Berns MW, Nelson JS. Laser applications in biomedicine—Part I: Biophysics, cell biology, and biostimulation. *J Laser Appl* 1989;1:34–39.
4. Ashkin A. Acceleration and trapping of particles by radiation pressure. *Phys Rev Lett* 1970;24:156–159.
5. Ashkin A, Dziedzic JM, Bjorkholm JE, Chu S. Observation of a single-beam gradient force optical trap for dielectric particles. *Opt Lett* 1986;11:288–290.
6. Ashkin A, Dziedzic JM. Optical trapping and manipulation of viruses and bacteria. *Science* 1987;235:1517–1520.
7. Tadir Y, Wright WH, Vafa O, Ord T, Asch RH, Berns MW. Micromanipulation of sperm by a laser generated optical trap. *Fertil Steril* 1989;52:870–873.
8. Berns MW, Wright WH, Tromberg BJ, Profeta GA, Andrews JJ, Walter RJ. Use of a laser-induced optical force trap to study chromosome movement on the mitotic spindle. *Proc Natl Acad Sci USA* 1989;86:4539–4543.
9. Steubing RW, Cheng S, Wright WH, Numajiri Y, Berns MW. Single beam optical trapping and micromanipulation of mammalian cells. In: Laser–Tissue Interaction SPIE Publ 1990;1202:272–280.
10. Willadsen SM. Cloning of sheep and cow embryos. *Genome* 1989;31:956–962.
11. Willadsen SM, Janzen RE, McAlister RJ, Shea BF, Hamilton G, McDermand D. The viability of late morulae and blastocysts produced by nuclear transplantation in cattle. *Theriogenology* 1991;35:161–170.
12. Seidel GE Jr. Embryo transfer: the next 100 years. *Theriogenology* 1991;35:171–180.
13. Pool R. Making light work of cell surgery. *Science* 1990;248:29–31.
14. Schierenberg E. Altered cell division rates after laser-induced cell fusion in nematode embryos. *Dev Biol* 1984;101:240–245.
15. Steubing RW, Weber G, Zimmermann K, Monajembashi S, Greulich K, Wolfrum J. Laser induced fusion of mammalian cells and plant protoplasts. *J Cell Sci* 1987;88:145–149.
16. Rorie RW, Pool SH, Prichard JF, Betteridge K, Godke RA. Production of chimeric blastocysts comprising sheep ICM with goat trophoblast for intergeneric transfer. *J Anim Sci* 1989;67(Suppl 1):401–402.
17. Godke RA, Beetem DD, Burleigh DW. A method for zona pellucida drilling using a compact nitrogen laser. In: *Proceedings Seventh World Congress on Human Reproduction*. Helsinki, Finland;1 1990:abstr 258.
18. Wanger EF, Stewart TA, Mintz B. The human β-globin gene and a functional thymidine kinase gene in developing mice. *Proc Natl Acad Sci USA* 1981;78:6376–6380.
19. Swanson LW, Simmons DM, Arriza J, Hammer R, Brinster RL. Novel developmental specificity in the nervous system of transgenic animals expressing growth hormone fusion genes. *Nature* 1985;317:363–366.
20. Malter HE, Cohen J. Embryonic development after microsurgical repair of polyspermic human zygotes. *Fertil Steril* 1989;52:373–380.
21. Chisari FV, Pinkert CA, Milich DR, Filippi P, McLachlan A. A transgenic mouse model of the chronic hepatitis B surface antigen carrier state. *Science* 1985;230:1157–1160.
22. Palmiter RD, Chen HY, Brinster RL. Differential regulation of metallothionein-thymidine kinase fusion genes in transgenic mice and their offspring. *Cell* 1982;29:701–710.
23. Walters L. The ethics of human gene therapy. *Nature* 1986;320:225–227.
24. Thompson S, Clarke AR, Pow AM, Hooper ML, Melton DW. Germ line transmission and expression of a corrected HPRT gene produced by gene targeting in embryonic stem cells. *Cell* 1989;56:313–321.
25. Constantini F, Chada K, Magram J. Correction of murine β thalessemia by gene transfer into the germ line. *Science* 1986;233:1192–1194.
26. Gordon JW. Approaches to germinal cell gene therapy. *J In Vitro Fert Embryo Transfer* 1990;7:191.

27. Isola LM, Gordon JW. Systemic resistance to methotrexate in transgenic mice carrying a mutant dihydrofolate reductase gene. *Proc Natl Acad Sci USA* 1986;83:9621–9625.
28. Tucker M, Cohen J. Micromanipulation for assisted reproduction. In: Sciarra JJ, Speroff J, eds. *Gynecology and obstetrics.* Philadelphia: JB Lippincott; 1991.
29. Willadsen SM. Micromanipulation of embryos of the large domestic species. In: Adams CE, ed. *Mammalian egg transfer.* Boca Raton: CRC Press; 1982:185–210.
30. Willadsen SM, Fehilly CB. The developmental potential and regulatory capacity of blastomeres from two-, four- and eight-cell embryos. In: Beier HM, Lindner HR, eds. *Fertilization of the human egg in vitro.* Heidelberg: Springer-Verlag; 1983:353–357.
31. Gardner RL. An investigation of inner cell mass and trophoblast tissues following their isolation from the mouse blastocyst. *J Embryol Exp Morphol* 1972;28:279–312.
32. Solter D, Knowles BB. Immunosurgery of mouse blastocysts. *Proc Natl Acad Sci USA* 1975;72:5099–5102.

Subject Index